TWINS AND HIGHER
MULTIPLE BIRTHS:

A Guide to their Nature and Nurture

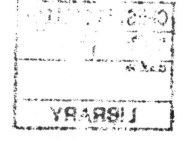

TWINS AND HIGHER
MULTIPLE BIRTHS:
A Guide to their Nature and Nurture

Elizabeth M Bryan
MD FRCP DCH

Honorary Consultant Paediatrician and
Senior Research Fellow
Queen Charlotte's and Chelsea Hospital
and Medical Director of the Multiple Births Foundation

Edward Arnold
A division of Hodder & Stoughton
LONDON   MELBOURNE   AUCKLAND

© 1992 Elizabeth Bryan

First published in Great Britain 1992

British Library Cataloguing in Publication Data

Bryan, Elizabeth M.
  Twins and Higher Multiple Births: Guide
  to Their Nature and Nurture
  I. Title
  305.9045

ISBN 0-340-54452-X

Typeset in 10/11 pt Palatino by
Rowland Phototypesetting Limited, Bury St Edmunds, Suffolk
Printed and bound in Great Britain for Edward Arnold, a division of
Hodder and Stoughton Limited, Mill Road, Dunton Green,
Sevenoaks, Kent TN13 2YA by St Edmundsbury Press,
Bury St Edmunds, Suffolk and Robert Hartnoll Limited, Bodmin, Cornwall

Preface

Twins invariably inspire interest and admiration. Each year most of the 8000 mothers who have twins in Britain are told how lucky they are, and not least by members of the medical profession. In some ways the parents of twins are indeed lucky, yet few doctors and nurses realise what is involved in caring for two babies at once.

While pursuing a study of placental function in multiple pregnancy in 1974, I had the chance to meet over 100 mothers of twins fairly frequently throughout the first year of the babies' life, often in their homes. Previously I had known nothing of the problems of having young twins. By the end I had learned a great deal.

Not only did I discover the immense practical, financial and, especially, emotional difficulties involved but also the paucity of support available to the mothers. They had been given little advice. They could find no written information. Their paediatrician and family doctor were largely unaware of the problems.

My first impressions of immense unmet needs have been amply confirmed by over 3000 families with twins with whom I have now talked, either through the Twins and Multiple Births Association or in my work as a paediatrician in the Multiple Births Foundation Twins Clinics. It is to the many helpful parents that I am indebted for most of the examples quoted in the text. I have preserved confidentiality by changing distinguishing details. I have mainly called the children 'him' because this clearly distinguishes the child from the mother.

This book is based on my book *The Nature and Nurture of Twins* published by Baillière Tindall in 1983. Much has happened since then, both in the study of twins and of course in the context of treatment for subfertility. The text has been updated and a lot of new material added. Much of this is concerned with higher order births, the number of which is rapidly increasing in many countries. It is also concerned with the ethical issues arising from new forms of treatment.

Although this book is primarily meant for paediatricians I hope that it will interest anyone concerned with helping families from conception onwards. Some sections, such as that on schooling, will more directly concern the doctor working in the community than the hospital paediatrician.

The book is not meant to be a detailed practical guide to the care of twins. Nor does it give technical guidance on obstetrical procedures or placental examinations, for which specialized textbooks are available. Rather, it offers a comprehensive overview of twinning and of twinship, of the effect of twins on the mother and the rest of the family, and on the growth and development of twins themselves from conception to adulthood.

As much as anything, I hope the book will give readers some insight into what it means to be a mother, father, brother or sister of twins—and not least to be a twin oneself.

E.M.B.

Acknowledgements

In writing on a subject that calls on so many disciplines I have needed help from very many people. Responsibility for the book's contents must be mine alone but I am especially indebted to Ilona Bendefy, Barbara Broadbent, John Buckler, Gerald Corney, Jane Denton, Alison Elliman, Robert Goodman, Judith Goodship, Rachel Hudson, William James, Julian Little, Ian MacGillivray, Frances Price, Jane Redshaw and Judith Richardson.

I thank Jane Gardiner for her care in typing the manuscript and also Christine Tomkins, Karen Broughton and Joshila Tailor. My literary agent, Carol Heaton, has given constant encouragement.

I owe much to my colleagues in the Multiple Births Foundation, particularly Faith Hallett, Barbara Read and Linda Hayward, and I am grateful to many members of the Twins and Multiple Births Association for their invaluable insights into the pleasures and problems of having twins, and more.

Throughout the gestation of the book I have been indebted to the literary skills of my husband, Ronald Higgins. Without his support I might never have undertaken the task.

The book is dedicated to the memory of my mother, Betty Bryan, who nurtured my early interest in medicine with such enthusiasm.

Contents

1

History of twins

The widespread interest in twins has its own psychological and even philosophical roots. Most cultures believe in the uniqueness of each human life and personality and are therefore bemused that some of us have, or seem to have, an identical copy. This is certainly seen as a marvel of nature, a cause of wonder, of magic or of humour.

Others see identical twinship as some sort of metaphysical insult. They feel that the very possibility of it not only subtracts from the idea of unique individuality but is a kind of insult creating a sense of existential unease. Many of these feelings, negative and positive, are expressed in mythology and in tribal customs associated with twinning.

Biblical twins

Twins plainly excited much interest in Biblical times. The most famous pair were Esau and Jacob, conceived as a result of Isaac's prayer for his barren wife, Rebekah. Esau and Jacob have often been described as dizygotic (DZ, see p. 18) because of their physical dissimilarity as adults—Esau being a 'hairy man' and Jacob a 'smooth man'. On the other hand, because Esau 'came out red' it has also been suggested that he was an example of the fetofetal transfusion syndrome (see p. 52) but as this only occurs in mono-zygotic (MZ, see p. 15) twins the two hypotheses are incompatible.

The idea of conflict between twins, so common in mythology, is ex-emplified by the struggle for the first birthright that Esau and Jacob were said to have had within the womb. Esau won this round but finally lost when Jacob tricked his father into giving the birthright to him.

Another pair of twins described in Genesis are Pharez and Zarah, the children of Tamai and Judah, who also competed to be delivered first. Zarah presented an arm which was labelled with a red string. Later, when the babies were born, the string was attached to the second baby, showing that Pharez had replaced Zarah in birth order.

Mythology

Twins abound in Greek and Roman mythology. Many were either gods themselves or the offspring of gods and as such had supernatural powers. Castor and Pollux, the heroic sons of Zeus and Leda, had powers over the wind and waves and were known as the seafarers' guardians. When Castor was killed in battle Pollux was so desolate that he begged his father to allow him to join his brother. They became the heavenly constellation, Gemini.

Romulus and Remus are probably the most famous twins in Roman mythology. These were the sons of Mars and one of the vestal virgins, Sylvia. The babies were to be drowned with their mother in the River Tiber but their cradle floated into the bank where they were found and suckled by a she-wolf. There are, of course, famous statues depicting them in both Rome and Siena (Fig. 1.1). When they grew up the two brothers wanted to found a great city but could not agree on a site. In the course of their dispute Romulus killed Remus and then went on to found the city of Rome, over which he ruled for many years.

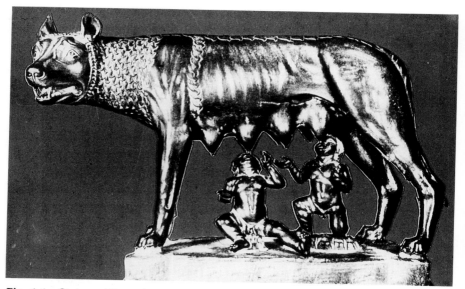

Fig. 1.1 Statue of Romulus and Remus being suckled by the she-wolf. By permission of the Capitoline Museum, Rome.

Narcissus is a much maligned mythological twin. It is sometimes forgotten that when he spent long hours looking at his reflection in a pool, he did so not out of vanity but to remind himself of his lost sister, to whom he was devoted.

Twins are often found amongst the gods of the Asiatic religions. Sometimes these are depicted as conjoined twins—a figure with two heads or one with several sets of limbs. The Acvin are twin gods in Indian mythology and are believed to look after the weak and oppressed.

In Mexico the ancient Aztecs worshipped the goddess of fertility, Xochiquetzal, whom they believed to be the first mother of twins.

Twins in the arts

Writers, poets and artists have all explored the theme of twinship and through their work we can learn much of its various aspects.

Many writers have, of course, exploited the similarity of twins and the confusion that can spring from it. In his play, *Menaechmi*, the Roman comic dramatist, Plautus, employed a theme that has since been the basis for countless dramas in many languages. A twin named Menaechmus, who was so like his brother that even their mother could not tell them apart, was lost at the age of seven. Many years later his twin brother, now renamed Menaechmus himself, sought out his lost twin. It was only when strangers started mistaking him for his brother that he realized his search would be successful.

Shakespeare had twins of his own—Hamnet and Judith—who were plainly DZ. In his drama, however, he concentrates on the confusion of identity between 'identical' twins. In the *Comedy of Errors* two masters, who appear to be MZ twins, each have one of an MZ pair as a servant.

Like many early writers, Shakespeare did not realize that male/female pairs could not be 'identical' twins. The most obvious example of his confusion is in *Twelfth Night*, where it was said, of Viola and Sebastian, 'an apple, cleft in twain is not more twin than these two creatures'.

Amongst children, Tweedledum and Tweedledee in Lewis Carroll's *Through the Looking Glass and What Alice Found there* must be the most popular pair (Fig. 1.2).

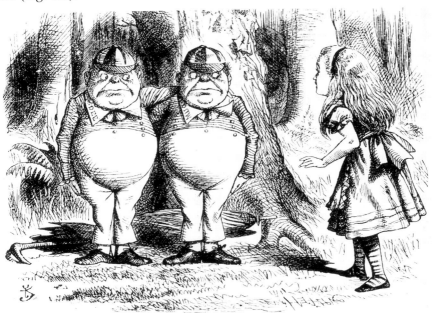

Fig. 1.2   Tweedledum and Tweedledee with Alice. From Lewis Carroll's *Through the Looking Glass and What Alice Found There*. By permission of Macmillan and Co.

The immensely close attachment and interdependence of twins are illustrated by Thornton Wilder in *The Bridge of San Luis Rey*. A pair of twins are so close that, when one falls in love, there is no space for a third person. The external relationship is so devastating to the twins that it has to be sacrificed. Both twins value their own bond above all. Later, Wilder movingly describes the desolation of the survivor after the death of his twin.

Cultural and religious beliefs about twins

Throughout history there have been strongly held cultural and religious beliefs about twins in many parts of the world (Gedda 1961; Corney 1975a). Many of these persist today, even if usually in modified and less extreme forms. Within the last 20 years an English paediatrician working in Zimbabwe was dismayed to find that one of a pair of premature twins who had been born and successfully nursed in hospital for several months was killed the day they were due to return to their own village. It was the custom of that tribe to kill twins.

Attitudes towards twins vary greatly in different parts of the world, and even between different tribes within quite small geographical areas. For some twins, therefore, the difference between being born on one side of the river rather than the other may be that between being welcomed (and even being regarded as having supernatural powers) and being rejected and killed.

Attitudes towards twins have been seen to change over time. Early this century a trader and his family were travelling through the Yoruba territory in Nigeria when his wife was delivered of twins. As he came from a tribe that respected twins the babies were allowed to survive. The trader prospered and it became clear to the Yoruba people that the twins had brought no ill-effect to the family. The Yoruba chiefs therefore decided to change their policy and from then on their own twins were welcomed.

The killing of twins was widespread and has been reported from many parts of Africa and Asia, as well as amongst Australian aboriginals and Eskimos. Ideas on the origin of this custom are varied and there are several theories as to why twins were disliked. One is that it is animal-like for a human mother to have more than one baby at a time. Another is that two babies must mean two fathers—the mother must therefore either have committed adultery or have conceived the second baby through an evil spirit.

There is often a functional side to the beliefs as well. In a nomadic tribe it is difficult for a mother to carry two babies for many miles and, when food is scarce, breast-feeding two babies may be impossible. Some tribes killed both babies, some just the second-born or, in mixed-sex pairs, the girl. In some tribes only male/female pairs were killed. These were condemned on the basis that incest was inevitable, either in intrauterine life or later. On the other hand the Bantu positively welcomed male/female pairs as newly wed couples and in parts of Japan and the Philippines such pairs were expected to marry each other.

Aversion to twins was not limited to primitive societies. They were commonly disliked in Japan; in noble families their arrival was kept secret and the second baby might be given to a courtier. Twins were also rejected in parts of South America.

Mothers of twins also suffered. 'May you become the mother of twins' was in some African tribes the strongest curse. Indeed, words were unnecessary: two fingers of the right hand pointed towards a woman could have the same terrible effect! In some tribes mothers were killed together with their babies or, if not killed, banished to a distant 'twin town', sometimes for life. When the presence of a second baby was discovered the mother was sometimes moved from the village, still in labour, so that she did not contaminate the area. When the second baby was born unexpectedly, elaborate rituals of purification were performed.

In parts of East Africa the mother was shunned until the babies had cut their first teeth.

On the whole, fathers of twins were let off lightly. Some North American Indians insisted on a period of abstinence from meat and fish, which must have been hard for a hunter. In parts of Peru the father had to abstain from salt, pepper and sexual intercourse for 6 months—an intriguing triad.

Customs associated with twins

In some parts of the world there are elaborate ceremonies and rituals associated with twins.

Twin images

Carved wooden images of twins are common in some parts of Africa, particularly in the Ibeji cult of the Yoruba. Ibeji, literally meaning 'to beget

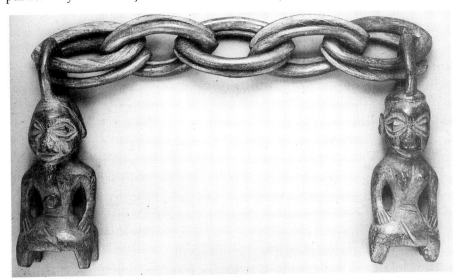

Fig. 1.3 Wooden twin images from West Africa, linked by chain. The whole is made from one piece of wood.

two', is used either as a general term for twins or specifically for Orisha, the goddess of twins. Through the traffic of slaves the Ibeji cult has spread to many parts of South America and the Caribbean. Some images are memorials to twins who have died. Often the twin images, sometimes in large numbers, are used for special rituals and kept in places of worship (Fig. 1.3).

Weather

Twins were often believed to have supernatural powers, both good and bad, over the weather. The Egyptian twin gods Shu and Tefnut were, respectively, the wind and rain god, and the powers of Castor and Pollux have already been mentioned (see p. 2).

In parts of eastern and southern Africa twins were thought to cause famine due to drought or flood and were therefore killed immediately to prevent such catastrophes.

Many North American Indians also held twins responsible for the climatic conditions. The Mohaves, for instance, believed that twins came from the sky using lightning, thunder and rain as their means of descent. When praying for a storm to abate, the Tsimshian would say 'calm down, breath of twins'. Many South American tribes attributed aspects of the weather to the mood and behaviour of twins. Indeed twins were used to forecast the weather according to their state of health. When they were feeling well, the weather would be clement. When they had a headache or indigestion, a storm was likely.

Death of a twin

It has been widely believed that a twin would rarely survive the death of the other. If a twin did survive he was thought likely to be exceptionally strong—the possessor of the vitality of both.

In Sussex it was thought that a single surviving twin had special healing powers: he or she could cure thrush, for example, by breathing into the mouth of the sufferer.

In some parts of Africa surviving twins carry a wooden image of their dead twin around their neck or waist. This gives company to the survivor and a refuge for the spirit of the dead.

Twin names

Twins in many African tribes are given fixed names. Amongst the Yoruba the firstborn twin is called Taiwo (he who has the first taste of the world) and the second called Kainde or Kehinde (he who lags behind). The younger sibling of twins is called Idowu (the servant of twins) and this name is also given to the third member of triplets. Subsequent children are called Alaba (the servant of Idowu) and Idogbe. In other parts of Africa twins are called Ochin and Omo, Tali and Bali, Buth and Duoth.

The children of twins may also have special names. In one tribe, for example, the firstborn is Dosu (girl, Devi), the second Dosavi (Dohnevi) and the third Donyo (Dosovi).

Conception

Certain foods are thought to help women who want twins. In parts of the Far East a double banana, chestnut or millet seed is added to her diet; in mediaeval Scotland a tumbler full of water from the well in St. Mungo was supposed to ensure a twin birth. Some North American Indians say twins occur if the mother lies on her back instead of on her side during labour, so enabling the fetus to split in two. Others believe that too much work during pregnancy can result in twins.

Fertility

Twins themselves are thought by some to induce fertility. In Wales they were often invited to weddings to ensure children for the newly weds.

Twins are evidence of high fertility in the mother and some tribes believe that this fertility can be transferred to the land. Mothers of twins may be required to join in elaborate rituals to ensure a good harvest.

Old wives' tales

False beliefs about the biology of twins have been rife throughout the centuries. In mid-seventeenth century Europe it was still thought that boy and girl twins could not coexist in the same uterine cavity because of the 'horror incestus'. Even today parents may be influenced by superstitions. An elderly midwife recalled how, when one of her patients was delivered of twins, the husband immediately sued for divorce on the grounds of adultery: two babies must have meant two fathers.

Parents of MZ girls may still sometimes worry about their children's fertility. One mother anxiously sought advice as to which of her 4-year-old girls would be infertile. Ever since their birth she had lived under the painful misapprehension that only one of her MZ twins would be able to bear children.

Those who have a boy and a girl are sometimes concerned about the fertility of the girl. The farmer father of a boy and a girl pair told me he assumed that his daughter would be infertile because he knew that when a cow gives birth to twins of different sexes the heifer is sterile. This so-called 'freemartin' is caused by virilization by hormones from the bull fetus. The farmer did not realize that the pattern of vascular anastomoses in human and bovine placentae is different.

The study of twins

Scholars and philosophers have long been fascinated by twins. Until recently, however, few scientists have shown the same interest. Hippocrates thought about twins and decided that they were conceived by the division of a sperm into two parts and that each part penetrated one of the uterine horns. A number of others, including Democritus, Empedocles and Aristotle had ideas on the origin of twins. Interest in obstetrical aspects was kindled in the Renaissance period and anxiety was expressed over the dangers of exsanguination of the second twin after the firstborn's cord had been cut.

It is perhaps surprising that the value of twins as a research tool was not appreciated until the second half of the nineteenth century. This may have been partly because the distinction between MZ and DZ twins was still not clearly defined. Accurate determination of zygosity has only recently become possible.

Twin research was revolutionized by Sir Francis Galton, who realized that twins could be of value in the study of the effects of heredity and environment on human development. His classic *The History of Twins as a Criterion of the Relative Powers of Nature and Nurture* (1875) is a memorial to his pioneering work.

Before Galton's time twins were regarded as an interesting phenomenon and an obstetrical challenge but of no material or substantial relevance to the rest of the population. Following Galton's work, twins have been increasingly used as a tool for genetic research but it is only in the last 15 years or so that interest has been shown in the special problems that twins themselves, and their families, may experience. The pleasures of being a twin or a parent of twins are readily recognized: many professionals are unaware of the problems. This book tries to explore the special situation faced by these families.

2

The biology of twinning

Long before sophisticated methods of determining the zygosity of twins were developed, it was recognized that at least two types of twins existed—identical (otherwise termed monozygotic (MZ), monozygous or uniovular) and fraternal (dizygotic (DZ), dizygous or binovular).

MZ twins arise from the early division of a single fertilized ovum (zygote). Evidence for this is provided in at least three ways: (i) by conjoined twins; (ii) by the single chorion found in some twin placentae; and (iii) from the typing of genetic markers.

DZ twins occur as the result of fertilization of two separately released ova and are no more alike than any two siblings.

There has been speculation as to the existence of a third type of twin (Mijsberg 1957; Bulmer 1970; Corney and Robson 1975). Such twins, it is thought, might arise from the division of an ovum whose resulting parts are then independently fertilized. These uniovular dispermatic twins would therefore be intermediate between MZ and DZ. The embryological possibility of this third type is clearly there and, after several fruitless lines of investigation, the first convincing supportive evidence has been provided by Nance (1981) who describes an acardiac twin fetus that was thought, on human leucocyte antigen (HLA)-typing and chromosome analysis, to have arisen from the fertilization of a polar body. The twins were thus monovular, but not monozygotic. An apparently normal monovular dizygotic twin might well remain unrecognized (Goldgar and Kimberling 1981). However, there is little doubt that this type of twin is rare. Were they not so the percentage of pairs with identical genetic markers in a population of non-identical twins would be higher than that expected if all dizygotic twins arise from different oocytes; this has not been shown to be so.

Prevalence of twinning

The true incidence of twins cannot be determined because many twin conceptions are unrecognized because of the loss of one twin early in intrauterine life (see p. 32). Furthermore, some multiple births may not have been recorded if a pair, one stillborn and one liveborn, was delivered before 28 weeks gestation (the limit has recently been lowered to 24 weeks). Under UK legislation the liveborn infant would have appeared in the records as a single birth. Finally, the prevalence of twins in the adult population is lower than that at birth because both perinatal and infant

Table 2.1 International variation in twinning rates[a]

Continent, country or area	Type of study[b]	Period of study	No. of twin maternities	Twinning rate (per 1 000)	Reference
Africa					
Algeria		1963	2 181[c]	13.3	Hollingsworth and Duncan (1966)
Ghana, Korle Bu	H	1954–56	291	52.4	
Libyan Arab Jamahiriya		1972–75	5 260	12.3	
Mali	H	1968	761	21.8	Imperato (1971)
Nigeria, lowest rate	H	1976–79	352	23.7	Harrison and Rossiter (1985)
highest rate	H	1964–68	216	45.1	Nylander (1969)
Seychelles		1972–76	236	27.2	
South Africa[d]		1963	2 784	16.8	
Tunisia		1972–74	10 972	27.9	
Uganda, Mbale	H	1971–80	1 104	16.3	Zake (1984)
America, North					
Antigua and Barbuda		1972–75	56	10.3	
Bahamas		1972–76	482	21.8	
Barbados		1960	80	11.1	
Canada		1972–76 and 1976–79	20 786[e]	9.0	
Costa Rica		1974	579	10.2	
Cuba		1973 and 75	5 871	14.1	
Dominican Republic		1972–76	28 626	32.5	
El Salvador		1972–76 and 1978–80	12 455[f]	9.6	
Greenland		1972–76·	59	13.2	
Jamaica		1960	1 652	25.7	
Mexico		1972–78	89 945[g]	5.3	
Nicaragua		1967	520	6.7	
Panama		1972–75 and 1977–80	6 899	16.2	
Former Canal Zone		1974–78	21	7.4	

		Years	Number		Reference
Trinidad and Tobago		1972–76	1 929	14.5	
USA		1972–75	116 464	9.2	
		1978–79	65 511	9.6	
America, South					
Brazil		1974–76	147 353	16.8	
Chile		1972–80	31 245	14.7	
Ecuador		1972–74 and 1976–77	22 109	18.7	
Venezuela		1963	3 439	9.7	
Asia					
Burma	H	1972–73	462	11.7	Kyu et al. (1981)
Cambodia, Pnom-Penh	H	1957–60	242	15.2	Olivier et al. (1965)
		1964	90	10.6	
Hong Kong		1972–77 and 1979–80	8 117	12.5	
		1963–73	2 564	16.0	Goswami and Wagh (1975)
India, sample of townships	H	1965–75	1 026	14.7	Bildhaiya (1978)
Ahmedabad		1966–75	154	9.0	Junnarkar and Nadkarni (1979)
Palgar Block sample townships		1969–75	96	8.6	Rao et al. (1983)
Tamilnadu		1969–73	81	9.8	Ghosh and Ramanujacharyulu (1979)
South Delhi		1983–84	149	8.4	Shah and Patel (1984)
Bombay	H	1961–64	1 769	9.7	Modan et al. (1968)
Israel		1972–80	6 309[h]	9.8	
Israel		1972–74 and 1976–80	82 647[i]	5.6	
Japan		1955–67	151 709	6.4	Imaizumi and Inouye (1984)
		1974	12 392	5.8	
Korea				9.7	Kang and Cho (1962)
Ryukyu Islands		1968	188	8.4	
Singapore		1972, 1973 and 1975–80	4 457	13.1	

Table 2.1 *Continued*

Continent, country or area	Type of study[b]	Period of study	No. of twin maternities	Twinning rate (per 1 000)	Reference
Singapore	H	1960–70	3 276	8.1	Tan et al. (1971)
Singapore	H	1969–70	174	7.9	Foong (1971)
	H	1970–72	234	7.5	Dawood et al. (1975)
Taiwan, Cheng-Chung whole country		1956–65	122	5.7	Lin and Chen (1968)
		1963–64	4 703	5.6	
Taipei		1972–77	?	4.5	Cheng et al. (1986)
Vietnam, Saigon	H	1952–62	1 266	10.7	Olivier et al. (1965)
Europe					
lowest: Spain		1951–53		9.1	Bulmer (1960a)
highest: East Germany		1950–55		12.4	
lowest: Bulgaria		1978	891	6.5	UN *Demographic Yearbook* (1981)
highest: Ireland		1977	800	11.6	
Cyprus		1972–77 and 1979–80	1 889	19.2	
Turkey, Ankara	H	1965–	149	14.9	Say et al. (1967)
Oceania					
American Samoa		1972	18	16.7	
		1976	10	9.2	
Australia		1973–79	15 455[i]	9.5	
Fiji		1976–81	802	7.6	Pollard (1985)
Guam		1972–79	393	15.9	
New Guinea, selected communities in west		?–1946[k]	790	10.3	Groenewegen and van de Kaa (1967)
New Zealand		1972–79	4 406[l]	9.8	*New Zealand Yearbook* (1982)
New Zealand Maoris			122	9.4	
Pacific Islands		1973,4,6,8,9	344	18.2	
Papua New Guinea	H	1970–71	421	19.1	Archer (1973)
New Britain		1953–67	87	31.2	Scragg and Walsh (1970)

Tonga	1975–78	64	17.9	Feĺszer (1979)
USSR				
Arctic region	1944–50		7.7	Kandror (1961)
Moscow	1956		11.9	
	1973		7.8	Lipovetskaya and Yampol'skaya (1975)

[a] Unless otherwise stated, data are from the United Nations *Demographic Yearbooks* (1975, 1981). Although these data are purported to relate to maternities, this is not always certain, as indicated in the notes below. Literature sources suggest that the rates in Japan and Australia are about half those indicated in the 1981 *Yearbook*, and hence the published figures have been taken as relating to babies (footnote i).

The figures obtained from the *Yearbook* for some other countries appear sufficiently high for it to be surprising that no reports appear to have been published, and the figures may therefore relate to babies rather than maternities. The countries involved are the Seychelles, Tunisia, Brazil, Chile, Ecuador, Cyprus, Singapore, Guam and the Pacific Islands.

These data from the *Yearbooks* mostly relate to pregnancies ending in live birth, whereas the data for which other references are given relate to maternities with delivery of live or stillborn babies.

[b] H—hospital series, otherwise deliveries in a defined geographical area.

[c] Includes maternities ending in births other than of known twins or singletons.

[d] UN *Demographic Yearbook* 1975 provides breakdown by 'race'; the method of classification is uncertain and therefore the figures have been pooled.

[e–h] Figures appear to change from maternities (M) to individual babies (B), or vice versa:

 Canada B → M in 1974
 El Salvador M → B in 1980
 Mexico M → B in 1976
 Israel   M → B in 1973; B → M in 1979; M → B in 1980
 New Zealand M → B in 1975

[g] According to the 1981 *Yearbook*, the data from Mexico relate to confinements ending in live births or fetal deaths for all years except 1976.

[i] Figures in 1981 *Yearbook* have been taken as referring to individual babies rather than to maternities.

[j] Excluding countries for which it is unclear whether figures relate to maternities or individual babies.

[k] All previous deliveries of women surveyed in 1945–1946 who were aged 15 or more.

[l] According to the 1981 *Yearbook*, the data from New Zealand relate to confinements ending in live births or fetal deaths in the period 1972–1974.

Source: From Little and Thompson (1988) by permission of the authors and John Wiley & Sons.

mortality are higher in twins than singletons (see p. 105). Thus, the prevalence of twins at a certain time is all that can be accurately estimated.

Twinning rates vary greatly in different parts of the world (Table 2.1)
largely due to wide variations in DZ twinning. MZ twinning rates appear to
be remarkably constant all over the world, at about 3.5 per 1000 maternities.

In the UK the prevalence of twin deliveries is now about 11 per 1000
(Registrar General 1989), whereas in parts of Nigeria it has been reliably
reported to be as high as 45 per 1000 (Nylander 1967, 1970a). In general it
appears that the negroid races have the highest incidence of twinning,
mongoloid races the lowest with Caucasians and Asian Indians being
intermediate. Occasionally, as for instance in parts of Finland (Eriksson and
Fellman 1973), an isolated community may have an unexpectedly high
twinning rate, presumably due to inbreeding in a genetically prone population.

Figures from many developing countries must be interpreted with caution
(Nylander 1975a). If the data are obtained from hospital records the twinning rates may be abnormally high because twin deliveries, together with
other high-risk pregnancies, are over-represented amongst hospital deliveries. Conversely, national records may underestimate the number of twins,
as babies may not be individually registered as twins, particularly in areas
where they are unwelcome or if one twin is stillborn. Twin taboos are still
strong in some African tribes (see Chapter 1).

Sex ratio

Although there are slightly more male than female twin births, the sex ratio
(male:female) is lower than in singletons. In triplets there is actually a
preponderance of females (Bulmer 1970; Czeizel and Acsadi 1971) (Table
2.2).

The higher incidence of females amongst multiple births compared with
single births is limited to MZ twins and the sex ratio falls with the timing of
the zygote division. The later the division, the lower the sex ratio (James
1980a). Amongst conjoined twins there is a significant excess of female pairs
(see p. 59). James (1988) has argued that this may be because a proportion
are formed as a consequence of anomalous X-inactivation (see p. 66).
Amongst DZ twins the sex ratio may be slightly higher than in singletons
(James 1986a).

Table 2.2   The sex ratio (male:female) in multiple births

Country	Single	Twin	Triplet
England and Wales	0.515	0.508±0.001	0.480±0.009
France	0.514	0.506±0.001	0.471±0.009
Italy	0.515	0.508±0.001	0.487±0.008
USA, white	0.514	0.507±0.001	0.498±0.006
USA, black	0.507	0.501±0.001	0.502±0.012
Japan	0.519	0.520±0.004	0.515±0.041

Source: From Bulmer (1970) by permission of the author and Oxford University Press.

MZ and DZ twins

The proportion of like- to unlike-sexed twins in a given population can be used to calculate the number of MZ and DZ twins. This is the basis for Weinberg's differential rule. Weinberg (1902) reasoned that, as the sex of each DZ twin is independently determined, there must be equal numbers of like-sexed and unliked-sexed DZ twins. The number of MZ pairs must, therefore, be the excess of like-sexed over unlike-sexed pairs. Similarly the number of DZ pairs would be twice the number of unlike sex. Thus the MZ and DZ twinning rates in a population may be calculated by the formulae:

$$MZ = \frac{(L - W)}{n}$$

$$DZ = \frac{2U}{n}$$

where L and U are the number of like- and unlike-sexed twin maternities in a total sample of n maternities. This does not allow for a sex ratio with the slightly higher incidence of males but apparently this minor discrepancy makes little difference to the overall figure (Bulmer 1970).

The validity of Weinberg's formula has been questioned on the basis that sexes among DZ pairs might not be determined independently. (James 1987) studied data from various twin surveys in which zygosity had been accurately determined. He found a significant excess of DZ pairs of like sex. James suggests that this could be due to the sex of the zygote being determined by the time of conception in relation to the menstrual cycle; DZ twins usually being formed close together in time. An excess of identically sexed pairs might therefore occur in this group. Conversely, a higher intrauterine mortality amongst male fetuses could lead to an underestimation of like-sex pairs. The need for amendment of Weinberg's rules has since been supported by the work of Orlebeke *et al.* (1989) but not by Vlietinck *et al.* (1988). The latter found that figures obtained from a population of over 2500 pairs of twins in which zygosity had been carefully determined agreed closely with those obtained by applying Weinberg's formula.

MZ twins

MZ twins arise from the splitting of a zygote during the first 14 days after fertilization. Correct identification of the placental membranes at delivery gives a good indication as to the stage of development at which this occurred (see p. 82). It appears that there may be a fundamental difference in the embryological mechanism involved in the formation of mono- and dichorial MZ twins (Leroy 1985).

Dichorial MZ twins

The mechanism of splitting may be more complex than a simple separation of the two cells deriving from the first division of the fertilized egg. If the two resulting blastomeres were enclosed in the same thick zona pellucida they would be unlikely to develop independently because they would just merge together again. If, on the other hand, the blastomeres were isolated from the zona pellucida they would not be able to survive.

The more likely explanation for the occurrence of dichorial MZ twins has emerged from the study of *in vitro*-cultured bovine ova (Ozil 1983). If the embryo hatches from the zona pellucida by progressive herniation rather than rapidly through a large slit, an hour-glass effect is produced, of which each part contains all cellular components. If there is then a rupture of the narrow connecting tissue, separate twin blastocysts can develop independently. Ozil (1983) produced MZ fetuses in the cow by bisecting a blastocyst after removal from the zona pellucida and then placing each 'half' into an empty zona pellucida. Similar results have been obtained in other mammals, including sheep and mice.

Monochorial MZ twins

Monochorial twins probably arise at the blastocyst stage through division or duplication of the inner cell mass within a single trophectoderm.

Monoamniotic twinning is thought to occur relatively late in development because it results from duplication of the embryonic rudiment of the germ disc (ectodermal plate). Armadillos offer a unique example of monoamniotic multiple embryogenisis—the embryonic disc splits regularly into several parts.

An MZ twinning rate of 3.5 per 1000 maternities appears to be constant world-wide, although there may have been a slight increase in the rate in the UK (Emery 1986) and in some other countries (Allen and Parisi 1990; Rydhstrom 1990a) since 1960. The introduction of infertility drugs (Derom *et al.* 1987) and oral contraceptives (Macourt *et al.* 1982) could both be contributory factors in this increase (see p. 17).

No predisposing factors have yet been recognized as definitely associated with MZ twinning. Some workers have found a slight increase in MZ twinning with maternal age (Bulmer 1970; Elwood 1978; Inouye and Imaizumi 1981; Harrison and Rossiter 1985; Bonnelykke 1990) but this has not been confirmed by others (Nylander 1975c). All fertile women appear to have the same chance of producing MZ twins and, unlike mothers of DZ twins, one set of twins does not increase their risk of having another set in a subsequent pregnancy. Having said this, there does now seem to be incontrovertible evidence of an occasional example of familial MZ twinning (Harvey *et al.* 1977; Segreti *et al.* 1978). Shapiro *et al.* (1978) describe a family with four sets of MZ twins, in which the twinning gene appears to be carried by both males and females.

Nevertheless, epidemiological studies have repeatedly shown that families with MZ twins do not have larger numbers of twin relatives than expected and that the MZ twinning rate is independent of race (Morton 1962). Unless a mother of MZ twins has a strong history of MZ twins in the family, she can be told that her chances of having twins again are not increased.

As implied, the causes of MZ twinning are unknown and, in view of the probable difference in embryological mechanisms involved in mono- and dichorial types, there may well be more than one cause.

Some researchers believe that MZ twinning is a form of congenital malformation caused by a developmental arrest early in embryonic life, before tissue differentiation has begun (Stockard 1921). The global uniformity of the human MZ twinning rate may be due to the relative constancy of an intrauterine environment. In the less stable embryonic environment of an egg (a trout's egg in Stockard's case) it has been shown that twinning can be increased by depriving the egg of oxygen and warmth (Stockard 1921).

No such results are available in mammals. However, it has been claimed that in the human the ratio between monochorial and dichorial placentation is particularly high amongst extrauterine twin pregnancies (Arey 1923) and it has been suggested that defective nutritional conditions might play a role in the formation of human MZ twins. Similar suggestions resulted from the finding of an increase in the incidence of MZ twins in multiple births arising from ovulation induction (Derom *et al.* 1987) and assisted conception (Edwards *et al.* 1966; see below). It is possible that the technical procedure itself could predispose to zygote division or that a less favourable intrauterine environment caused both subfertility and zygote division.

It has also been suggested that MZ twinning can result from exposure to teratogenic insult at a particularly sensitive stage of gestation. Kaufman and O'Shea (1978) produced MZ mouse twins after exposure to vinicristine. The higher incidence of congenital malformations in MZ twins (Little and Bryan 1988) may support this theory. On the other hand, the malformations could be secondary to the MZ twinning process itself: monochorionic placentation may well provide less favourable conditions for development. It remains to be shown whether congenital malformations are more common in monochorionic than dichorionic MZ twins (see p. 87).

Another possible predisposing factor to MZ twinning may be over-ripeness of the ovum before ovulation or delay in its fertilization. It has been reported that mothers of MZ twins exhibit significantly more prolonged and irregular menstrual cycles than mothers of DZ twins. Such abnormal ovulatory conditions might correspond to oöcyte overmaturation (Harlap *et al.* 1985).

It has been suggested that the changes in MZ twinning rates in the UK could be related to the use of oral contraceptives (Emery 1986). Results from earlier studies on the effects of these drugs were conflicting but a large study from Australia showed that significantly more MZ pregnancies occurred in pregnancies that took place soon after stopping oral contraceptives than occurred in pregnancies in non-users (Macourt *et al.* 1982). It has been suggested that the changes in the fallopian tubes and endometrium caused by these drugs may be such as to delay implantation of the zygote and, as in the armadillo (Benirschke 1981), cause it to divide. This theory has yet to be substantiated but supportive evidence comes from Japan, where few oral contraceptives are used and no change has been seen in the MZ twinning rate (Imaizumi and Inouye 1984).

In higher order pregnancies it is more common than would be expected to find a combination of MZ and DZ offspring. It has been suggested that blastomeres are more likely to split to produce MZ twins when several blastocysts are present and this happens particularly after ovulation induction and embryo transfer (Atlay and Pennington 1971). Derom's study of triplets resulting from treatment for infertility confirmed the earlier finding of a higher than expected number of monozygotic pairs within sets (Derom *et al*. 1991). The incidence of dizygotic triplets amongst induced pregnancies was 16 per cent, showing a zygote splitting rate three times that found in a normal population. As some of the mothers with DZ triplets had received ovulation-stimulating drugs for problems other than infertility, the authors concluded that the drugs themselves were likely to be responsible for the increased splitting rather than the subfertility itself.

It appears that there is now enough technical knowledge available to allow the deliberate production of human MZ twins. However, the ethical issues involved are profound. Some would argue that this procedure would be justified where the twin could be used for the cytogenetic and diagnostic analysis before deciding whether the second twin should be allowed to develop further (Kaufman 1985). Many however, would find this degree of interference unacceptable.

DZ twins

DZ twins result from the fertilization of two independently released ova. The number of DZ twin births can therefore be affected by the frequency of double ovulation, by sperm activity or by the rate of abortion (see p. 34). The first is probably the most important factor, although the role of sperm activity may have been underestimated (James 1978a).

Superfecundation

When two babies of apparently different ethnic origin are born in the same maternity, superfecundation (the conception of twins as a result of two coital acts in the same menstrual cycle) should be suspected (Archer 1810). Different paternities have since been confirmed by blood grouping in several cases (Geyer 1940; Gedda 1961; Sorgo 1973; Majsky and Kohl 1982) and more recently by HLA-typing (Terasaki *et al*. 1978; Majsky and Kohl 1982). Many other causes of superfecundation have been falsely suspected, as indicated by Mauriceau (1721): ' . . . another woman, who likewise had two children—the one like her husband, and the other like the gallant. But this does not prove superfoetation because sometimes different imaginations can cause the same effect.'

Further evidence of superfecundation is provided by the discordance for teratogenic malformations sometimes seen in DZ twins. If the twins are at different stages of development at the time of the teratogenic insult it follows that they were probably conceived at different times (see p. 68).

Not surprisingly, in our monogamous Western society, the frequency of superfecundation is unknown.

Superfetation

It used to be thought, on the grounds of differences in birth weight, that twins were often conceived in separate menstrual cycles—superfetation.

But weight is, of course, a poor indicator of gestational age and even MZ twins may have large intrapair weight discrepancies. Superfetation in man is rare, although Rhine and Nance (1976) describe an interesting family that, they suggest, has a dominant gene for superfetation. In four generations, six pairs of twins (at least three of unlike-sex) were born with marked weight discrepancies. In five of the pairs the smaller twin died in the perinatal period. A more extensive study in the US and Italy added more evidence of hereditary superfetation and the authors suggest that the dominant gene is expressed in the placenta, where it acts to reverse the normal placental inhibition of the female menstrual cycle (Nance *et al.* 1978).

Causes of DZ twinning

No single cause of DZ twinning is known but, unlike MZ twinning, at least some of the associated factors have been recognized. It has been estimated that between 11 and 27 per cent of Caucasian women are twin-prone (Wyshak and White 1965), a far greater number than those who actually produce twins. Lazar *et al.* (1981) have devised a scoring system (using seven maternal characteristics found to be associated with twinning) by which the probability of a twin pregnancy for a particular woman can be predicted (see p. 31). We are still, however, far from being able to predict accurately which women will have twins, and research on this subject is much needed.

Genetic and racial factors

It is widely believed that twins 'run in families' (which in the case of DZ twins is true) but there are still many falsely held beliefs, for example that twins usually occur in alternate generations.

Family studies have now shown that the genetic determinant for DZ twinning comes directly through the female line (Weinberg 1902; Bulmer 1960; White and Wyshak 1964; Nylander 1975a) but may well not be expressed in each generation. There is no doubt that the main genetic determinant for DZ twinning is maternal, but whether paternal genes have any influence is still being hotly debated. Early reports of an increased incidence of twins on the paternal side of the family (Davenport 1927; Greulich 1934) are now thought to have been due to under-reporting of singletons (Nylander 1975a).

Two studies of twinning in inter-racial marriages also suggest restriction of the carrier gene to females in that the DZ twinning rates depended on the mother's race (Morton 1962, Khoury and Erickson 1983). However, conflicting results come from Parisi *et al.* (1983), who found a paternal influence in their study of 950 unselected twin pairs of known zygosity. They also found a relationship between the two types of twinning on the basis of a significantly increased frequency of DZ twins among maternal relatives of MZ twins.

It appears that the gene concerned influences gonadotrophin production, which in turn stimulates double ovulation. Nylander (1973) found that in three groups of Nigerian (Yoruba) mothers, one with singletons, another with one set of twins and a third with two sets of twins, there was a positive correlation between serum follicle-stimulating hormone (FSH) levels and twinning, with a difference between each of the three groups. Similarly, Nigerian mothers of singletons had higher levels of FSH (Nylander 1978) than mothers of singletons in Japan, where there are particularly low rates of twinning (Soma *et al.* 1975).

No amount of bias in reporting could account for the vastly disparate twinning rates found in different ethnic groups throughout the world. The chance of a woman from the Yoruba tribe in Nigeria having twins is about eight times that of one from Taiwan (Ping and Chin 1967) and five times that of most Caucasians. Indeed, similar disparities are found in inter-racial populations where the accuracy of twin statistics in all groups is probably similar (Morton 1962). In the United States the non-white population has a consistently higher twinning rate than the whites (Bulmer 1958), although not as high as most African groups. This may be due to the introduction of some Caucasian genes by inter-racial marriages, or to environmental differences.

All negroid races have a relatively high twinning rate, although there is still considerable variation between ethnic groups, as Nylander found in his study of the various tribes in Nigeria (Nylander 1971a; Nylander and Corney 1977). Unusually high rates have also been found in some isolated Caucasian groups, such as those in the remote Finnish islands of Åland (Eriksson and Fellman 1973). The high incidence amongst isolated groups is likely to be the result of endogamy. The increasing number of immigrant marriage partners in Åland has been reflected in a falling twinning rate since the beginning of the twentieth century (Eriksson and Fellman 1973).

Theoretically, both the familial and the racial determinants of DZ twinning could be essentially environmental. In support of this idea is Nylander's finding of a much lower incidence of twins in Yoruba women living in towns than in rural villages. This could not be accounted for by age or parity differences alone. Nylander suggests that the traditional diet of this tribe may contain some hormone-stimulating substance, possibly in the yam, which is eaten less by those living an urban and therefore more westernized life (Nylander 1978, 1979). However, Morton's (1962) findings in Hawaii, and Khoury and Ericksson's (1983) in the US, contradict a purely environmental determinant because in inter-racial marriages, both parents (presumably) share the same environment, including diet. It is likely that both genetics and environment play a part in DZ twinning.

Maternal age and parity

An older mother with an already large family is most likely (and often least eager) to have twins. Many authors (Anderson 1956; Bulmer 1959a; Millis 1959; Eriksson and Fellman 1967; Elwood 1978; Nylander 1981; Bonnelykke 1990) have reported that the incidence of twins increases with age, reaching a peak at 35–39 years (Fig. 2.1). Nylander (1975b) suggests that this is due to increasing ovarian activity until the late thirties and it has now been shown that levels of these hormones in ovulating blood do increase with maternal age (Guyton 1981). Thereafter, the graafian follicles become exhausted as the menopause approaches.

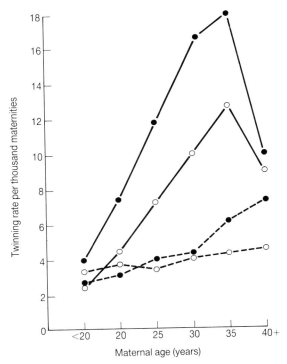

Fig. 2.1 The twinning rate among American whites and blacks, by maternal age. From Bulmer (1958) by permission of the author and editors of *Annals of Human Genetics* and Cambridge University Press, o---o white, monozygotic; ●---● black, monozygotic; o——o white, dizygotic; ●——● black, dizygotic.

Earlier studies related to Caucasian populations but Nylander (1971b, 1975b) has found the same pattern in Nigeria, except that here the peak is reached earlier—at 30–34 years. Women start childbearing earlier in West Africa and it may be that the ovaries then reach maximal activity earlier than Caucasians.

DZ twinning rates increase with parity independent of maternal age (Bulmer 1970; Nylander 1975b; Fig. 2.2). This is scarcely surprising as both DZ twins and a large family are signs of high fertility. Other indications that mothers of twins conceive easily is the high twinning rate amongst illegitimate births (in women over 25 years) (Eriksson and Fellman 1967; Campbell *et al.* 1974), as well as those conceived in the first 3 months of marriage (Bulmer 1959a; Allen 1981). There was a rush of twin births in the United States in 1946, probably due to a twinning tendency in those women who conceived most quickly following the return of the fathers at the end of the Second World War (Allen and Schachter 1970). However, in the last three instances, coital rates are likely to be high and it could be that more frequent sexual intercourse accounted for the high twinning rate by increasing the chances of superfecundation (James 1972).

It has also been suggested that frequent coitus may cause an increase in

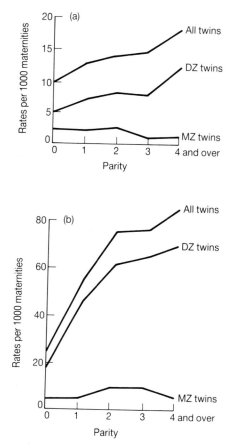

Fig. 2.2 Influence of parity on the incidence of twinning in (a) Aberdeen and (b) Nigeria. From Nylander (1975c) by permission of the author and WB Saunders Co. Ltd.

the release of gonadotrophins as a result of the erotic responses, thus further increasing the chances of DZ twinning (Hollenbach and Hickock 1990).

Maternal height and weight

More tall women than small have twins (Anderson 1956; Campbell *et al.* 1974; Corney *et al.* 1979; MacGillivray *et al.* 1988b). Similarly, weight appears to have a positive correlation with DZ twinning (Campbell *et al.* 1974). Both height and weight are indices of nutrition. Bulmer (1959b) found that in countries where there was severe shortage of food in the Second World War (e.g. France, the Netherlands and Norway) twinning rates fell, whereas in countries in which there was no undernourishment (e.g. Sweden and Denmark) they were unchanged during the war.

Other maternal factors

Women who have borne twins tend to differ from mothers of singletons in their menstrual and reproductive histories. It has been found that women with irregular menstrual cycles are less likely to have twins (Hemon *et al.* 1979) and that there is a positive correlation between twinning and both early menarche (Skerlj 1939; Wyshak 1981) and short menstrual cycles (Wyshak 1981). Likewise Wyshak (1978) found that mothers of twins have an earlier natural menopause than mothers of singletons.

It appears that the introduction of hormone-suppressing agents for contraception may well have affected the pattern of DZ twinning. There appears to be an increased chance of a multiple pregnancy immediately after stopping oral contraception, probably due to a rebound effect on the previously suppressed pituitary hormones (Rothman 1977; Bracken 1979). On the other hand, the overall chances of a multiple pregnancy in women who have previously used oral contraceptives are less than in those who have never taken hormone suppressing drugs (Rothman 1977; Hemon *et al.* 1979).

Seasonal variation

Timonen and Carpen (1968) reported a marked seasonal variation in twinning rates and suggested that the higher rate of twin conceptions in the summer months in Finland might be due to the increased hours of daylight. Several other authors (Edwards 1938; Knox and Morley 1960; Kamimura 1976; Elwood 1978; Imaizumi *et al.* 1980; James 1980b; Cheng *et al.* 1986; Nakamura and Miura 1987) have reported seasonal variations in twinning. Some have related these to climatic conditions in their countries, but no regular pattern emerges.

Social class

There are conflicting reports on the effect of social class on twinning rates. This may be partly due to the definitions used but also because of the other related factors, such as family size and maternal height. Finally, there are major problems in unravelling the real association of different factors with twinning, the incidence of which is constantly changing in a setting of changing marital and family-life patterns, as well as revolutionary development in economic and environmental conditions (MacGillivray *et al.* 1988b).

Golding (1986), in a European multicentre review, found an association between increased twinning rates, low educational attainment and agricultural labour; he also found decreased rates in the professional classes. However, Myrianthopoulos (1970) found higher rates in upper socioeconomic groups in both whites and blacks in the USA. Amongst the Yoruba tribe in Nigeria the incidence of twins is much higher among the lower socioeconomic, usually rural, population than among the higher, more urban, socio-economic groups (Marinho *et al.* 1986). Diet may be a factor here (see p. 20).

Treatment for infertility

The use of gonadotrophic hormones and clomiphene citrate in the treatment of anovulation is responsible for a number of DZ twins and of higher order multiple pregnancies. Multiple embryo and gamete transfer to the uterus is responsible for a 23 per cent rate of multiple pregnancies in those pregnancies resulting from assisted conception (Interim Licensing Authority 1990) and the average number of babies per delivery is correlated with the number of embryos or ova transferred (Fig. 2.3). Overall, as many as 17 per cent of multiple births in the UK may be the result of treatment for infertility.

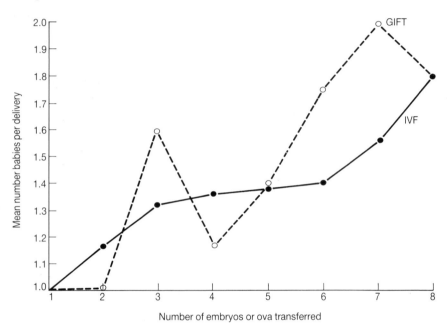

Fig. 2.3   Mean number of babies per delivery according to the number of embryos (for *in vitro* fertilization (IVF)) or ova (for gamete intra-fallopian transfer (GIFT)) replaced. From Beral et al. (1990) by permission of the authors and the *British Medical Bulletin*.

Until treatment for infertility becomes better regulated, the contribution of this source to the overall population of DZ twins is likely to increase as the number of new treatment centres rapidly increases.

Boklage (1986) has recently challenged the long-held assumption that MZ and DZ twins arise from entirely unrelated processes. He has believed that MZ and DZ twinning share some of their causes, including at least some heritable factors contributing to non-righthandedness (NRH), to midline symmetry malformations and to patterns of brain and body asymmetry. He has found that twinning is familially related to NRH and that both MZ and DZ twins, their siblings and their parents have an equal excess of NRH over members of families without twins. Similarly, twins and their relatives have excesses of certain malformations, and singletons with these same malformations have a greater than expected number of NRH parents, and indeed of parents who are twins. He suggests that disturbances of oöcyte development may be responsible for this whole system of twinning-related anomalies. Clearly these suggestions need further study.

Secular trends in twinning rates

In recent years many developed countries, including the USA, many parts of Western Europe, Australia, New Zealand, Japan, Hungary (Czeizel and Acsardi, 1971), Poland (Rola-Janicki 1974) and Canada (Elwood 1973), have reported a change in their twinning rates (James 1986b). The oft-quoted figure of 1 in 80 deliveries in the UK is now outdated and should be revised regularly. In many countries a decline in twinning rates started in the 1950s and continued until the late 1970s. In the UK the rates levelled off at 1 in 105 and then started to rise again (Fig. 2.4); in 1989 the rate was 1 in 90. Where the decline has been analysed it appears to be confined to DZ twins. It started and finished earlier in the USA (Jeannerret and Macmahon 1962), possibly because the trend has been counteracted by ovulation-stimulating drugs (James 1978a) and other forms of treatment for infertility.

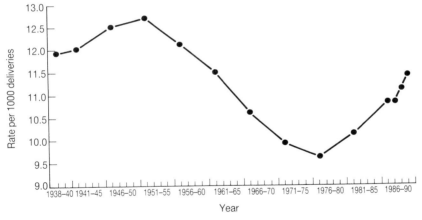

Fig. 2.4   Twinning rates in England and Wales 1938–1989.

The cause of the fall in twinning rates is unknown. Earlier childbearing and smaller families are not the full explanation (James 1975). Use of oral contraceptives and pesticides has been suggested, so has the rise in levels of air, water and soil pollution (Eriksson *et al.* 1976). James (1978a) suggested that reduced sperm activity may be responsible, as there is evidence, at least in the US, that sperm counts had fallen in the years immediately before his study (Nelson and Bunge 1974; Rehan *et al.* 1975).

From developing countries we have only the reports from parts of Nigeria (Nylander 1975b); here the rates have fallen more recently (Marinho *et al.* 1986).

Determination of zygosity

Most parents of twins are anxious to learn the zygosity of their twins as soon as possible. Few are satisfied by the assurance that this is likely to become apparent by the children's second birthday. It is natural that they should want to know all there is to know about their children. In addition, many parents say they feel foolish not being able to answer the question most commonly asked. The children themselves often want to know. Finally, and for some, the most important, both the mother and any daughter (be she a twin or sibling) may like to know what their chances of having twins are. For many, the knowledge that these chances are greatly increased by dizygosity will influence decisions about further pregnancies, or at least their timing. Quite apart from the advantages to medical and scientific research, these are ample reasons for determining as accurately as practicable the zygosity of all newborn twins (Bryan 1986).

Where the children's sex differs there is, of course, no problem. Also taking placentation into account, the zygosity of over half of Caucasian twins can be determined in the delivery room. Yet, too often, the zygosity is not considered at birth, so that invaluable information from the placental membranes is lost and blood samples become harder to collect.

Physical features

Physical features in older children and adults are a relatively good means of establishing zygosity (Cohen *et al.* 1975; Kasriel and Eaves 1976; Eisen *et al.* 1989) unless, of course, one twin is discordant for a major congenital anomaly or for a disability, such as cerebral palsy. A study of 200 pairs of Swedish twins Cederlof *et al.* (1961) found that 72 affirmed in a reply to a mailed questionnaire that they had grown up 'as alike as two peas'. Of these, 71 were subsequently found to be alike for the five blood groups tested. But appearances are of little help in newborn twins. Intrauterine influences may well be stronger than genetic ones, particularly in cases of the fetofetal transfusion syndrome (see p. 52), when MZ twins may have large intrapair weight discrepancies.

Ear form has been suggested as a useful guide (Dahlberg 1926), but comparing two tiny ears is not easy. Nor is the comparison of finger and palm prints. The ridge count on fingers is thought to be genetically determined and thus the counts can give some indication of zygosity (Smith and Penrose 1955; Holt 1968). The sum of the left and right maximal ATD palmar angles can also be used (Holt 1968). As the overlap between MZ and DZ is considerable, these methods are only useful as adjuncts to others.

Later, the pattern and timing of teeth eruption as well as the forms of teeth may be helpful (Fearne, J. personal communication) as may their pattern of body growth.

Sex

One-third of all twins are of unlike sex and all these must be DZ, with the exception of an extremely rare case of heterokaryotypic chromosomal anomaly (see p. 65).

Placentation

For many years it was believed that all MZ twins had a single chorion. Indeed, some medical textbooks still categorically state this and some paediatricians still appear to believe them (Partridge 1987). Parents may still present their indistinguishable four- or five-year-old twins and declare that they are fraternal because they had two placentae (Lykken 1978; King *et al.* 1980). From early in the pregnancy parents may be misled by radiographers and obstetricians on the evidence of two placentae seen on ultrasound.

It is now known that those MZ twins whose zygote has divided before the sixth day after fertilization have separate chorions. This, as well as the method of examination of placental membranes, will be discussed more fully in Chapter 4. Suffice it to say here that only about two-thirds of MZ twins will have monochorionic placentae. In these, a definite diagnosis of monozygosity can be made, as no convincing report of a monochorionic placenta in a DZ pregnancy has been offered.

Nearly half of Caucasian twins have dichorionic placentae and are of like sex. For these, other lines of zygosity determination are necessary.

Laboratory investigation

As MZ twins are derived from one zygote they must be alike for all genetically determined characters, whereas DZ twins originating from two zygotes are no more alike than other siblings. Zygosity can be determined by studying common population variants known as polymorphisms. These include blood groups, serum proteins, enzyme polymorphisms and DNA polymorphisms. For example, if the father of twins is AB for the AB0 blood group and the mother is group 0, the offspring may be group A or group B. If one twin is group A and the other group B they are clearly DZ. If both twins are group A they could be MZ or DZ. There is a 1 in 2 chance of these parents producing an A zygote that goes on to form MZ twins and a 1 in 2 × 1 in 2, i.e. 1 in 4 chance of producing two A zygotes. In calculations this is usually shown as the relative chance of dizygosity: monozygosity, which in this case would be ¼:½, or 0.5:1.

The laboratory often receives samples from the twins without accompanying parental samples. If the parental genotypes are not known then the likelihood of DZ twins having the same genotype depends on the frequency of each allele in the population. The relative chance of dizygosity can be calculated for the genotypes of many marker systems on the basis of their gene frequencies, as shown in Table 2.3. Gene frequencies for markers vary for people from different geographical or ethnic backgrounds and this should be taken into account when using these tables (Race and Sanger 1975).

The relative chance of dizygosity for different marker systems can be combined in Bayesian calculations, as shown in Table 2.4. Many of the blood group and biochemical markers that are used do not on their own provide a great deal of zygosity information. Ideally, marker systems that give maximum information, i.e. where the father has alleles A and B and the mother C and D, should be used so that the relative chance of dizygosity if the twins have the same genotype is 0.25:1. Locus-specific DNA probes that detect

Table 2.3 Biochemical genetic markers used at MRC Human Genetics Unit, University College, London, in the determination of zygosity in newborn twins. Relative chances in favour of dizygosity are given for each genetically determined character

Enzyme or serum protein system	Twin pair of like phenotype	Relative chance in favour of dizygosity
Tissue enzymes typed on placenta		
Placental alkaline phosphatase	1	0.7006
Pl	2-1	0.5606
	2	0.3856
	3-1	0.4678
	3	0.2938
	3-2	0.3417
Phosphoglucomutase, locus 3	1	0.7569
PGM_3	2-1	0.5962
	2	0.3969
Red cell enzymes		
Acid phosphatase, locus 1	A	0.4624
ACP_1	BA	0.5937
	B	0.6320
	CA	0.3615
	CB	0.4248
	C	0.2756
Phosphoglucomutase, locus 1	1	0.7788
PGM_1	2-1	0.5899
	2	0.3813
Adenylate kinase	1	0.9555
AK	2-1	0.5215
	2	0.2730
Adenosine deaminase	1	0.9409
ADA	2-1	0.5282
	2	0.2809
Esterase-D	1	0.9054
ES-D	2-1	0.5438
	2	0.3008
Glutamic-pyruvic transaminase	1	0.5646
GPT	2-1	0.6250
	2	0.5588
Serum proteins		
Group-specific component	1	0.7569
Gc	2-1	0.5962
	2	0.3969
α_1-antitrypsin	M	0.9555
Pi	MS*	0.5215
	S*	0.2730
Haptoglobin (sometimes developed in the newborn)	1-1	0.4761
Hp	2-1	0.6178
	2-2	0.6561

*S or other non-M types.
Source: From Corney and Robson (1975) by permission of the authors and W. B. Saunders Co. Ltd.

Table 2.4 An example of the determination of the chances of dizygosity in a pair of twins alike for all blood group and biochemical markers and of the most common phenotype at all loci, using the tables of Smith and Penrose (1955) and Race and Sanger (1975)

Marker system	Phenotype	Relative chance of dizygosity for a particular system	Relative chance of monozygosity for a particular system
Initial odds		0.7000	0.3
Sex	Female	0.5000	1.0
ABO	A	0.6945	1.0
MNSs	MS	0.5161	1.0
Rh	R_1r	0.5400	1.0
Kell	K−	0.9548	1.0
Secretor	Sec	0.8681	1.0
Duffy	Fy(a+)	0.8099	1.0
Kidd	Jk(a+)	0.8616	1.0
Dombrock	Do(a+)	0.8094	1.0
Xg	Xg(a+)	0.9573	1.0
Pl	1	0.7006	1.0
PGM_3	1	0.7569	1.0
ACP_1	B	0.6320	1.0
ADA	1	0.9409	1.0
ES-D	1	0.9054	1.0
GPT	2-1	0.6250	1.0
Gc	1	0.7569	1.0
Pi	M	0.9555	1.0
Combined chance after testing		0.0056	0.3
Chance of dizygosity = 0.0056/0.3056 = 0.0183			

P, *Yt* and *Hp* have not been used as they are not fully developed in the newborn, and *Lu*, *PGM₁* and *AK* because they are linked to *Sec*, *Rh* and *ABO* respectively.
Source: From Corney and Robson (1975) by permission of the authors and W. B. Saunders Co. Ltd.

variable numbers of tandem repeats fit this pattern. Information from these can be included in a Bayesian calculation in the same way as the blood groups and biochemical markers. Even more informative than these polymorphisms are the patterns detected by DNA fingerprinting (Derom *et al.* 1985; Hill and Jeffreys 1985) where many loci are tested at the same time, building up a pattern that is unique to the individual. MZ twins have identical DNA fingerprints (Fig. 2.5) but the probability that DZ twins have the same DNA fingerprint has been calculated as 3×10^{-14} making this approach the most accurate laboratory method for zygosity testing.

DNA fingerprinting has the added advantage that only small volumes of blood (or placental tissue) are needed. Placental tissue is easily obtained, even when one or both twins are stillborn, and analysis can be done satisfactorily on specimens that have been frozen. The disadvantage is that the test is expensive.

If cord blood samples have not been taken, blood can be taken from the babies later. However, this sampling will need to be postponed for at least 6

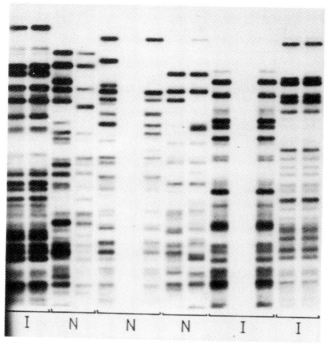

Fig. 2.5 DNA fingerprint band patterns of MZ and DZ twins. N, dizygotic; I, monozygotic. By permission of Cellmark Diagnostics.

months if blood transfusions have been given during the neonatal period.

Unless there are medical indications (or the children require venepunctures for some other reason) an inessential and painful procedure should not be imposed on children over the age of 12 months or so—it should wait until the children are old enough to freely agree to it themselves. It is sometimes difficult to persuade parents of this.

Intertwin acceptance of skin grafts is often stated to be the ultimate confirmation of monozygosity. However, the situation is complex, incompletely understood and therefore difficult to quantify (Corney and Robson 1975). Skin grafting in twins as a means of determining zygosity is, in any case, both unjustified in practical terms and unethical, particularly in the newborn.

Methods of zygosity determination are comprehensively reviewed by Burn and Corney (1988).

3

Multiple pregnancy

A mother may learn that she is expecting two babies, not one, as early as the sixth week of her pregnancy. On the other hand, she may occasionally have no suspicion about the second baby until after the delivery of the first. At whatever stage the twin is discovered, most parents have a time of shock followed by readjustment. It is clearly better for this process to be completed before the mother has to look after the two babies. Several mothers have described their difficulties in relating to two fetuses when they had already developed a deeply felt relationship with what they thought was one baby. This difficulty is especially felt when twins are discovered only in the third trimester.

The medical hazards, as well as the practical and psychological problems, that may confront a mother of undiagnosed twins, are now well known. In centres where ultrasound scanning is not routinely practised there may be a place for selective screening of predictably high-risk cases such as a mother with a family history of twins (Michels and Riccardi 1978). Other criteria for screening can be deducted from Chapter 2.

As a result of their study of a large number of French mothers of twins, Lazar et al. (1981) suggested a scale for preconceptional prediction of twins using six maternal features—age, parity, twins in her family, regularity of menses, blood groups 0 and blood group A.

Diagnosis

Before the advent of screening with ultrasound scanners an unexpected second baby was not uncommon and in some centres 50 per cent of mothers who had twins went into labour before the twins had been diagnosed (Farooqui et al. 1973; MacGillivray 1975a; Grennert et al. 1976). Where the twins had been detected earlier the diagnosis rested on clinical suspicion followed by radiological confirmation. Possible indications of a multiple pregnancy include an inappropriately large uterus, an unusually rapid weight gain, the palpation of multiple fetal parts or the mother's reports of increased fetal movements. In obstetric units with no routine screening procedures most multiple pregnancies are not diagnosed until after the 30th week—long after the time at which a mother should be having special care, supervision and extra rest.

Cheaper and more readily available methods of screening for multiple pregnancy than ultrasound may be more appropriate as first lines of investigation in some developing countries. These methods include measurements of maternal serum alphafetoprotein (AFP), human chorionic gonadotrophin (hCG), trophoblast proteins, human placental lactogen (hPL) and swangerschaftsprotein (these last two have proved useful in the early detection of a multiple pregnancy (Grennert el al. 1976, Jandial *et al.* 1979)). In developing countries the most efficient method of detecting a multiple pregnancy is likely to be an accurate clinical measurement, such as the fundal height. Leroy *et al.* (1982) found that 90 per cent of multiple pregnancies had a fundal height above the 90th centile for a single pregnancy by the 20th week and 98 per cent by the 28th week.

Alphafetoprotein

Maternal serum AFP is routinely measured in many antenatal clinics as a screening test for fetal neural tube defects. Two fetuses increase the total AFP production and this is reflected in the maternal serum. One study showed that nearly 80 per cent of maternal AFP levels in multiple pregnancies were above the 90th centile for a single pregnancy (Knight *et al.* 1981). Thus a mother with a raised serum AFP may have a period of intense anxiety only relieved by the discovery that her raised AFP is due to nothing worse than twins. AFP values in twin pregnancies, however, vary over a wide range so that some cases will still fall well within the normal limits for a single pregnancy. Thom and colleagues (1984) found that AFP levels were higher in MZ than DZ pregnancies, possibly due to the difference in placentation.

Ultrasound

With routine screening of all pregnancies for twins some centres now approach a detection rate of 100 per cent (Grennert *et al.* 1976; Patel *et al.* 1984) and the average stage of pregnancy at which the diagnosis is made is substantially earlier. In one unit the average time of diagnosis fell from 33 weeks to 19 weeks over a 6-year period following the introduction of ultrasound screening (Grennert *et al.* 1976; Fig. 3.1). However 12–16 weeks—the stage of pregnancy at which routine scanning is often carried out—is not the easiest time to detect twins and in less experienced hands the second fetus may be missed. In one study, one-fifth of all multiple pregnancies in which an ultrasound scan was carried out had at least one false-negative report (Jarvis 1979). Some patients have had three scans and have still been surprised by a second baby at delivery.

Two gestational sacs can be detected as early as 6 weeks by abdominal ultrasound and even earlier by the vaginal approach (D'Alton and Mercer 1990). With these very early diagnoses a major question is whether to tell the parents immediately and risk a later disappointment (see p. 169), or whether to delay until the risk of losing a fetus is less; this risk is much higher than generally recognized. There is evidence that in 50 per cent or more of twin pregnancies one fetus is lost (Robinson and Caines 1977)—the 'vanishing twin syndrome' (Fig. 3.2). Indeed Levi (1976) found that only 29 per cent of twin pregnancies diagnosed before the 10th week ended up with two live

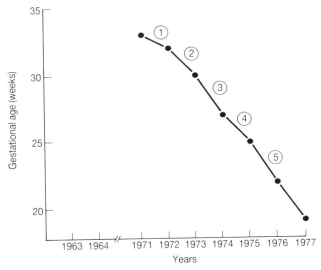

Fig. 3.1 Average gestational age at diagnosis of twin pregnancy in relation to introduction of diagnostic facilities. By permission of L. Grennert (personal communication). 1, Introduction of ultrasonic facilities; 2, ultrasonic screening of selected population; 3, ultrasonic and HPL screening of all gravidae attending the antenatal clinic; 4, ultrasonic and HPL screening of all gravidae within the district; 5, screening of entire population.

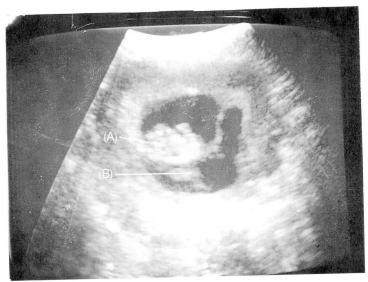

Fig. 3.2 Ultrasonic scan of twin pregnancy at 13 weeks' gestation showing one normal fetus (A) and one empty sac (B). Vaginal blood loss occurred at 12 weeks. By permission of Dr Valerie Farr.

babies. The majority of mothers had one full-term baby. However, later research has questioned the very high number of twin pregnancies and suggested that some may be mistaken diagnoses as, in some cases, it is not always easy to differentiate between a second gestational sac and the early separation of embryonic membranes (Landy *et al.* 1982, 1986; Ramzin *et al.* 1982).

Schneider *et al.* (1979) made an interesting observation in relation to ovulation-induced twin pregnancies. In the 11 cases in which clomiphene had been taken, ovular resorption occurred in 7, whereas in the 12 pregnancies induced by gonadotropins all 12 resulted in the delivery of two babies.

X-rays

X-rays, once the mainstay of diagnosis of multiple pregnancy are used much less often now and are being superseded by ultrasound scans. There are, however, still times when they are needed, particularly in centres with less sophisticated ultrasound scanning techniques. For example, an X-ray may be indicated when ultrasound scanning gives an equivocal result, if more than two fetuses are suspected (Fig. 3.3) or in the case of suspected fetal bony abnormalities (Fig. 3.4). Radiography for assessing the position of the fetuses has now been largely superseded by ultrasound.

Breaking the news

Recent studies have highlighted the importance of breaking the news of a multiple pregnancy sensitively (Spillman 1985; Macfarlane *et al.* 1990a). Many mothers have been caused quite unnecessary anxiety about an abnormality because of the obvious interest that staff have shown in their ultrasound followed by a delay in giving them information while further consultation is undertaken.

Other couples, particularly those being told of higher multiple pregnancies (see p. 191), have complained about medical staff's unthinking jokes in giving information to parents, which at best will shock and at worst devastate them.

As soon as a couple have been told the diagnosis they should be given information about a multiple pregnancy and the telephone number of an individual or organization that can provide them with information about parenting twins. Many couples suffer weeks of unnecessary anxiety through ignorance about available sources of help.

Abortion

Spontaneous abortions of twins are often missed, especially in early pregnancy when the fetuses are not easy to distinguish. It follows that figures on the incidence of twin abortions should be interpreted with caution. Incidences of up to 20 per cent have been recorded but in two large studies, each of approximately 2000 abortions, the incidence of twins was only 1.2 per cent (Javert 1957) and 0.3 per cent (Benirschke and Driscoll 1967). However, in a

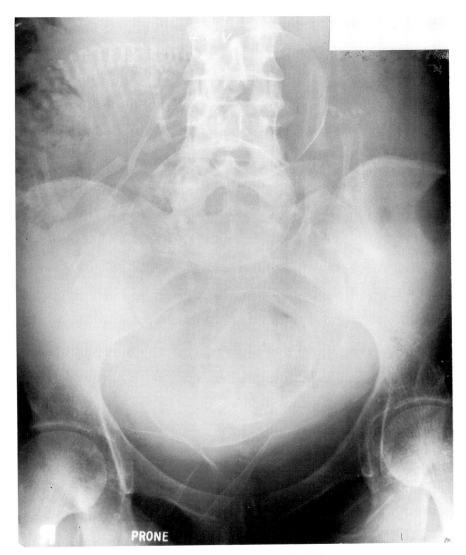

PRONE

Fig. 3.3 X-ray showing triplets. By permission of J. Malvern.

more recent study in which 1939 spontaneously aborted embryos and fetuses were examined in detail, the incidence of twin abortions was 3 per cent—approximately three times greater than would be expected (Livingstone and Poland 1980). The authors distinguished between embryos (less than 30 mm crown–rump length) and fetuses and found the same increase in both groups when compared with singletons.

Amongst aborted twins there is a striking preponderance of monochorionic twins (Livingstone and Poland 1980). Disturbances of the

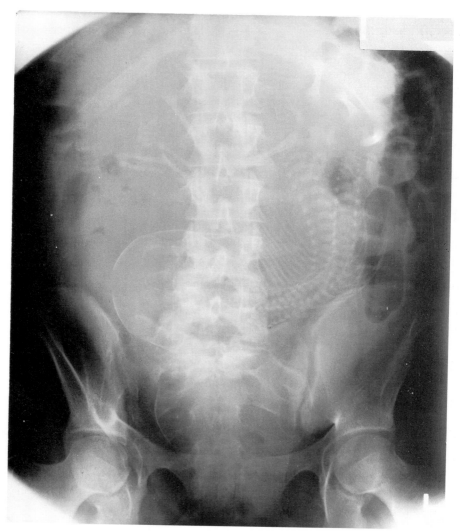

Fig. 3.4   X-ray of conjoined twins.

fetofetoplacental circulation are probably responsible for many abortions in this group. Out of 26 fetuses examined by Livingstone and Poland definite evidence of the fetofetal transfusion syndrome was found in eight. Javert (1957) found that there were relatively fewer malformed fetuses amongst twins and attributed this to the disproportionately high incidence of circulatory disturbances. Perhaps surprisingly, Livingstone and Poland did not confirm this finding. They found a similar proportion of malformations amongst both twin embryos and fetuses as singletons.

The death of just one fetus, which may or may not be aborted, is quite common. This is shown by the relatively high incidence of twins found in first-trimester ultrasound scans (see p. 32) compared with the number of twins actually delivered. Similarly, on routine ultrasound screening, it is not unusual to find an empty second gestational sac. In one large study this was found in 0.8 per cent of all pregnancies (Ramzin *et al*. 1982). Evidence of a blighted twin may also be seen in some cases of first-trimester bleeding with continuation of a normal single pregnancy (Finberg and Birnholz 1979). However, an accurate estimation of the incidence is difficult, first, because first-trimester ultrasound scans are not routinely carried out, and second, because of the risk of false-positives in early pregnancy, as described earlier (see p. 32). Threatened abortions appear to be 3–4 times as common in twin pregnancies as in single pregnancies (Patel *et al*. 1984).

Heterotopic pregnancy

A simultaneous intrauterine and extrauterine pregnancy is said to occur once in 30 000 pregnancies (Reece *et al*. 1983) and predisposing factors include pelvic inflammatory disease, surgery to the fallopian tubes, ovulation-stimulating drugs and assisted conception. Molloy *et al*. (1990) found that assisted conception resulted in a 300-fold increase in the risk of a heterotopic pregnancy, with an incidence of 1 in 70 for gamete intrafallopian transfer (GIFT) patients and 1 in 130 for *in vitro* fertilization (IVF).

Tubal pregnancies have been described in association with triplets where there are two intrauterine fetuses (Snyder *et al*. 1988; Molloy *et al*. 1990) or two ectopic fetuses (Porter *et al*. 1986).

The diagnosis of a heterotopic pregnancy is commonly made after termination of the pregnancy, although a higher percentage are now being diagnosed preoperatively by vaginal ultrasonography (Rempen 1988). Assays of β-HCG can suggest the diagnosis, which should then be confirmed by ultrasonography. As long as the diagnosis is made early and the extrauterine fetus is either removed by salpingectomy or a selective feticide is performed, the outcome should be good for the intrauterine twin. There have been extremely rare instances where infants from both the intrauterine and extrauterine pregnancy have survived. In 1990 Dahniya and colleagues reviewed the 14 cases reported in the world literature up to that time.

Management of multiple pregnancy

The role of some measures thought to promote fetal growth and prevent premature onset of labour, such as bedrest, cervical cerclage and β-sympathomimetic drugs remains controversial and in their review of the literature MacGillivray and Campbell (1988) found no measures that had had significant effects on preventing preterm labour, low birth weight, pre-eclampsia or in reducing perinatal mortality. The risks to the mother of a multiple pregnancy compared to a single one are increased, especially if she has a medical condition, such as cardiac, renal or metabolic disease. Discussions on these and other aspects of management are beyond the scope of this book and the reader is referred to MacGillivray *et al.* (1988a) and to textbooks on obstetrics.

Bedrest

The role of bedrest is one that has provoked particular controversy. There have been numerous studies on the effects of bedrest but a review of those carried out in the last 30 years found no convincing evidence of a beneficial effect (MacGillivray 1986). Even when mothers at particularly high risk of preterm labour are selected, no beneficial effect of bed rest has been demonstrated (Crowther *et al.* 1989).

Whatever the medical arguments for and against bedrest, there are considerable disadvantages in terms of financial cost to both the family and the health services (Patel *et al.* 1984) as well as the disruption to the life of the mother, her partner and her existing children (Powers and Miller 1979, Tresmontant and Papiernik 1983). It can, for example, be particularly distressing for an older child if his mother first deserts him and then returns with two babies who distract attention from him.

The problems may also be emotional. In one study 62 per cent of mothers who had bedrest found it a stressful experience (Hay *et al.* 1990); it can be particularly so if they are worrying about an older child. The same authors found that 30 per cent of mothers with an older child reported depression in the last trimester, compared with 6 per cent of those where it was the first pregnancy.

It may well be that the most successful way to reduce the complications of a multiple pregnancy and the long-term risk to twin children is by offering more home-based professional support and advice. The results of such a strategy in France have been encouraging (Tresmontant and Papiernik 1983; Papiernik *et al.* 1985).

Complications of multiple pregnancy

The high perinatal mortality associated with twinning is largely due to complications of pregnancy, such as premature onset of labour, fetal intra-uterine growth retardation and difficulties of delivery. The management of multiple pregnancy is thus concerned with the prevention, early detection and treatment of these complications.

Pre-eclampsia

Pre-eclampsia, an important complication of pregnancy, is generally recognized to occur more often in multiple pregnancy. The incidences reported inevitably vary according to the diagnostic criteria adopted. Several authors have found at least a three-fold increase compared with singletons (Gutmacher 1939; Bender 1952) but the increase in incidence of the severe form may be higher still (MacGillivray 1984). Pre-eclampsia is characteristically a disorder of primagravidae but MacGillivray (1958) found that the chances of the severe form developing in a second (twin) pregnancy if the first (single) had been normal were 130 times that in a second single pregnancy.

Studies of multiple pregnancies give no convincing support to the theory of an immunological basis for pre-eclamptic toxaemia. Were it so, the disease would be more common in DZ pregnancies than in MZ. However, Campbell *et al.* (1977), in their study of over 300 multiple pregnancies, found no higher incidence of either the mild or the severe form of pre-eclampsia in mothers of DZ twins.

Polyhydramnios
The volume of amniotic fluid present in multiple pregnancy is particularly difficult to assess because the bulk of two fetuses can give the false impression of an increased amount of fluid. As with pre-eclampsia, differences in criteria largely account for the varying incidences reported and, as amniotic fluid is rarely accurately measured, it is usually a subjective diagnosis. With these reservations, however, comparisons within a single centre are probably valid and most authors agree that polyhydramnios is more common in multiple pregnancy. The incidence of polyhydramnios in the 1983 Scottish Twin Study (Patel *et al.* 1984) was 6 per cent in twin pregnancies compared with 0.3 per cent in singleton pregnancies; in Aberdeen it was 2.4 per cent versus 0.4 per cent. There is, of course, a high perinatal mortality associated with polyhydramnios. Law (1967) found that twins from a multiple pregnancy complicated by polyhydramnios had almost three times the risk of a perinatal death as those from pregnancies without increased volumes of amniotic fluid.

Perhaps surprisingly this increase in the occurrence of polyhydramnios affects DZ as much as MZ pregnancies (Guttmacher 1939; Nylander and MacGillivray 1975). However, a higher incidence of acute polyhydramnios was found in MZ pregnancies by Gaehtgens (1936). None of the other studies differentiated between the two forms of polyhydramnios.

At least some of the MZ cases of polyhydramnios are the results of the fetofetal transfusion syndrome (see p. 52) where the recipient twin's hypervolaemia results in polyuria and a consequent increase in amniotic fluid. Kloosterman (1963) suggested that the hypervolaemia, in turn, is due to an increase in maternofetal transfer of fluid in response to high fetal plasma proteins. The fetofetal transfusion syndrome, together with cases secondary to congenital malformations, at least partially explains the increased perinatal mortality associated with polyhydramnios (Tow 1959; Farooqui *et al.* 1973).

The high incidence of polyhydramnios in DZ pregnancies is harder to explain unless the increased intrauterine load somehow impedes the circulation and reabsorption of amniotic fluid.

The rare condition of acute polyhydramnios with its high fetal wastage appears to be confined to MZ twin pregnancies. Weir *et al.* (1979) found eight cases in over 30 000 deliveries. Two of these were in monoamniotic pregnancies and the remaining six were monochorionic diamniotic. All occurred in the second trimester between the 21st and 28th weeks and ended in a premature delivery within a few days. Apart from a pair of campomelic dwarfs the fetuses were normal, which suggests that a disturbance in the fetoplacental circulation was the most likely cause.

Acute polyhydramnios is a rapidly progressive disorder precipitating a premature delivery within a few days of onset. Repeated amniocenteses to remove the fluid may prevent the onset of labour long enough to produce a viable baby (Mahoney *et al*. 1990). Bender's (1952) patient had eight taps over 7 weeks. If polyhydramnios in twins is associated with a fetal abnormality it may in certain circumstances be possible to stop fluid accumulation by feticide of the affected twin (see p. 42), allowing the pregnancy of the normal twin to continue. Spontaneous abatement seems to occur only if one fetus dies (Bender 1952).

When polyhydramnios occurs in one sac, the other sac is frequently severely oligohydramniotic and the fetus may suffer from the so-called 'stuck twin' phenomenon (Mahoney *et al*. 1985). On ultrasound scan the stuck twin is seen in a relatively fixed position against the abdominal wall, even with changes in the mother's position.

Other complications

Other, less serious, complications occur in multiple as in single pregnancies but the symptoms are often more severe. Such a large uterine load may cause many symptoms, including breathlessness, indigestion and backache. These can be distressing and worrying to a mother. Even if the discomfort cannot be alleviated she will feel much better if reassured that these symptoms are a normal, if unfortunate, part of a twin pregnancy.

Prenatal diagnosis

Although the general management of a multiple pregnancy is rarely the concern of the paediatrician until near the time of delivery, there are some aspects about which both obstetricians and patient may value his advice—prenatal testing for fetal abnormalities is one of these.

Prenatal diagnosis by amniocentesis is now widely available and other methods such as fetal blood sampling, chorion villus sampling and fetoscopy are provided in specialist centres.

A multiple pregnancy, however, alters the risk of some abnormalities. For instance, trisomy 21 is less common in twins, whereas some neural tube defects are more common. On the other hand, concordance for neural tube defects, even in MZ twins, is unusual and Down syndrome, although usually concordant in MZ twins, rarely affects both of a DZ pair (see p. 65). However, with two fetuses the combined risk of at least one being affected is higher than a single pregnancy. Some would argue that amniocentesis should be offered to women at a younger age with multiple pregnancies (Rodis *et al*. 1990; Fig. 3.5).

Amniocentesis

Amniocentesis presents a particular problem with multiple pregnancy (Hunter and Cox 1979). It is technically more difficult and in many units the risks of inducing an abortion are greater. In addition, the results may pose a

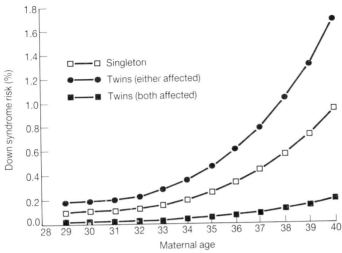

Fig. 3.5 Live-born Down syndrome risk versus maternal age in singleton and twin gestations. From Rodis *et al.* (1990) by permission of the author and editors of *Obstetrics and Gynaecology.*

far greater dilemma for parents of twins than singletons, as the chances of both twins being abnormal are small.

Amniocentesis is now offered to many older mothers for the detection of chromosomal abnormalities, and to others with a personal or family history of neural tube defects or some genetically determined disorder.

Although some centres report excellent results (Elias *et al.* 1980; Tabsh *et al.* 1985) others find it technically difficult to aspirate fluid from both amniotic sacs. Some parents are thus faced with making a decision on the findings from only one specimen.

Inadvertent double amniocentesis of one sac may also occur but various methods for determining whether both sacs have been sampled have been suggested, including injection of dyes, estimation of cell counts, determination of AFP and other protein concentrations and determination of other enzyme activities (Elejalde and Elejalde 1984; Filkins *et al.* 1984; Farge *et al.* 1985). An ultrasound scan or fetoscopy can provide the answer when the fetuses are of different sex or one has an anatomical defect.

Chorionic villus sampling

There has been success in multiple pregnancies with chorionic villus sampling with forceps under ultrasonic guidance (Kaplan and Eidelman 1983). The procedure is easier with dichorionic placentae, especially when the placental tissue is well separated.

If the trophoblast samples show an identical genotype (for example on karyotype or haemoglobin analysis) additional studies are necessary to ensure that trophoblast tissues from both twins has been obtained (Monni *et al.* 1986).

Fetal blood sampling

Rodeck and Wass (1981) recommend the single uterine puncture method for multiple pregnancies because it is less traumatic and should reduce the risk of preterm labour. The sampling needle is inserted through the septum into the second sac with the aid of the fetoscope. In dichorionic cases, where the septum is too opaque for direct visualization, the fetoscope may also be inserted into the second sac.

Fetoscopy

Direct visualization of the fetus in multiple pregnancy can be satisfactorily performed by fetoscopy. In monochorionic multiple pregnancies the second fetus can be seen through the amniotic membrane. Sometimes it is also possible to see it through a dichorionic septum but if this is too opaque the fetoscope will need to be passed through the septum into the second sac (Rodeck 1984).

Selective feticide

Many couples who would not hesitate to have a pregnancy terminated for a single abnormal fetus cannot agree if it means the sacrifice of a normal baby at the same time. The killing of one fetus is now an option available to parents who have a multiple pregnancy in which one of the fetuses has a serious anomaly.

Selective feticide has been performed for a number of anomalies where only one twin is affected, including trisomy 21 (Beck *et al*. 1981; Kerenyi and Chitkara 1981; Rodeck 1984), Tay–Sachs disease (Petres and Redwine 1981), Hurler syndrome (Aberg *et al*. 1978), Turner syndrome (Gigon *et al*. 1981), microcephaly, spina bifida, haemophilia, Duchenne muscular dystrophy, epidermolysis bullosa (Rodeck 1984), thalassaemia (Antsaklis *et al*. 1984) and cystic fibrosis (Bryan 1989). Severe cases of the fetofetal transfusion syndrome (Wittmann *et al*. 1986) may also indicate selective feticide (see p. 54), as may heterotopic pregnancy (see p. 37).

Methods

The advantage of hysterotomy (Beck *et al*. 1981; Gigon *et al*. 1981) is that the mother is spared the distressing experience of carrying a dead baby. (She also avoids the theoretical risk of disseminated intravascular coagulation resulting from a macerated fetus, although this has yet to be reported). However, most would consider that the degree of uterine disturbance involved in this operation creates an unacceptable risk of precipitating labour.

Other methods include injection of air into the umbilical vein of the affected fetus (Rodeck 1984) and cardiac puncture with exsanguination of the fetus (Aberg *et al*. 1978, Kerenyi and Chitkara 1981).

The risks involved

Selective feticide is rarely indicated in a monochorionic pregnancy because of the risk to the surviving twin of exsanguination (into the dead fetus; Donnenfeld *et al.* 1989) or disseminated intravascular coagulation (DIC) (p. 71).

When parents are offered the option of selective feticide they must be made aware of the potential risks attached to the procedure. These include precipitating an abortion or preterm labour, an incorrect selection of the target fetus when no anatomical markers are available and the introduction of infection. Failure to kill the fetus has also been reported (Petres and Redwine 1981).

The decision to proceed with selective feticide should depend not only on the severity of the abnormality (and this can be difficult to estimate in conditions with variable degrees of mental retardation, as in Turner or Klinefelter syndrome) but also on whether the child is likely to die at or soon after birth or survive as a burden to himself, his twin and his family for many years. A further consideration is the safety of the unaffected twin. An abnormal fetus may actually jeopardize the life of the healthy child, as in cases where an anencephalic causes polyhydramnios, and thus induces premature labour.

Parents will need a great deal of support and counselling both when making their decision and throughout the pregnancy; some may need this support for many years afterwards (see Chapter 14).

Follow-up

A follow-up study of the first 12 mothers in the UK to have a selective feticide for discordant anomalies in their twins, found that all 12 said they felt they had made the correct decision but that many thought their loss had been underestimated or even forgotten, and that bereavement support had been inadequate (Bryan 1989). Several also felt the fetus had not received the respect it deserved (see p. 170).

The bereavement was generally felt more deeply by those who had discovered that one of their much-wanted twins had an unexpected anomaly, such as Down syndrome or anencephaly, than by those who had known all along that they might have to lose the entire pregnancy because of a genetic disorder, such as cystic fibrosis or haemophilia (Bryan 1989).

Preparation for twins

For a mother expecting her first, single baby there are endless sources of advice and information. In addition, whether she likes it or not, she will be deluged with stories of experiences that others have been through before her. In contrast, a mother who is told that she is having twins often knows no mother of twins to whom she can turn with all the questions and worries that quickly arise. In one study only one of 23 mothers who heard that they were expecting twins knew another mother of twins well enough to contact her (Bryan 1977b). Many others are upset by misleading old wives' tales about the difficulties of twin labours and the frailty of twin children. All will have questions and fears; all too often these are not voiced, partly because of the discouraging bustle of the antenatal clinic and also because others seem to think that parents should just be delighted with twins (Chang 1990).

Many professionals are not aware of the special needs of families with twins and it has been shown that parents are often ill-prepared and do not have realistic expectations of how the birth of twins will affect their family (Hay *et al.* 1990). Mothers are often unrealistically optimistic about the outcome. Twenty-three per cent were not at all worried about the work involved and 29 per cent were not worried about the babies' health. Similarly, many were not prepared for the impact the birth of twins would have on the relationship with their partner. Only 14 per cent were concerned about this during their pregnancy and yet 91 per cent, for example, were unable to get out together during the first 3 months after the birth (Hay *et al.* 1990).

It is well-recognized that an older child is likely to be more disturbed by the arrival of twins than of a single child (see p. 130). It is therefore essential to prepare the older child for the arrival while there is still time to give her or him a lot of attention. Mothers need to be warned; one study showed that only 31 per cent of mothers had been concerned about problems with the older child, whereas 64 per cent later reported experiencing significant problems (Hay and O'Brien 1984).

In the US (Malmstrom *et al.* 1988), Australia (Hay *et al.* 1990) and the UK (Hallett 1991) efforts are now being made to educate professionals and to inform couples of the special needs of twins and their families. However, parents often have to be persuaded of the need for help. Many couples have unrealistic expectations as to what life with young twins will be like and parents should be encouraged to explore carefully the help that could be available from relatives and friends as well as from paid and voluntary services.

Several parent organizations have produced videos and literature for prospective parents. In the UK, prenatal meetings are given by the Multiple Births Foundation with illustrated talks and the opportunity to meet parents with twins of different ages, and to readily see all the literature available (Appendix 1).

Emotional and practical support can best be provided by other mothers of twins. As is clear, few medical staff have the appropriate empathy or practical knowledge. Most areas in the UK now have a local parents of twins club, members of which are happy to make immediate contact with an expectant mother. Failing this, the national Twins and Multiple Births Association (TAMBA) gives contact addresses of individual families in the area, as well as providing literature on practical aspects of multiple pregnancy and the care of twin children. Similar organizations have been started in other countries (see Appendix 2).

Much of the practical advice from other mothers of twins will save the parents money at a time when they are likely to be unusually pressed. For example, some equipment useful for one baby is inappropriate to duplicate. It is wise to discourage mothers from actually buying a twin pram before the babies are born and seen to be well. It is often possible to reserve a pram through shops, or a second-hand one through the twins club. Should one or both babies die the parents would have avoided having an expensive and painful reminder of their loss.

4

The twin fetus

From the moment of fertilization the development of the human fetus depends on the intrauterine environment. Any given twin fetus, however, is affected not only by these innumerable environmental factors but also by its interaction with the second fetus. At best it must compete for nutrition, at worst it may be severely, even lethally, damaged by its co-twin.

Intrauterine growth

It is no wonder that newborn twins tend to be smaller than singletons. The twin fetus has to share, often very unequally, the maternal supply of nourishment and, in monochorionic twins, there is the additional handicap of an energy-wasting 'third circulation'.

Surprisingly, a twin fetus does usually manage to grow at the same rate as

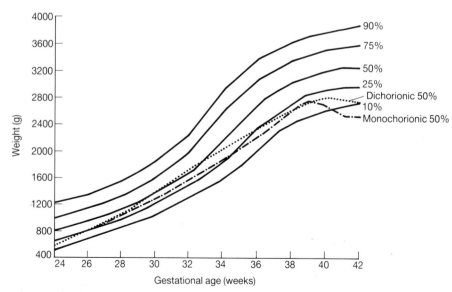

Fig. 4.1 Birth weights of live monochorionic and dichorionic twins compared with singletons. From Naeye *et al.* (1966) by permission of the authors and the editors of *Pediatrics.* Copyright American Academy of Pediatrics 1966.

a singleton for the first two trimesters (McKeown and Record 1952; Naeye *et al.* 1966, Fliegner and Eggars 1984; Fig. 4.1). The few that do not are likely to be the much lighter twins in grossly weight-discordant pairs (Crane *et al.* 1980).

From the 26th to 28th week onwards the rate of growth decreases in comparison to that of a singleton. The average weight of a newborn twin is about 800 g less than a singleton although, if allowance is made for differences in gestational age, the discrepancy is reduced to 500 g (Hemon *et al.* 1982). As a result of their study of over 2000 liveborn twins between 24 and 42 weeks gestation, Naeye *et al.* (1966) produced the centile charts shown in Figure 4.2. They found that monochorionic twins were, in general, lighter than dichorionic for the period of gestation and that their intrapair variation in weight was greater.

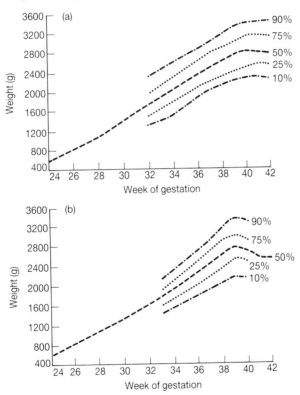

Fig. 4.2 Birth weights of live (a) dichorionic, and (b) monochorionic twins. From Naeye *et al.* (1966) by permission of the authors and the editors of *Pediatrics*. Copyright American Academy of Pediatrics 1966.

As in many animal species, the growth of the human fetus is influenced by litter size, and the deceleration in growth rate that occurs at about 36 weeks in singletons takes place correspondingly earlier in twins and higher multiple births. McKeown and Record (1952) suggests that this deceleration occurs when the total litter weight reaches a critical level—about 3 kg in man.

The typical pattern of intrauterine growth of twins is similar to that of growth-retarded singletons in that the weight falls away disproportionately more than the occipitofrontal circumference or the length (Fenner *et al*. 1980). Factors associated with intrauterine growth retardation in singletons, such as maternal size and smoking, apply equally to twins (Hemon *et al*. 1982). There are, of course additional, and partly unexplained, factors operating in a multiple pregnancy.

The mechanical restraint of uterine overcrowding seems unlikely to be a significant factor. The work of Morris *et al*. (1955) suggests that uteroplacental perfusion is reduced in multiple pregnancy. Indirect evidence of a reduced oxygen supply to the twin fetus is provided by the higher cord blood haemoglobin levels found in twins and also the fact that in twin pairs of discordant weight the smaller tends to have the higher haemoglobin level (Clemetson 1956; Walker and Turnbull 1965).

Zygosity

Even when allowance is made for length of gestation, MZ twins are lighter than DZ. This difference in weight was originally attributed to the reduced efficiency of a monochorionic placenta. However, Corney *et al*. (1972), while confirming the findings of others of a weight discordance between the two types of twins, showed that this could not be explained by the effects of placentation (nor indeed by a number of other variables). That is to say that even MZ twins with two chorions and, therefore, separate circulations, were lighter than DZ twins. There was no obvious reason for this weight difference but the authors offered three possible explanations. The first was that the low weight could be related to events in early embryonic development when the cell mass is reduced by its division into two embryos. Second, the explanation may be immunological—the antigenic differences between DZ twins could beneficially affect intrauterine growth. Third, maternal factors may play a part. The mothers of DZ twins are, on average, taller and their levels of hormones higher than mothers of MZ twins.

Placenta

The growth of the twin fetus is affected by the site of implantation of the placenta in the uterus (see p. 83), the site of umbilical cord insertion into the placenta (see p. 84), the absence of an umbilical artery (see p. 85) and, in monochorionic twins, by the haemodynamic effects of the 'third circulation' (see p. 87).

There is debate as to the importance of the placenta in limiting fetal growth. McKeown and Record (1953) and Grunewald (1970) found higher placental indices at all gestations in multiple pregnancies, whereas Bleker *et al*. (1979) found lower placental indices until 37 weeks; thereafter they were higher than singletons. However, at equivalent relative placental weight, twins were still lighter than singletons, even when allowing for gestational age. The percentage of placental weight reduction in twins (12 per cent) is less than their relative body weight deficit (20 per cent). Therefore twins' growth retardation cannot be totally accounted for by impaired placental development.

Intrapair discordance in growth

Discrepancies in birth weight are more common and larger within MZ pairs. This is mainly due to the cases of fetofetal transfusion syndrome, when the haemodynamic imbalance results in transfer of nutrition from donor to recipient (see p. 52). Another cause of unequal fetal growth in mono-chorionic twins is eccentric insertion of one of the two umbilical cords into the placental disc (see p. 84). One twin fetus may then receive less of the available maternal nutrition than its co-twin (Figs. 4.3 and 4.4).

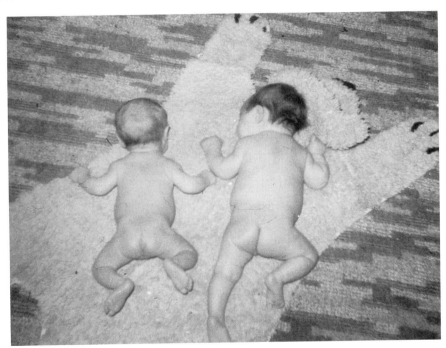

Fig. 4.3 MZ twin girls showing continuing growth discrepancy at 6 weeks. Twin 1 (right): birth weight 3.18 kg. Twin 2 (left): 1.55 kg.

Dichorionic twins, although less often, can be grossly discordant in size. This is more common when the placentae are separate than when they are fused (Fujikura and Froehlich 1971).

When a single umbilical artery is found in twins it is most often the smaller twin that is affected. Whether the absence of an artery, by reducing fetomaternal circulation, is responsible for the poor fetal growth or whether some other detrimental factor disturbs both growth and umbilical artery development is unknown.

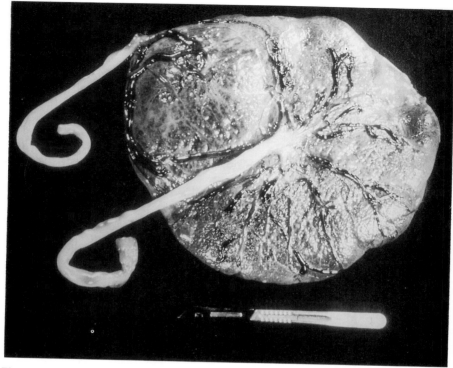

Fig. 4.4 Monochorionic placenta of infants shown in Fig. 4.3 with eccentric insertion of one umbilical cord.

Monitoring fetal growth

The monitoring of fetal development by ultrasound scan has given us a new insight into the growth of the living fetus. Before ultrasound was introduced, studies had necessarily been limited to dead or prematurely delivered fetuses that were to some degree abnormal.

There have now been a number of studies on fetal biparietal diameters (BPD) in twin pregnancy (Fig. 4.5). These measurements are technically more difficult in multiple pregnancies but nevertheless provide useful information (D'Alton and Mercer 1990). Schneider (1978) found that the 50th centile for twins is nearer the tenth centile for singletons. However, Crane *et al.* (1980) showed that if discordant twins (those whose birth weight differed by over 25 per cent) were excluded then the BPDs of twins were the same as those of appropriately grown singletons. In discordant pairs the BPD of the heavier twin was similar to that of both concordant twins and of singletons, whereas the lighter twin had, in many cases, a BPD well below the normal range (Fig. 4.6).

Discordance in BPD, which can be detected during the second trimester, is most likely to be due to the fetofetal transfusion syndrome and carries a high mortality. Diverging BPD after the 30th week, however, has a better

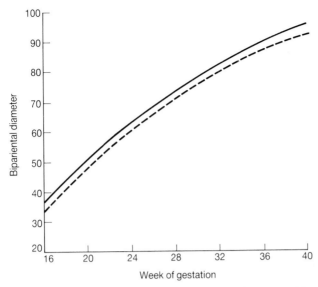

Fig. 4.5 Mean twin and singleton biparietal diameters between 16 and 40 weeks' gestation. From Leveno *et al.* (1979) by permission of the author and the editors of the *American Journal of Obstetrics and Gynaecology.* — Singleton; --- twin.

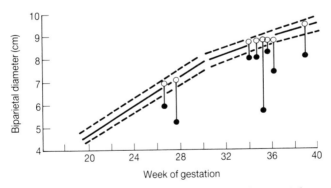

Fig. 4.6 Biparietal diameters in eight pairs of discordant-weight twins plotted against the normal range for singletons. The measurements were the last taken before delivery. From Crane *et al.* (1980). Reprinted with permission from The American College of Obstetricians and Gynaecologists. ○ Larger discordant twin; ● smaller discordant twin.

prognosis and is probably a reflection of unequal maternofetal transfer to the two fetuses (Crane *et al.* 1980).

It has been suggested that other ultrasound measurements may give more reliable indications of fetal growth. Neilson (1981) found that the product of the crown–rump length and the trunk area identified all growth-retarded twin fetuses whereas, in an earlier study, 44 per cent had been missed on BPD measurements.

Some workers report that the abdominal circumference may be a more reliable measurement (Chitkara *et al.* 1985; Storlazzi *et al.* 1987; Blickstein *et al.* 1989). The value of Doppler umbilical flow monitoring in multiple pregnancies is still to be evaluated. Results have so far varied but it is clearly an area where rapid development is to be expected (D'Alton and Mercer 1990).

Alphafetoprotein

Maternal serum AFP levels may also give some indication of fetal wellbeing. As with singletons (Wald *et al.* 1977), a negative correlation has been shown between mean birth weight of a twin pair and maternal AFP levels measured between the 11th and 24th weeks (Wald *et al.* 1978). Wald *et al.* (1979) offered this as an explanation for their later finding of higher AFP levels in MZ than DZ twin pregnancies; MZ twins are, on average, lighter than DZ.

However, Brock *et al.* (1979) suggested that the results could predict two separate groups of low birth weight twins. They found that high AFP levels were associated with preterm delivery whereas a low AFP provided a warning of early intrauterine growth retardation.

The effects of a shared blood circulation

One in four pairs of twins have an important additional influence on their intrauterine development—a shared circulation (see p. 87). In many instances monochorionic twins harmoniously share a 'third circulation' without apparent ill-effect. Occasionally, as in the case of acardia (see p. 62), the fetus is actually dependent on this intrapair circulation for survival. In other instances, as in the fetofetal transfusion syndrome, the results may be disastrous.

The chronic fetofetal transfusion syndrome

The chronic fetofetal transfusion syndrome is the result of an intrauterine blood transfusion between a pair of monochorionic twins. It is the cause of some of the greatest disturbances in twin fetal development. Not only may unequal growth occur but the effects of anaemia and polycythaemia may be so profound as to cause death to one or both fetuses.

It is a more common condition than is generally realized, occurring in at least 15 per cent of monochorionic pregnancies (Rausen *et al.* 1965; Dudley and D'Alton 1986).

The severe growth retardation frequently seen in the donor twin shows that the transfusion is a chronic process often lasting many weeks (Fig. 4.7). Indeed the syndrome has been recognized as early as the 10th week of pregnancy in a pair of aborted twin fetuses (Benirschke 1972).

The donor twin is usually smaller—invariably so when there are large intrapair weight discrepancies. (When the twins are of similar weight they

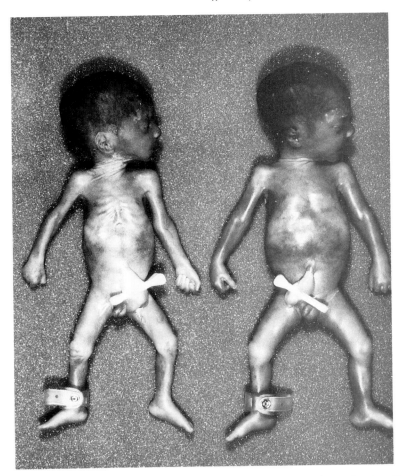

Fig. 4.7   Fetofetal transfusion syndrome in 24 weeks gestation aborted twins. Donor (left): weight 670 g; Hb 11.8 g/100 ml; recipient (right): weight 830 g; Hb 17.5 g/100 ml.

are likely to be examples of the acute type of fetofetal transfusion syndrome (see p. 77).) The poor growth of the donor is due to the loss of nutrients and haemoglobin (Hb) to the co-twin. There may also be reduced maternofetal transfer of amino acids across the grossly abnormal and oedematous placenta (Bryan 1977b).

Differences in the weights of some of the fetal organs may be even greater than those of the body as a whole. Most information has been provided by Naeye (1963, 1964a,b, 1965; Naeye and Letts 1964) who found that all organs of the recipient were significantly larger than those of the donor and that the donor's were like those of a singleton suffering from intrauterine malnutrition. Sparsity of lymphoid tissue in spleen and thymus was typical and changes in the cardiovascular system were particularly striking. The cardiac mass of the recipient was sometimes twice that of the donor. Histologically there was hyperplasia of myocardial fibres and an increase in muscle mass in both systemic and pulmonary arteries. The recipient's renal glomeruli were more mature not only than their donor's but also than those of singletons. This acceleration in development may occur in response to the increased blood volume that, in turn, probably accounts for the high fetal urine production which may cause gross polyhydramnios. This increase in amniotic fluid is often the first clue to a disturbance in the fetofetal haemodynamic balance.

It has also been suggested that high concentrations of atriopeptin, which have been found in recipients, may contribute to the excess amniotic fluid by affecting renal function and causing a diuresis (Nageotte *et al*. 1989).

Recent advances in both the prenatal diagnosis and treatment of the fetofetal transfusion syndrome (Fisk *et al*. 1990) include ultrasound, which may show discordant fetal growth and amniotic fluid volume in the two sacs, and Doppler studies of umbilical artery flow, which are often unhelpful in establishing a diagnosis (Giles *et al*. 1990) but in some cases the donor twin may show signs of poor placental perfusion (Fisk *et al*. 1990). However, none of the ultrasound appearances are specific for the syndrome.

Even in severe cases, fetal blood samples collected in the mid-trimester have shown that, unlike at birth, the haemoglobin and haematocrit level of donor and recipient are not very dissimilar, although the donor's blood film shows marked evidence of increased haemopoiesis. Similar findings have been reported in a monochorionic triplet pregnancy with two donors and one recipient (Fisk *et al*. 1990).

The diagnosis can be conclusively confirmed by the infusion into the donor of a safe biological marker (such as adult packed red blood cells) and later testing for its presence in the recipient. The prognosis for mid-trimester fetofetal transfusion syndrome is poor: most fetuses die either from prematurity, as delivery is precipitated by polyhydramnios, or from cardiac failure with hydrops. Serial amniocenteses may help in some cases (Urig *et al*. 1990; Radested and Thomassen 1990). Hydrops in the recipient twin has responded to digoxin given to the mother in some cases.

In more severe cases, a number of intrauterine therapies has been attempted. Laser ablation of placental anastomoses identified by direct vision through a fetoscope has been performed on several occasions (De Lia and Cruishank 1990, De Lia 1991). Selective feticide—the donor being killed to save the life of the recipient—is a difficult choice but may be thought preferable to the almost certain loss of both (Wittman *et al*. 1986). However, the possibility of damage to the survivor must also be considered. Brain, liver and kidney lesions are found in a significant minority of monochorionic twins whose siblings die *in utero*.

Reversal of hydrops in the recipient has been reported after haemorrhage from a chorionic plate that was punctured inadvertently at amniocentesis. This was presumably due to a blood-letting of the recipient, which reduced the high haematocrit. Another possibility is an intrauterine serial give-and-take transfusion from the recipient to the donor, although this is likely to provide only very temporary relief.

Pregnancies in which the fetofetal transfusion syndrome becomes apparent only in the third trimester have a much better prognosis and the give-

and-take transfusion prior to delivery may greatly improve the condition of the newborn infants (see p. 100).

Chimerism

Occasionally a DZ twin has two distinct blood groups. He is then known as a chimera and must have received blast cells from his twin during intrauterine life. This condition can occur only in the rare situation of placental ana- stomoses in a fused (dichorionic) placenta (Nylander and Osunkoya 1970; Corney 1975b). Such twins are, at least partly, immunologically tolerant of each other and will, for instance, accept each other's skin grafts (Benirschke and Kim 1973). Blood chimerism has no ill-effect in humans, unlike some animals, such as the freemartin bovine fetus, who are made sterile by the sexual maldevelopment caused by male cells in the female's tissues.

Congenital malformations

The study of congenital malformations in twins is beset with special prob- lems (Little and Bryan 1988). Definitions of congenital malformations vary from one study to another and the method of ascertainment may vary greatly; these factors may affect the validity of comparisons between twin and singleton populations for different studies. On the one hand it is difficult to collect a large enough sample if a geographically defined popula- tion is studied, but on the other, if the study is limited to malformed twins, there tends to be an over-representation of concordant pairs. Furthermore, if one twin has died *in utero*, a malformed survivor may not be recognized as one of a twin pair (Carter 1965).

Prevalence at birth and concordance rates of anomalies in twins vary greatly between studies. This variation may reflect differences in study methods, including the gestation criterion used for defining stillbirth, the range of anomalies studied, opportunities for and thoroughness of examina- tion, variation in demographic factors, such as maternal age and zygosity distribution, and chance variation because the number of affected twins studied is often small.

Congenital malformations are more common in twin than in singleton births. This has been demonstrated in most, but not all, studies (Bryan *et al.* 1987; Table 4.1). It is not yet known whether the incidence of anomalies in multiple conceptuses is also higher or if the difference in prevalence at birth reflects differential fetal loss. The increase is confined to like-sexed pairs (Stevenson *et al.* 1966; Hay and Wehrung 1970). More recent studies in which zygosity has been determined by a direct method have demonstrated that the MZ group is responsible for the increase (Myrianthopoulos 1975, 1978; Myrianthopoulos and Melnick 1977; Schinzel *et al.* 1979, Cameron *et al.* 1983; Corney *et al.* 1983).

A number of major and multiple malformations, which are likely to be the result of an insult in early embryonic life, are over-represented amongst MZ twins whereas defects of later origin, such as cleft palate, are as common in both types of twins (Schinzel *et al.* 1979).

Table 4.1   Comparison of prevalence at birth (live and still) of congenital anomalies between twins of different types and singletons

Study population	Period of study	Population (P) or hospital (H) series	Method of ascertainment[a]	Singletons Number with anomalies	Singletons Rate (%)	RR[b] T:S	Total Number with anomalies	Total Rate (%)	Twins like sex Number with anomalies	Twins like sex Rate (%)	Unlike sex Number with anomalies	Unlike sex Rate (%)	RR[c] LS:US	Reference
Australia, Melbourne				210	1.8	1.1	6	1.9	4	1.9	2	1.7	1.1	
Brazil, Sao Paulo	1961–64	H	N	222	1.6	1.3	9	2.1	8	3.1	1	0.6	5.2	Stevenson et al. (1966)
Chile, Santiago				219	0.9	1.1	5	1.0	5	1.5	0	0.0	∞	
Colombia, Medellin				218	1.1	2.6	11	2.9	8	3.1	3	2.3	1.3	
Czechoslovakia				344	1.7	0.7	4	1.2	3	1.4	1	0.8	1.8	
Czechoslovakia, Prague	1929–62	H	M	67	1.3	2.0	132	2.6	–	–	–	–	–	Onyskowova et al. (1971)
Egypt, Alexandria				106	1.2	0.5	5	0.6	5	1.1	0	0.0	∞	
Hong Kong	1961–64	H	N	112	1.2	0.7	2	0.8	1	0.5	0	0.0	∞	Stevenson et al. (1966)
India, Bombay				335	0.9	0.6	5	0.5	5	0.7	0	0.0	∞	
India, Bombay	1982–83	H	?	280	1.6	1.7	8	2.7	5	2.4	3	3.4	0.7	Shah and Patel (1984)
India, Calcutta				58	0.3	0.7	1	0.2	0	0.0	1	0.5	0.0	
Malaysia, Kuala Lumpur	1961–64	H	N	161	1.0	1.6	6	1.6	5	1.7	1	1.2	1.4	Stevenson et al. (1966)
Malaysia, Singapore				336	0.9	1.2	7	1.1	6	1.2	1	0.8	1.5	
Mexico City				353	1.5	1.3	11	1.9	5	1.3	6	2.9	0.4	
Netherlands, Dordrecht	1981–83	H	?	29	1.2	3.5	5	4.2	4	9.3	1	1.4	6.6	Ceelie, 1985
Nigeria, Zaria	1976–79	H	N	247	1.1	2.0	35	2.3	–	–	–	–	–	Harrison et al. (1985)
Norway[e]	1967–79	P	B	23 424	3.0	0.9	426	2.8	306	2.9	123	2.5	1.2	Windham and Bjerkedal (1984)
Panama City				324	2.1	0.8	5	1.7	3	1.5	2	2.1	0.7	
Philippines, Manila				246	0.8	2.1	6	1.7	6	2.2	0	0.0	∞	
S. Africa, Cape Town				26	0.9	0.0	0	0.0	0	0.0	0	0.0	∞	
S. Africa, Johannesburg	1961–64	H	N	241	2.2	2.0	11	4.4	10	5.4	1	1.6	3.4	Stevenson et al. (1966)

								MZ		DZ		RR	
Location	Years	Method[a]	N	Rate (%)	Ratio[b]	Number with anomalies	Rate (%)	Number with anomalies	Rate (%)	Number with anomalies	Rate (%)	MZ:DZ	Reference
(continued from previous page)	—	—	—	—	—	—	2.3	24	3.1	6	1.4	2.2	Stevenson et al. (1966)
UK, Birmingham	1950–52	N, HV, 5	1 204	2.2	1.3	41	2.6	26	2.8	15	2.4	1.2	McKeown and Record (1960)
UK, Northern Ireland[f]	1974–79	M	6 340	4.0	1.3	172	5.2	115	5.2	51	4.8	1.1	Little and Nevin (1988)
USA, Atlanta[g]	1969–76	M, 1	6 767	3.3	1.5	181	4.9	115	4.9	28	2.5	2.0	Layde et al. (1980)
USA, Cleveland	1955–63	N	?	3.3	3.2	80	10.6	—	—	—	—	—	Hendricks (1966)
USA, New York	1950–56	N	3 698	4.0	1.7	182	6.9	—	—	—	—	—	Guttmacher and Kohl (1958)
Yugoslavia, Ljubljana		?	163	1.9	1.3	8	2.5	5	3.7	3	3.3	1.1	}
Yugoslavia, Zagreb	1961–64	N	106	1.3	0.5	1	0.6	1	1.0	0	0.0	∞	} Stevenson et al. (1966)
USA, multicentre	1959–65	P, 7	8 288	15.6	1.2	219	18.3	90	24.1	91	14.8	1.6	Myrianthopoulos (1978)
Belgium, Ghent	1964–67	?	—	—	—	17	2.4	9	3.1	8	1.9	1.6	Cameron et al. (1983)
UK, Birmingham	1963–67	?	—	—	—	66	3.1	24	4.0	42	2.7	1.5	Corney et al. (1983)
UK, North-east Scotland	1968–79	N	—	—	—	57	4.3	20	5.3	26	3.7	1.4	Corney et al. (1983)

[a] Method of ascertainment: B, review of birth notification records; M, review of routine records from multiple sources; N, neonatal examination; P, physical examination; HV, health visitor. Number following letter denotes age in year to which infants followed-up, e.g. 1 to first year.
[b] Ratio of prevalence rate at birth of anomalies in twins to rate in singletons.
[c] Ratio of prevalence rate at birth of anomalies in twins of like sex (LS) to rate in twins of unlike sex (US).
[d] Only a sample of singletons was examined.
[e] Rates are adjusted for maternal age and parity.
[f] Follow-up of variable length to a maximum of 5 years according to year of child's birth and type of anomaly; bias of ascertainment as between singletons and twins thought to be unlikely.
[g] Live births only.
Source: From Little and Bryan (1988) by permission of John Wiley & Sons.

Why MZ twins should have an increased frequency of malformations, particularly those originating in early embryonic life, is not clear. Many authors favour the idea that MZ twinning is in itself a form of congenital malformation and that the unknown agent responsible for the twinning process (see p. 15) may also cause the structural anomaly (Little and Bryan 1988). In support of this theory is the fact that conjoined twins have a particularly high frequency of malformations (unrelated to their conjoined state) and they may even be discordant for these.

Other workers have suggested that the shared placental and fetal circulation of monochorionic twins provides a less favourable environment for fetal development (Bulmer 1970). However, studies by Melnick and Myrianthopoulos (1979) and Corney *et al.* (1983) have failed to show a higher incidence of malformations amongst MZ twins with monochorionic placentation than with dichorionic. Melnick and Myrianthopoulos (1979) have offered another explanation. They suggest that the disruption of the developmental genetic clock of the embryo caused by the zygote division and the temporary reduction in cell number could cause a numerical and temporal biochemical disadvantage in the two 'new' embryos. This might make them more susceptible to the action of subtle environmental agents. However, the results of these studies do not exclude the possibility that some specific anomalies, notably certain types of congenital heart disease, may occur more commonly in monochorionic twins (Cameron *et al.* 1983; Burn and Corney 1984).

There is a higher concordance for all malformations amongst MZ than DZ twins. For instance, a twin with cleft palate from a like-sex pair is at least five times more likely than an unlike-sex twin to have an affected co-twin (Douglas 1958; Metrakos *et al.* 1958; Hay and Wehrung 1970; Little and Bryan 1988).

Nevertheless, for most malformations MZ twins are still more likely than not to be discordant. The twinning process itself may well influence fetal development and thus be responsible for discordance in anomalies being the norm (Little and Bryan 1988). Placental anastomoses with an unusual fetoplacental circulation may be one explanation. Unequal splitting of the zygote has been suggested as another. Finally, twin embryos may reach different stages of development at a particular gestational age and thus be more or less susceptible to teratogenic insults at that time. Even syndromes with multiple anomalies, such as Klippel–Feil, Goldenhar, De Lange and Rubinstein–Taybi are often discordant (Schinzel *et al.* 1979).

No specific malformation with invariable MZ concordance has been reported. The Prader–Willi syndrome is the one malformation complex in which all reported cases have been concordant. However, of a total of five cases at least one showed a marked difference in severity (Schinzel *et al.* 1979).

Anomalies unique to multiple conception

Conjoined twins

This tragic malformation is a form of MZ twinning and is thought to result from the imperfect division of the embryo after the formation of two embryonic discs (Zimmerman 1967; Potter and Craig 1976). The cause is unknown but is assumed to be the same as for MZ twins in general (see p. 15).

In view of its rarity it is not surprising to find that reports on the incidence of conjoined twinning vary. The figure given by Bulmer (1970) of 1 in 100 000 maternities is probably too low; twice this frequency is more likely (Hanson 1975), i.e. 1 in every 200 MZ twin maternities. There are no known predisposing factors although there have been occasional reports of geographical (Bhettay *et al.* 1975; Viljoen *et al.* 1983; Zake 1984) and temporal (Kaplan and Eidelman 1983; Viljoen *et al.* 1983; Harrison and Rossiter 1985) clustering and also of seasonal (Milham 1966) and racial (Jaschevatsky *et al.* 1980) variation.

All studies have reported a low sex ratio (Milham 1966; Benirschke and Kim 1973; Zake 1984). Indeed, in Milham's (1966) study of 22 cases, 20 were female. There has been only one report of a second set of conjoined twins in a family (Hamon and Dinno 1978) and, as would be expected with MZ twinning, a family history of twins is not particularly common. Conjoined pairs occur more frequently in triplet sets than would be expected (Schinzel *et al.* 1979). In at least one case the normal fetus has had its own amniotic sac, which suggests that zygote division must have taken place on two separate occasions (Vestergaard 1972).

An interesting finding in Milham's (1966) study was that of a high stillbirth rate in previous pregnancies. Seven of a total of 33 pregnancies had ended with the delivery of a stillborn infant.

The site and extent of fusion of the fetuses is infinitely variable. Thoracopagus is the most common form of fusion and accounts for over 70 per cent of cases (Rudolph *et al.* 1967; Edmonds and Layde 1982; Fig. 4.8). Pyopagus is the next most common. The full range of conjoined twins is listed in Table 4.2 (Guttmacher and Nichols 1967).

In thoracopagus twins there is a high incidence of congenital heart disease, which therefore seems related to the degree of union. The anomalies are similar to the defects described in Ivemark's syndrome, including anomalous pulmonary venous return, common atrium, single ventricle, conotruncal abnormalities and endocardial cushion defects (Noonan 1978). In one study, 90 per cent of such twins shared a common pericardium and 75 per cent had conjoined hearts (Nichols *et al.* 1967).

Edmonds and Layde (1982) noted that 40 of their 81 sets of conjoined twins had malformations that were not obviously associated with the site of junction. Some of the malformations, such as imperforate anus and diaphragmatic hernia, could be explained mechanically. Others seemed related to a more fundamental disturbance of embryogenesis.

Primary discordance, i.e. malformations occurring in only one of the pair's unjoined organs, is rare. Cases discordant for meningomyelocele,

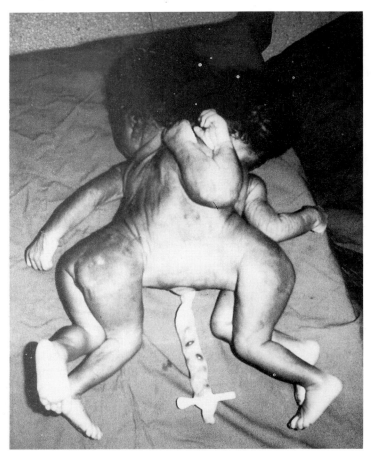

Fig. 4.8   Newborn thoracopagus conjoined twins.

Table 4.2   Types of conjoined twins

Inferior conjunction
Diprosopus—two faces with one head and body
Dicephalus—two heads and one body
Ischiopagus—inferior sacrococcygeal fusion
Pygopagus—posterolateral sacrococcygeal fusion

Superior conjunction
Dipygus—two pelves and four legs
Syncephalus—facial ± thoracic fusion
Craniopagus—cranial fusion

Mid conjunction
Thoracopagus—thoracic fusion
Omphalopagus—fusion from umbilicus to xiphoid cartilage
Rachipagus—vertebral fusion above sacrum

---

anencephaly and cleft lip have, however, been reported (Ornoy *et al.* 1980; Seller 1990). Cases of differing sex are probably due to pseudohermaphroditism (Szendi 1939; Milham 1966; Khanna *et al.* 1969). On the other hand, secondary discordance is a common finding—different defects of parts of joined organs belonging to each of the twins.

The feasibility of separating conjoined twins obviously depends on the site and extent of fusion and the degree to which organs are shared, as well as the availability of appropriate surgical expertise and intensive care facilities. Unfortunately the diagnosis of conjoined twins is too often made only after the onset of labour. Thus the mother is not able to have an elective caesarean section, which would reduce the risk of damage to herself and the babies. Nor is she likely to be in a hospital equipped to deal with such rare and complicated cases. Suspicion of conjoined twins should be aroused in all cases of polyhydramnios in multiple pregnancies and also in those where an X-ray or ultrasound reveals an abnormal fetal posture (Rudolph *et al.* 1967).

Nowadays many conjoined twins can be successfully separated. Obviously prognosis depends on the extent of union and the nature of additional anomalies. Nichols *et al.* (1967) concluded that more than 50 per cent of twins joined by the mid-portion would survive following surgical separation, but Edmonds and Layde (1982) found that overall, less than one-quarter of conjoined twins would survive long enough to be potential candidates for surgery. Several detailed descriptions of separating conjoined twins are given in the comprehensive review edited by Bergsma (1967). In the same volume Pepper (1967) considers the ethical dilemma presented by conjoined twins, first in considering initial resuscitation of the infants at birth and then of surgical separation, particularly if the survival of one is likely to be at the expense of the other. Finally, he discusses the long-term psychological adjustment of those who have been separated, as well as those who remain fused.

A number of conjoined twins have lived surprisingly full and active lives (Gedda 1961). Some—both men and women—have married and had children. Many have shown different tastes and temperaments, which at times have led to intrapair tensions. Perhaps it is more surprising that others have managed to live together in harmony.

Masha and Dasha, a pair of Russian twins now approaching their forties (*Sunday Times* 1989) share a single lower half to their body but are entirely separate from the waist upwards. They have had to learn to accept their differences. Dasha is the spokesperson whereas Masha is quieter, and more easily upset. They spent most of their childhood disagreeing, even fighting. They had different tastes for television, music and exercise. Now they have learnt to compromise and take turns over the choice of activities.

Many physiological responses of a conjoined pair may be autonomous. Heart rhythms may differ and change independently in response to external stimuli. If one of a pair becomes pregnant the other may continue to menstruate.

The xiphopagus pair, Chang and Eng (1811–74) were the original 'Siamese twins'. They married two sisters and one had 12 children and the other ten.

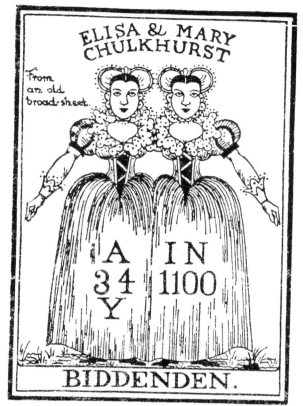

Fig. 4.9   The Chulkhurst sisters—conjoined twins.

One of the earliest and most famous English pairs were Elisa and Mary Chulkhurst from Kent, who are depicted on the village sign as 'The Biddenden Maids' (Fig. 4.9). Born in 1100, they were laterally joined in the scapular and gluteal regions. After their death at the age of 34 the Chulkhurst Charity was established. Part of this includes the distribution each Easter of biscuits embossed with their figures.

In all cases of unseparated twins the death of one is quickly followed by the death of the other, even if there is no structural cause for this. It is likely that thromboplastin from the dead twin crosses into the survivor's circulation and causes disseminated intravascular coagulation.

In both the 'Siamese' and the Chulkhurst pairs one twin died a few hours before the other. On both occasions the survivor is said to have chosen to die rather than accept an attempted surgical separation.

Acardia

Acardia or chorioangiopagus parasiticus, the most severe of all malformations, occurs in about 1 in 30 000 deliveries (Benirschke and Kim 1973). Such cases are confined to monochorionic pregnancies, as survival of the fetus is dependent on a shared circulation with the (usually normal) co-twin. However, in one instance a triploid twin acardiac with a 70XXX+ 15 karyotype was delivered with a co-twin with a normal male karyotype and a monochorionic placenta (Bieber *et al.* 1981). The sex discordance may be due to polar body twinning.

There is some suggestion that acardia may occur more often in triplet pregnancies (Frutiger 1969; James 1978b; Schinzel *et al.* 1979).

Acardiac fetuses vary from a mass of amorphous tissue to an incomplete but well-formed fetus weighing up to 3.5 kg. They are usually attached to a monochorionic placenta by an umbilical cord with only one artery.

The sex ratio in acardiac twins is lower than in twins in general (James 1978b). The mean maternal age is higher (Frutiger 1969), consistent with the finding that some acardiacs are trisomic (Kerr and Rashad 1966, Scott and Ferguson-Smith 1973) and it appears to be more common in monoamniotic placentae (James 1978b).

There are two theories as to the mechanism by which acardia develops. First, a primary failure of cardiac development has been suggested by the finding of a general disturbance of morphogenesis. It is not uncommon for specific abnormalities present in the acardiac twin to occur in the co-twin as well. In one study, 10 per cent of 85 acardiac twins had a pump twin with a similar congenital anomaly (Schinzel *et al.* 1979). An acardiac conjoined twin has also been reported (Geeves 1928) as has a fetus-*in-fetu* (Junquiera and Pinto 1951). In another study, six out of 12 acardiac cases had abnormal karyotypes, with a normal karyotype in each pump twin. No consistent chromosomal anomaly has been demonstrated (Van Allen *et al.* 1983).

The second mechanism suggested is that the heart atrophies as a result of passive perfusion and reversal of circulation. The early pressure flow in the placental artery of one twin exceeds that of the other and results in a reversal of flow at the artery-to-artery anastomosis. The recipient twin is perfused with low pressure hypoxic blood via the umbilical and iliac arteries. This circulation supplies the lower segment relatively more than the cranial, often resulting in a preferential development of the lower part of the body. This hypothetical mechanism has been named the twin reversed arterial perfusion (TRAP) sequence (Van Allen *et al.* 1983).

The hazards to the pump twin are often overlooked. Not only is it at greater risk of a congenital anomaly but there is a high mortality rate, usually due to the combination of intrauterine cardiac failure and prematurity (Van Allen *et al.* 1983; Moore *et al.* 1990). Preterm delivery and therefore the perinatal outcome of the pump twin appear, however, to be related to the size of the acardiac twin compared to the pump twin. Moore *et al.* (1990) found that the mean birthweight ratio in twins born before 34 weeks was 60 per cent, whereas in those born after 34 weeks it was 29 per cent. Thus, prenatal estimation of the relative weights can provide some indication of the likely outcome and may effect counselling and management.

The perinatal management of these infants should be greatly improved now that the problem can be foreseen by routine ultrasonic examination and intrauterine treatment can be given for cardiac failure.

Fetus-*in-fetu*

Sometimes a fetus or parts of a fetus may be lodged within another fetus. This is known as a fetus-*in-fetu*, and is considered to be an MZ twin. It may well have a similar origin to that of an acardiac twin (Janovski 1962; Grant and Pearn 1969) as may another form of twinning, the sacrococcygeal teratoma (Gross *et al*. 1951). The frequency of fetus-*in-fetu* is unknown. The parasitic fetus is most commonly attached near the origin of the superior mesenteric vessels, and usually in the upper retroperitoneal space, although other sites of attachment have been reported.

The parts of a single fetus are most commonly found but there have been reports of two (Gross *et al*. 1951, Eng *et al*. 1989), three (Lee 1965) and, one of the most notable cases, a cerebral tumour containing five fetuses (Kimmel *et al*. 1950). Some other anomalies, such as sirenomelia and related anomalies, may be due to the maldevelopment of the caudal region such as the VATER association. (Schinzel *et al*. 1979, Jones and Benirschke 1983). This acroynm stands for Vertebral defects, Anal atresia, Tracheo-Eosophageal fistula with atresia and Radial upper limb hypoplasia.

Hall *et al*. (1983) found that 11 of 135 cases (8 per cent) of amyoplasia (a form of arthrogryposis) were probably MZ twins. In each case only one twin was affected. Disruption by the twinning process itself may be a factor. An unequal share of cells committed to the formation of the somites from which skeletal muscle is derived is one of the possible explanations.

Anomalies not unique to multiple conception

A number of anomalies are not unique to twins but are of particular interest in multiple conceptions.

Congenital heart disease

A number of workers have found congenital heart disease to be more common in like-sexed twins than in singletons (McKeown and Record 1960; Hay and Wehrung 1970; Mitchell *et al*. 1971; Myrianthopoulos 1975; Layde *et al*. 1980; Cameron *et al*. 1983; Burn and Corney 1984; Little and Nevin 1989). Most studies report low overall concordance rates.

MZ twins appear to account for this increase. Anderson (1977) found that 58 per cent of twins in his study were MZ and similar trends have been reported by others (Campbell 1961; Kenna *et al*. 1975; Noonan 1978; Bryan *et al*. 1987). Concordance rates reported amongst MZ twins are highly variable, ranging from 6.8 per cent to 46 per cent (Campbell 1961; Nora *et al*. 1967; Jorgensen t al. 1971; Anderson 1977; Bryan *et al*. 1987). However, the concordance rates in the larger and more reliable studies tend to be low. Burn found a concordance rate of 8 per cent from 88 MZ pairs (Bryan *et al*. 1987). The reason why only one MZ twin is commonly affected is not clear. It has been suggested that haemodynamic differences in early fetal life could affect the development of the cardiovascular system.

Burn suggests that a disturbance of laterality is a more likely explanation in many cases. There is a variety of embryological evidence to support the concept of a left–right gradient. As the bend to the right of the early heart tube is crucial to subsequent development it is important that the embryo should distinguish left from right. Laterality is thought to be determined from the left side (Corballis and Morgan 1978). Late twinning could cause the 'right half' of the pair to lose its point of reference so, while the other twin determined laterality clearly and correctly, the affected twin was not able to clearly differentiate left from right. The resultant disturbance of the rightward bend of the heart could lead to maldevelopment (Burn 1988).

Positional defects

Twins would be likely to suffer from more positional defects due to the intrauterine congestion and relative restriction of movement. Minor foot deformities and skull asymmetry may be more common in twins (Schinzel *et al.* 1979) but usually resolve quickly and spontaneously. They are rarely mentioned in twin studies. True talipes equino varus and congenital dislocation of the hip appear to have a strong genetic component (Idelberger 1929, 1951).

Chromosomal anomalies

Most known chromosomal anomalies have been reported in twins (Benirschke and Kim 1973). These are usually discordant in DZ twins and, surprisingly, also occasionally in MZ (Riekhof *et al.* 1972; Scott and Ferguson-Smith 1973). The twins are then known as heterokaryotes. Instances of mono- or trisomy may be explained by chromatid non-disjunction at cell division. In the case of heterokaryotic twins it is thought that abnormal chromosome segregation would have occurred at early embryonic cleavage rather than during gametogenesis, but at all events before the splitting of the conceptus.

Heterokaryotes XY/XO are the explanation for the occasional pair of MZ twins of different sexes. Indeed, discordance is common in Turner syndrome (Riekhof *et al.* 1972; Karp *et al.* 1975; Pedersen *et al.* 1980; Perlman *et al.* 1990). Unlike Down syndrome and Klinefelter syndrome, where most, but not all (Scott and Ferguson-Smith 1973; Rogers *et al.* 1982), are concordant in MZ twins. Phenotypically dissimilar twins may have similar chromosome mosaicisms in blood (lymphocyte) cultures, due to the shared fetal circulation in a monochorionic placenta, but show different karyotypes in fibroblast cultures (Potter and Taitz 1972; Uchida *et al.* 1983). As most cytogenetic studies are done on lymphocytes it is likely that some heterokaryote twins will go unrecognized.

Unlike other congenital malformations, trisomy 21 (Down syndrome) is not increased in twins. Indeed, the prevalence at birth is actually lower in twins of like sex than in singletons (Keay 1958; MacDonald 1964; Hay and Wehrung 1970; Layde *et al.* 1980; Windham and Bjerkectal 1984; Doyle *et al.* 1991). It has been suggested that this low frequency may be due to a higher early loss of affected MZ embryos due to the combined insult of zygote cleavage and chromosomal imbalance.

Not surprisingly, concordance in DZ twins is unusual, as two separate chromosomal anomalies would be necessary. Nevertheless, several authors have reported a somewhat higher frequency of Down syndrome than would be expected, even allowing for maternal age (MacDonald 1964; Bulmer 1970; Avni *et al*. 1983). This suggests that some women may have a predisposition to the chromosomal anomaly.

Klinefelter syndrome (XXY) appears to be more common than expected not only in twins but also in their relatives (Hoefnagel and Benirschke 1962; Ferguson-Smith 1966; Soltan 1968; Nielsen 1970). The reason for this is not known. The increase seems to be particularly pronounced amongst siblings of affected DZ twins but is not associated with maternal age. Hoefnagel suggests that there may be a relationship between the chromosomal error and the twinning process.

There also appears to be an increased frequency of twins amongst people with Turner syndrome (Lemli and Smith 1963; Lindsten 1963; Nance and Uchida 1964; Pescia *et al*. 1975; Carothers *et al*. 1980) and also amongst their (normal) family members (Nielsen and Dahl 1976). Carothers *et al*. (1980) suggest that there may be a postzygotic mechanism common to twinning and X-chromosome loss.

Another example of discordance in chromosome pattern is provided by a case of girl twins where only one suffered from muscular dystrophy (Burn *et al*. 1986). The twins were MZ on the basis of physical similarity, placentation and blood grouping, tissue type and serum polymorphism but discordant for Duchenne muscular dystrophy. Investigation of the X inactivation pattern showed that the affected girl was using exclusively the maternal X while only a paternal X was active in her twin. This was attributed to chance asymmetry in the X inactivation process in the cells of the inner cell mass at the blastocyst stage.

Neural tube defects

The association of neural tube defects (NTD) with twinning is complex and still ill-understood. Reports vary as to the incidence. In a comprehensive review of the literature Elwood and Elwood (1980) found that the number of twins with NTD was slightly lower than expected. Pooling of data from a wider range of populations suggests that the frequency of anencephalus in twins is slightly higher than in singletons, while the converse applies for spina bifida (Little and Bryan 1988).

In view of the known familial incidence of neural tube defects it might be expected that concordance in MZ twins would be high; in fact the reverse is true. Concordance is rare and no higher amongst MZ than DZ twins. Elwood and Elwood (1980) in their literature review found a concordance rate for anencephalus of 4.1 per cent and for spina bifida of 5.1 per cent. The highest reported concordance rate in the literature on NTD is 8.3 per cent for anencephalus (Imaizumi 1978).

Another aspect of the relationship between neural tube defects and twinning has been explored by Knox (1970, 1974). In his epidemiological study of neural tube defects, Knox showed a general association between the frequency of anencephaly and dizygotic twinning rates. He suggested that neural tube defects could arise as a result of interaction between two fetuses. Maternal tissues might accept less easily two antigenically different and competing trophoblasts. Contact between the two trophoblasts might lead to an interaction in which one fetus was destroyed and the other left with a neural tube defect.

Further support for the idea of an association between twinning and neural tube defects has been provided by Le Marec *et al*. (1978). They found a significantly higher frequency of twins amongst the parents of 155 children with neural tube defects.

Gastrointestinal and urogenital systems

Oesophageal atresia, with or without tracheo-oesophageal fistula, appears to occur more commonly in twins (Van Staey *et al*. 1984). Fraser and Nora (1975) found a five-fold increase and also found that 95 per cent of the twin pairs were discordant for the anomaly.

There have been reports of excesses of urogenital anomalies (Layde *et al*. 1980), although this has not been confirmed in a more recent study (Windham and Bjerkedal 1984). There are reports of higher than expected frequencies of twins in cases of symmelia and extrophy of the cloaca, both of which are anomalies of midline structures (Nance 1981).

Intrauterine infections

Intrauterine infections usually affect both twins, although occasionally only one twin suffers the teratogenic insult. However, in at least one of the cases reported it was shown that the other twin had in fact been infected (by the rubella virus) but suffered no lasting damage (Forrester *et al*. 1966). It may be that these two fetuses were infected at a slightly, but critically, different stage in their embryological development (see below).

Such discordance is difficult to explain in the rare cases with MZ pregnancies (Penrose 1937; Montgomery and Stockdell 1970; Menez-Bautista *et al*. 1986; Wang *et al*. 1990), particularly if they are known to have had a monochorionic placenta and, therefore, a shared fetal circulation (Wang *et al*. 1990).

In their review of congenital acquired immune deficiency syndrome (AIDS) Thomas and her colleagues (1990) found an unexpectedly high incidence of twins amongst the affected infants. In three cases there was apparent discordance for human immunodeficiency virus (HIV) infection, whereas in all the others there was some degree of discordance, both in type of symptoms and in their severity.

The authors suggest that the tendency to twinning amongst infected mothers may be due to the HIV virus itself, or to the effect of drug abuse. Alternatively, the high incidence of twins amongst young infected infants may just be because twins demonstrate their symptoms earlier.

Later in pregnancy the presenting twin could, theoretically, be at greater risk of infection from organisms in the genital tract. Benirschke and Driscoll (1967) found that chorioamnionitis was invariably associated with the first twin when only one sac was involved. However, there have been no reports of an increased incidence of such infections in firstborn twins. Nevertheless, the finding of higher levels of the fetally synthesized immunoglobulins M and A in firstborn twins does suggest that the ascending organisms may have provided antigenic stimulation for the synthesis of these immunoglobulins (Bryan 1976).

Teratogenic effects of drugs

As with infections it appears that there may be intrapair differences in susceptibility to the teratogenic effects of drugs, including alcohol. One twin may be severely affected whereas the other may have only minor signs or no signs at all (Mellin and Katzenstein 1962; Lenz 1966; Loughnan *et al.* 1973; Christoffel and Salafsky 1975; Schmidt and Salzano 1980). These differences were demonstrated in a trizygotic triplet pregnancy where the effects of maternal epanutin were expressed differently in each infant (Bustamante and Stumpff 1978).

Lenz (1966) suggested that, at least in the case of thalidomide, the teratogenic effect of which is sharply limited, this occasional discordance in a pair of twins could be due to the insult acting at the very beginning or end of the sensitive period. As DZ twins may be conceived several days apart, one embryo may be relatively retarded or accelerated in development by a few days and therefore escape unharmed.

While there is no evidence that ovulation-inducing therapy or new techniques in assisted conception increase the risk of delivery of congenital anomaly (Scialli 1986), these procedures lead to a high incidence of multiple pregnancies in previously subfertile women. Even if there was no association between subfertility and fetal anomaly, anomalies would be expected to occur at the 'background' rate in a group of women who would not otherwise have maintained their pregnancies and who are at higher risk.

Rhesus isoimmunization and hydrops fetalis

Rhesus isoimmunization occurs in twins, as it does in singletons. Management, however, is often much more complicated. Not only is it technically more difficult to perform amniocenteses and intrauterine blood transfusions in a multiple pregnancy but decisions on management may be far more difficult. The life of one fetus may have to be sacrificed, or at least risked, for the sake of the healthy survival of the other (Nylander and MacGillivray 1975). The risk of an intrauterine death of the more severely affected fetus if the pregnancy is allowed to continue often has to be weighed against the chances of losing both infants from the complications of prematurity if the babies are delivered too early. Selective intrauterine transfusion is possible only in skilled hands.

With dizygotic twins only one may be affected (Beischer *et al.* 1969). Even if both are Rhesus sensitized, the degree may differ according to their ABO blood grouping. Fetuses with the same ABO blood group as their mother tend to be more severely affected than those with different ones. There are instances where severe oedema (hydrops fetalis) has occurred in only one of

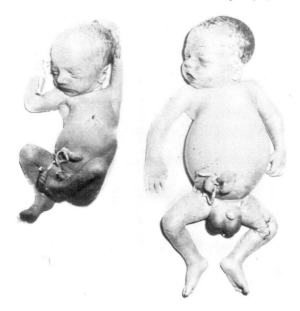

Fig. 4.10 Monozygotic twins with severe Rhesus isoimmunization. The smaller baby survived after two exchange transfusions while the hydropic one died after 15 minutes. From Kloosterman (1963) by permission of the author.

MZ Rhesus-immunized twins (Kloosterman 1963; Fig. 4.10). Here genetic differences cannot be responsible and differences in placental function become the most likely explanation. Differences in the placental transfer of the maternally derived immunoglobulin G, fetal plasma levels of albumin and colloid osmotic pressure may all be of importance (Barnes *et al.* 1977).

Amongst the vast array of causes of hydrops fetalis are a number specific to multiple pregnancy. Either or both twins in the fetofetal transfusion syndrome may become hydropic (Hibbard 1959; MacAfee *et al.* 1970) the recipient as a result of cardiac failure due to hypervolaemia and increased blood viscosity and the donor as a result of anaemia and hypo-albuminaemia, but surprisingly this is less common.

The abnormal circulation of an acardiac twin may cause oedema and the co-twin may also become oedematous due to cardiac failure from the increased load of a second fetal circulation.

Intrauterine death

Fetus papyraceus

Occasionally the compressed remains of a fetus, often embedded in the surface of the placenta, is seen together with a healthy single baby (Benirschke and Driscoll 1967; Fig. 4.11). This fetus is known as a fetus

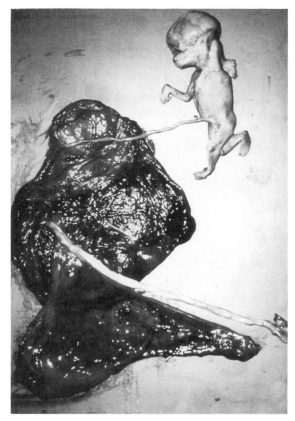

Fig. 4.11   Fetus papyraceus attached to a twin placenta. The twin was normal. By permission of H.G. Kohler.

papyraceus and the mother and the medical staff may have been unaware that she ever had a twin pregnancy. A fetus papyraceus probably occurs as rarely as 1 in 12 000 live births (Saier *et al*. 1975) or 1 in 200 twin pregnancies (Baker and Doering 1982). It has occasionally been reported in higher multiple pregnancies (Aiken 1969; Skelly *et al*. 1982). Most of these fetuses are the result of death in the second trimester. Before the second trimester a dead fetus is usually reabsorbed (p. 32), but in the third trimester the fetus that dies becomes macerated but not compressed. Mummification indicates that the death occurred at least 10 weeks before delivery (Saier *et al*. 1975).

The fetofetal transfusion syndrome and knotting of umbilical cords in monoamniotic twins account for the deaths of some of these fetuses. However, a large number of fetus papyraceus are dichorionic twins (Kindred 1944) so other explanations, such as separation of the placenta or blood group incompatibility, must be sought.

Later intrauterine death

About twice as many twins are stillborn as singletons. There are several reasons for this high fetal mortality. The maternal supply line is more likely to fail when two fetuses have to be sustained. One fetus often receives more nutrition than the other, but monitoring of individual fetal welfare may be difficult. Signs of fetal distress may be missed and the opportunity for active intervention lost. In other cases the life of one fetus may be deliberately risked if an induced premature delivery would jeopardize the chances of survival for the other (healthier) twin. This situation may arise in cases of blood group incompatibility. Finally, there are the added hazards, peculiar to twins, of interfetal vascular disturbances, such as the fetofetal transfusion syndrome.

Single intrauterine death

The intrauterine death of one fetus during the second and third trimester is between 0.5 per cent and 0.8 per cent of multiple pregnancies (Burke 1990).

Most twins survive the intrauterine death of their co-twin physically, at least, unharmed. However, in monochorionic twins, who share a placental blood circulation, the survivor may have severe problems, thought by many authors to be due to disseminated intravascular coagulation. Thromboplastin from the macerated fetus transfers to the live twin and causes intravascular coagulation with all its complications, such as haemorrhage, anaemia and jaundice. Clots and debris from the dead fetus form emboli, which may cause ischaemia and necrosis to organs, particularly the brain and kidney (Reisman and Pathak 1966; Moore *et al.* 1969; Koranyi and Kovacs 1975; Durkin *et al.* 1976; Melnick 1977; Yoshioka *et al.* 1979; Yoshida and Matayoshi 1990).

Review of pooled data on 53 cases suggests that disruption of the central nervous system is the most common complication (72 per cent) followed by gastrointestinal (19 per cent), kidneys (15 per cent) and lungs (8 per cent) (Szymonowicz *et al.* 1986).

If one fetus dies early in pregnancy, emboli may disrupt the development of the survivor. Schinzel *et al.* (1979) suggest that some congenital deformities, such as aplasia cutis, hydranencephaly, porencephaly and intestinal atresia may sometimes result from such ischaemic insults in a twin pregnancy. In a study of 113 cases of aplasia cutis, Mannino *et al.* (1977) found that as many as 15 had an MZ fetus papyraceus twin.

In some cases it is thought that the surviving twin may be damaged by a hypotensive episode that killed the co-twin (D'Alton *et al.* 1984; Fusi and Gordon 1990). Alternatively, the death of one twin may lead to a catastrophic fall in the blood pressure of the other, as blood drains from the survivor into the dead twin, in whom the vascular resistance has fallen.

Whether immediate obstetric intervention is indicated following the intrauterine death of one twin is now being questioned. Rydhstrom (1991) studied all twin pregnancies in which one twin had died *in utero* after the 27th week gestation in Sweden over a 10-year period. The perinatal mortality for the surviving twin was high at 10 per cent. There were no instances of coagulation disorders in the mothers.

Sixty-eight of the total number of 129 surviving twins were followed up. Only three suffered from serious disability, one with cerebral palsy alone, one with mental retardation alone and one with combined cerebral palsy and mental retardation. Thus disability was present in only 4.5 per cent of the sample, suggesting that the rate of disability in survivors is much less than previously indicated. These findings, together with the new theory as to the origin of any damage in the survivor, suggest that routine premature delivery of the surviving twin should not necessarily be recommended, as no intervention by an obstetrician, however rapid, would be likely to affect the outcome for the surviving fetus.

5

Twin delivery

The delivery of twins has added hazards not only due to likely prematurity but because abnormal presentation of the fetus is more common. For these reasons a twin delivery should, whenever possible, take place where full consultant obstetric, anaesthetic and paediatric staff are available.

Parental anxieties

Parents are usually aware of the real risks. They may also have unnecessary fears and misconceptions and these should be recognized and allayed wherever possible. This is particularly important for parents who have only recently discovered that they are having twins and have had little time to gain information.

Many mothers fear a longer and more painful labour. Indeed, some have started labour in the belief that they must go through the whole process twice over. In fact, there is no evidence that labour is prolonged in a multiple pregnancy (see p. 75). It is often more uncomfortable, owing to abdominal distension, but the contractions themselves are no more painful.

Parents are anxious too about the outcome for their babies and this anxiety may be reinforced by the number of medical personnel that gather as the time for delivery approaches. The mother may well think that such medical manpower means that something serious is afoot. She—and her partner—should therefore be told beforehand that some staff are there to watch and learn. She should have the option of reducing the audience should she so wish; few mothers do.

As paediatric staff should always be involved with a twin delivery it is helpful if the paediatrician can meet the mother during the antenatal period or, at least, during the early stages of labour. She may well welcome the opportunity to ask questions at this time.

Labour

Onset

The greater the number of fetuses, the earlier is the labour likely to start. Many studies have shown that the average length of gestation for twin pregnancies is approximately 260 days (McKeown and Record 1952; Karn and Penrose 1952; Guttmacher and Kohl 1958; Butler and Alberman 1969;

Stucki *et al.* 1982) compared with 280 days for singletons. The incidence of preterm delivery (less than 37 weeks gestation) is approximately 30 per cent, with reports ranging from 10 to 50 per cent (MacGillivray and Campbell 1988) compared to 5–10 per cent for singletons. Preterm delivery is higher amongst primigravidae (Kauppila *et al.* 1975; Khoo and Green 1975; Weekes *et al.* 1977a) and younger mothers (Weekes *et al.* 1977c).

Preterm labour is more common amongst MZ than DZ pregnancies (MacGillivray and Campbell 1988), and is particularly common in monochorionic MZ pregnancies. Thus, it appears that both zygosity and placentation are significant factors in the onset of labour. Uterine distension caused by polyhydramnios due to the fetofetal transfusion syndrome in monochorionic placentae is likely to account for some of the increase. Interestingly, MZ boy twins are more likely to be delivered prematurely than MZ girls, but this sex difference has not been shown amongst DZ twins (MacGillivray and Campbell 1988).

The causes of the onset of labour are uncertain. Uterine overdistension can be at most a contributory factor. In his ultrasound study of uterine growth in twin pregnancy, Redford (1982) found that there was no relation between uterine distension and onset of preterm labour. Indeed, preterm delivery was more often preceded by impaired than accelerated uterine growth. Were uterine distension alone responsible, labour would start much sooner—when the combined weight of the fetuses equalled that of the average term singleton.

The timing of labour in a multiple pregnancy may well be affected by the increase in circulating hormones of the fetal pituitary/adrenal system. Effacement of the cervix may also play a part in the early onset. The cervix may be prematurely effaced in a multiple pregnancy, possibly due to the increased pressure from the presenting fetus.

As prematurity is the single most important cause of the high perinatal mortality in twin pregnancies, prevention of an early onset of labour is of paramount importance. Unfortunately, attempts to do this with twin pregnancies have, so far, been relatively unsuccessful.

Oral doses of β-sympathomimetic drugs over several weeks have been tried but in most cases results have been disappointing (O'Connor *et al.* 1979; MacGillivray and Campbell 1988). In view of the premature cervical dilatation in many multiple pregnancies cervical suturing could theoretically be of benefit, although this has not been demonstrated (Weekes *et al.* 1977b). Indeed, some workers consider it to be contraindicated (Sinha *et al.* 1979).

Until more is known of the pathogenesis of preterm labour in multiple pregnancy the main means of reducing the perinatal mortality must be early diagnosis and to ensure intensive care facilities are readily available.

If the woman's home is at some distance from a specialist centre, it is highly desirable that she should be accommodated in the hospital (or preferably in a nearby hostel or with friends or relatives) from the beginning of the third trimester. Alternatively, a careful assessment of the state of the cervix should be carried out to detect effacement so that transfer to the central hospital can be arranged when necessary.

Duration

The relative duration of labour in single and multiple pregnancies is no longer open to valid assessment because, in current obstetric practice, slow labour is so often accelerated. However, earlier studies showed, perhaps surprisingly, that labour was no longer in multiple than in single pregnancies (Bender 1952; Danielson 1960; Garrett 1960). In addition Garrett (1960) found that the proportion of labours that were prolonged beyond 36 hours was no greater. Eastman (1961) suggested that this was due to prelabour cervical dilatation resulting in a shorter latent phase. Thus, despite the longer active phase needed to overcome the relative uterine inertia caused by overdistension, the total length of labour was not increased. Friedman and Sachtleben's (1964) findings in 184 twin pregnancies later confirmed Eastman's theory.

Although her labour is not prolonged and the contractions are not necessarily any more painful, the mother of twins is often distressed. Her general discomfort may be quite severe due to the distension and weight of the uterus. Her distress is often increased by her justifiably greater level of anxiety, and the anxiety that she picks up from the staff. This emphasizes the need for her to have a full and generally reassuring discussion beforehand.

Presentation

Up to one-third of twin infants present by the breech (Portes and Granjon 1946; Guttmacher and Kohl 1958)—with all the well-known risks that accompany this position—in contrast to 3.5 per cent of singletons. Kauppila *et al*. (1975) found that the perinatal mortality was twice as high in breech as opposed to vertex-delivered twins.

In only 40–50 per cent of cases do both babies present in the most favourable way—by the vertex (Portes and Granjon 1946; Potter and Fuller 1949; Guttmacher and Kohl 1958; Zuckerman and Brzezinski 1961; Farooqui *et al*. 1973; Campbell and MacGillivray 1988). In 30–40 per cent of cases one will be vertex and one breech (Portes and Granjon 1946; Guttmacher and Kohl 1958; Farooqui *et al*. 1973; Campbell and MacGillivray 1988) and in this group the vertex-presenting twin is born first in three out of four instances (Portes and Granjon 1946). Overall, about 75 per cent of firstborn twins will present by the vertex (MacGillivray and Campbell 1988).

One baby may have a transverse lie and the other vertex (5 per cent) or breech (1.5 per cent). Very occasionally, both may have a transverse lie. These less favourable forms of presentation inevitably lead to an increased incidence of instrumental deliveries and caesarean sections—the incidence varying according to the practice of different centres.

Mode of delivery

Opinions on the best mode of delivery vary greatly in time and place. The incidence of caesarean section has risen in both Europe and the US over the past 30 years. In Aberdeen there was a nine-fold increase in caesarean sections in twin pregnancies to nearly 27 per cent, compared with a three-fold increase amongst singleton pregnancies (MacGillivray and Campbell 1988). However, this rate, and that found in most European countries, is much lower than in the US, where it reaches over 80 per cent in some units (Cetrulo 1986). The European approach does not appear to have any less favourable outcome (MacGillivray and Campbell 1981; Rydhstrom and Ohrlander 1985; Olofsson and Rydhstrom 1985). Indeed, in Sweden Rydhstrom (1990b) found that caesarean sections appeared to have made no impact on the relative rate of morbidity or mortality amongst twin infants under 1500 g during a 10-year period when the caesarean section rate had increased almost ten-fold. Morales *et al.* (1989) found no advantage in caesarean section for non-discordant twin gestations under 1500 g but there was an increase in the incidence of respiratory distress syndrome.

The main indications for an elective caesarean section seem to be a breech presentation. Some obstetricians favour a caesarean section if either of the infants are presenting by the breech. Others will only be concerned if the first is in this position.

Complications of delivery

In addition to the complications of malpresentation there are a number of hazards peculiar to a twin delivery.

Locking

Because of the potentially catastrophic effect of locking of the twins, obstetric textbooks tend to devote a disproportionate amount of space to this complication. The impression gained is that it is not uncommon; in fact it is extremely rare—about 1 in 1000 twin deliveries.

Reviewing the literature up to 1957, Nissen (1958) found 69 cases; others have been reported since (Adams and Fetterhoff 1971; Khunda 1972, Mucklow 1990). Nissen divided the cases into four groups according to the different means of locking (Fig. 5.1). The first is *collision*, where contact of fetal parts between the twins prevents engagement of either. The second is *impaction*, where the impaction of fetal parts of one twin into the body of the other forces partial engagement of both. The third is *compaction*, where the presenting parts of both fetuses become fully engaged in the pelvis and prevent further descent. The fourth, *interlocking*, is where the underside of both chins are in such close apposition as to prevent delivery of the firstborn breech.

The cause of locking is unknown but has been variously ascribed to the small size of the fetuses in relation to the mother's pelvis, to oligohydram-nios, to premature rupture of the amniotic membranes, to hypertonicity of the uterus and to the use of oxytocins. All of these may be contributory factors. The condition is much more common in primigravidae (Nissen 1958; Khunda 1972) and may occasionally be associated with uterine abnor-malities (Parmar and Mulgund 1968; Theron 1969). It is probably more

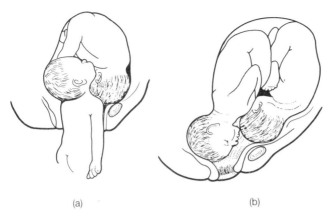

(a)   (b)

Fig. 5.1   Locking of twins (a) chin-to-chin; (b) collision of two heads. From Mac-Gillivray (1975b) by permission of the author and WB Saunders Co. Ltd.

common in monoamniotic pregnancies as Nissen (1958) found seven cases in his series of a total of 69 pairs of locked twins.

Unfortunately, locking is rarely appreciated until part of the presenting fetus has already delivered. This makes vaginal disentanglement extremely difficult. Even with caesarean section the mortality rate is high—43 per cent in Nissen's (1958) series and 31 per cent in Khunda's (1972). Both authors found that the risk was much higher to the leading baby.

The acute fetofetal transfusion syndrome

In contrast to the more generally recognized chronic fetofetal transfusion syndrome (see p. 52), this condition, also confined to monochorionic twins, actually occurs during labour. Blood is transfused from one fetus (the donor) to the other (the recipient) as a result of a haemodynamic imbalance in the fetoplacentofetal unit. Presumably this is due to changes in intravascular pressures across the large-vessel anastomoses (see p. 87) secondary to the changing uterine pressures of labour. One fetus becomes acutely hypervolaemic and later polycythaemic and the other fetus becomes hypovolaemic and then anaemic. Both fetuses may die of cardiac failure if not treated immediately (see p. 103).

Exsanguination of the second twin

As the great majority of monochorionic placentae, if not all, have vascular communications between the two sets of umbilical vessels, haemorrhage from the unclamped placental end of the umbilical cord of the first twin can cause severe blood loss to the second. It is now general practice to ligate both ends of the cord so this complication should no longer occur.

Vasa praevia

Whitehouse and Kohler (1960) reported six cases of vasa praevia (when blood vessels traverse the placental membranes in front of the presenting fetal part) in multiple pregnancy. All were associated with monochorionic placentae and thus rupture of the vessels could exsanguinate not only the first but both babies.

As a velamentous insertion is much more common in twin pregnancies (Benirschke and Driscoll 1967) it would not be surprising if vasa praevia also occurred more frequently. Strong and Brar (1989) found an incidence of 0.55 per cent in multiple pregnancies compared with 0.31 per cent in singleton pregnancies.

Monoamniotic twins

A few MZ twins share an amniotic sac and, as a result, their intrauterine life is particularly hazardous. Monoamniotic twins are thought to result from the later splitting of the developing zygote when the amniotic membrane has already developed. It is possible, however, that some cases are due to the disintegration of an amniotic septum. Triplets may also include a monoamniotic pair (Wharton *et al.* 1968).

Earlier authors reported an incidence of single amnions in twin pregnancies of less than 1 per cent (Quigley 1935; Potter 1963) but more recent studies suggest these were underestimates. Incidences of between 1 and 3 per cent are now more common (Wharton *et al.* 1968; Fujikura and Froehlich 1974).

Females are much more common in monoamniotic pregnancies than in twins in general. James (1977) suggests that this may be because the sex of the zygote is associated with the time within the menstrual cycle that it is formed.

The main hazard to a monoamniotic fetus is entanglement of the umbilical cords (Fig. 5.2). This tends to occur before the 25th week when the fetal movements are less confined (Barss *et al.* 1985). Foglmann (1976) found that this occurred in 60 per cent of over 200 cases of monoamniotic twins. It may lead to umbilical vessel occlusion with a high risk of anoxic death for both fetuses. Occasionally the cord of one twin may become tightly entwined around the neck of the other (Tagawa 1974). As the first twin is delivered it may not immediately be appreciated that the cord around its neck is that of the co-twin rather than its own.

Inevitably the incidence of knotting, and indeed death, in these twins is likely to be overestimated because healthy twins with no cord entanglement may not be noticed to be monoamniotic. Certainly, early reports gave extremely high mortality rates. In reviewing 109 cases in 1935, Quigley found a 68 per cent mortality rate, and in only 17 pairs did both babies survive. More recent studies have shown a perinatal mortality rate between 30 and 50 per cent (Benirschke and Driscoll 1967; Wharton *et al.* 1968; Tagawa 1974). Carr *et al.* (1990) found that this high perinatal mortality was limited to the very preterm deliveries. After 30 weeks the perinatal mortality rate in monoamniotic twins was no higher than in other twins.

Unless amniography has had to be performed for other reasons (which is unlikely) the diagnosis of monoamniotic twins is rarely made until after the birth of the first twin. The absence of an amniotic membrane may then be noticed or, less commonly, a knotted cord may be apparent on the first twin

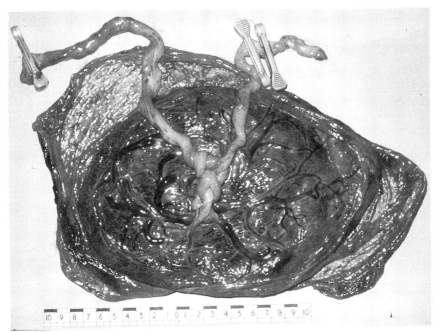

Fig. 5.2 Placenta of monoamniotic twins showing knotting of umbilical cords. By permission of Dr J. Pryse-Davies.

(Goplerud 1964). The number of unsuspected monoamniotic twins will be greatly reduced when membrane relationships can be accurately determined by ultrasound scanning. Promising results with echography of the amniotic membranes have now been reported (Bessis and Papiernik 1981). If the diagnosis of a monoamniotic pregnancy is made in time many obstetricians prefer to deliver the twins by caesarean section to reduce the risk of entanglement.

The undiagnosed twin

An unexpected second baby presents real problems, especially for medical staff who may be at once inexperienced and ill-prepared for the complications of a twin delivery. The problems for the mother (and father) however, will be no smaller. At the height of her exhaustion and stress she has to cope both with shock and the sudden need to relate to a second baby.

Undiagnosed twins are now rare in developed countries but there are still many centres in developing countries where a substantial proportion of twin pregnancies will not be detected prior to birth (see p. 31).

The main dangers to the undiagnosed twin are those of a precipitate delivery before its presence has been realized or, more commonly, retention and fetal anoxia due to contraction of the uterus following administration of oxytocin.

Birth interval

In the past it was generally agreed that the hazards to the second fetus of a delay in delivery beyond 30 min outweighed any risks of active intervention. Many considered the optimal time to be between 10 and 20 min (Spurway 1962; Benirschke and Kim 1973; Farr 1975) and believed that greater haste was harmful and associated with a significantly higher perinatal mortality rate (Farrell 1964). Others, however, felt the sooner the delivery, the better (Corston 1957; Muller-Holve *et al.* 1976) and would recommend rupturing the second amniotic sac immediately after delivery of the first baby to prevent the cervix contracting again.

However, the advent of reliable monitoring of fetal wellbeing in labour may be altering obstetric practice. Some obstetricians now consider that active intervention should only be undertaken if there are signs of fetal distress and that the actual duration of birth interval does not matter, although, from the mother's point of view, undue delay is undesirable.

Occasionally there is a long interval between the deliveries of both twins and triplets. Prolonged delivery intervals of between 35 and 131 days have been reported (Abrams 1957; Drucker *et al.* 1960; Banch 1984; Simpson *et al.* 1984; Brion *et al.* 1986). Unlike some other cases of prolonged intervals in which the mother had uteri didelphys (Williams and Cummings 1953; Dorgan and Clarke 1956; Green *et al.* 1961; Mashiach *et al.* 1981), these cases all had normal uteruses.

In some circumstances the interval is therapeutically prolonged for several weeks to allow the second fetus to mature (Conrad and Weidinger 1982; Feichtinger *et al.* 1989). Thomsen (1978) describes a case in which the first baby was delivered at 27 weeks' gestation weighing 680 g. Labour-inhibiting drugs were then given and a cervical cerclage inserted. Labour did not recur for another 4 weeks, at which time a 1192 g infant was delivered, and survived. There were two separate placentae but both were retained until after the birth of the second baby. Infection was not a problem.

Intervals of more than an hour or so are now uncommon, except in developing countries. Reports from some of these areas have confirmed the greatly increased risk run by the retained fetus. Adeleye (1972) studied 106 second twins in Nigeria who were retained for over 30 min. Many of the firstborn twins had been born outside the hospital. Retention was thought to be due to malpresentation in about half of the cases and to uterine inertia in the remainder. The perinatal mortality in the second twin was three times that of the first and, more significantly, rose to ten-fold (47 per cent) in those retained for over 2 hours.

Anaesthesia

No medical team prepared for the delivery of twins can be complete without an experienced anaesthetist. General and epidural analgesia are frequently required, sometimes, in the case of the second twin, at short notice.

Nearly all mothers will require some form of analgesia because of the greater discomfort of a twin labour. Those that cause respiratory depression, such as pethidine, should be avoided, particularly for the sake of the second twin who may already be embarrassed by reduced levels of oxygen.

Epidural analgesia is now the analgesic and anaesthetic of choice for twin deliveries. Amongst other things it has the advantage that the mother is already prepared for any manoeuvres such as an internal version, instrumental delivery or caesarean section, that may be necessary for the second twin. The delay caused by preparation and induction of a general anaesthetic is avoided and, not least, the mother can still have the pleasure of seeing her babies as they are born.

Several workers have found that, with epidural analgesia, the metabolic balance of both babies compares favourably with other forms of analgesia (James *et al.* 1977; Jaschevatzky *et al.* 1977; Weekes *et al.* 1977c). The acid-base status of the second twin is also as good as that of the first born, which is much less likely to be the case in deliveries conducted without epidural anaesthesia (Crawford 1987). Likewise, neither the length of labour nor the incidence of instrumental deliveries was increased by the use of epidural analgesia (Weekes *et al.* 1977c). Crawford (1975) actually found the delivery interval to be shorter with this form of analgesia.

Maternal hypotension due to aortocaval compression is a real danger and can lead to severe oxygen deprivation to both babies—precautions must be taken to avoid this.

Risks to first and second twin

Almost all studies show a higher perinatal mortality rate for the secondborn twin than the first (MacGillivray and Campbell 1988). Although many individual studies have been inconclusive, in that the difference between the two babies has not been statistically significant, when analysed cumulatively the evidence is overwhelmingly in favour of the firstborn. In reviewing the literature on over 23000 infants Wyshak and White (1963) found a perinatal mortality rate of 57.1 per 1000 for firstborn and 74.6 for second. In the 28 studies they analysed only two showed the reverse trend.

If one twin dies *in utero* the live twin is generally delivered first. However, even if macerated stillbirths are excluded from the figures the loss of the second twin is still higher than that of the first (Guttmacher and Kohl 1958; Potter 1963; Koivisto *et al.* 1975).

In good obstetric units, where delay in the delivery of the second twin is avoided, the difference in the fate of the two infants is now becoming steadily smaller.

The leading twin has to dilate the cervix, and is therefore at greater risk than the second of intracranial haemorrhage from birth injury, particularly if premature (Griffiths 1967). Theoretically, the risk of infection ascending from the genital tract is also greater, although there is scant evidence to support this (see p. 67).

Weighted against the chances for the second twin is the risk of fetal anoxia, particularly when delivery is delayed (Adeleye 1972) or when the second twin is undiagnosed. The second twin is then in danger of being trapped *in utero* or conversely catapulted out with undue speed if oxytocin is given. Further hazards are added by the greater likelihood of malpresentation or of a breech delivery requiring instrumental intervention. The respiratory distress syndrome may occur in the second twin alone or, if both are affected, the second twin is usually more severely affected and more likely to succumb (see p. 103).

6

The twin placenta

Placentation may have a profound effect on the long-term development of twins. Yet all too often details about it are recorded carelessly and the value of many twin studies is greatly reduced by lack of information on this vital factor.

Types of placenta

There are three types of placenta—single, fused and separate. The type found in a particular pregnancy is determined by three factors, the site of implantation in the uterus, the zygosity and, in MZ twins, the timing of zygote division. As DZ twins arise from two zygotes they always have individual placentae. Depending on their site of implantation these may remain entirely discrete or, if close, will fuse together partially, or completely, to form an apparently single placental disc. The relative frequency of these two types of dichorionic placentation cannot be determined satisfactorily from the literature; the criterion for fusion varies in different studies from a loose membranous attachment to firm adherence of placental tissues.

The type of placenta found in MZ twinning gives a good indication of the stage of development at which the zygote divided (Fig. 6.1). Of the two membranes surrounding the fetus the chorion develops towards the end of the first week while the amnion, which lines the chorion and directly surrounds the fetus, is not differentiated until the second week. If division of the conceptus occurs in the first week (about 34 per cent) the twins will develop separate amnions and chorions, as is the case with all DZ twins. If the embryonic mass divides before the formation of the amnion the result will be a common chorion and separate amnion. About 66 per cent of MZ twins have monochorionic placentae. Finally, if the division takes place after differentiation of the amnion, twins will not only share a common chorion but will also be contained in a single amniotic sac (1–2 per cent)—monoamniotic twins.

An interesting, but as yet unexplained, finding is that mothers of MZ twins with monochorionic placentae were younger than those with dichorionic placentae (MacGillivray et al. 1988b).

Several workers (Potter 1963; Nylander 1970b; Fujikura and Froehlich 1971), although not all (Corney et al. 1972), have found that MZ dichorionic placentae are more likely to be fused than DZ. Fujikura and Froehlich (1971) suggest that this is due to an increased chance of adjacent implantation

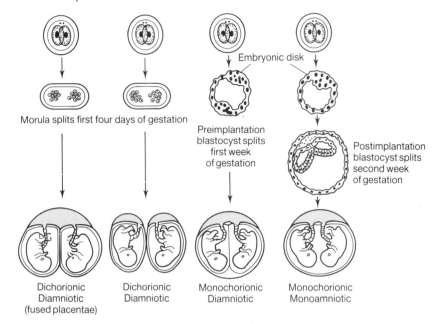

Fig. 6.1   The development and placentation of monozygotic twins. From Fox (1978). By permission of the author and WB Saunders Co. Ltd.

when the two zygotes come from the same fallopian tube, which, of course, they always do in MZ twins.

There is probably no difference in function between fused and separate placentae *per se* but as placental function may be affected by the site of implantation it would not be surprising if discrepancies in fetal growth in like-sexed DZ twins are greater in those with separate placentae, and this was found to be the case by Fujikura and Froehlich (1971). If one placenta is sited on the posterior wall of the uterus and the other, for instance, near the cervix, the first will receive a greater uteroplacental blood flow and thus better nutrition for that fetus. However, in two studies it was found that twins with a fused dichorionic placenta had greater birth weight discordancy than those with separate placentae. Clearly this subject needs further study.

The umbilical cord

Apart from some conjoined twins and the extremely rare case of monoamniotic twins with a forked cord, all twins have an individual umbilical cord. The cords may vary greatly in size and also in site of insertion into the placenta, and both these factors may affect fetal nutrition (see Fig. 4.4).

Abnormally inserted umbilical cords are more common in twin placentae (Benirschke and Driscoll 1967; Strong and Corney 1967) and intrapartum haemorrhage associated with a velamentous insertion contributes to the high perinatal mortality of multiple pregnancy.

Monochorial twin placentae have abnormal cord insertions much more commonly than dichorial. The orientation of the egg at implantation may be the explanation for this difference (Leroy 1985). In single pregnancies the attachment of the umbilical cord in the centre of the placenta reflects the primary site of implantation. In monochorial twins one of the two inner cell masses will be at opposite poles of the blastocyst. Inevitably one will be orientated away from the endometrial surfaces. A higher frequency of marginal insertions of the umbilical cord is therefore not surprising.

Marginal and velamentous insertions of the umbilical cord are more common in fused dichorionic than in separate placentae, and are even more common amongst higher order pregnancies. It is likely that the competition for space as the placentae develop is the cause for this. This may also be the explanation for the high incidence of single umbilical arteries in twins (see below), which are particularly associated with eccentric insertion of the umbilical cord (Benirschke 1990).

The umbilical vessels, as in singletons, usually spiral in an anticlockwise direction but this is variable and Edmonds (1954) found that the direction may differ within a pair of twins.

Most workers have found that single umbilical arteries (SUA) are more common in twins. In a review of 13 prospective studies Heifetz (1984) found an incidence of SUA of 2.3 per cent in twin infants—between three and four times the incidence found in singletons. As in singletons, malformations were more common in the twins with SUA but, apart from acardia, these malformations do not appear to be of a particular type. There is some indication that SUA is more common amongst MZ than DZ twins (Strong and Corney 1967; Boyd and Hamilton 1970) but the numbers are too small for a definite conclusion to be reached.

It is rare for twins to be concordant for SUA and, in general, the anomaly occurs in the smaller of the two infants (Heifetz 1984). This agrees with the finding of a higher incidence of SUA amongst small-for-dates singleton babies (Bryan and Kohler 1974).

Placentation and zygosity (Fig. 6.2)

For many years it was believed that MZ and DZ twins could be distinguished by the number of chorionic membranes. Unfortunately this belief dies hard. It later became evident that some MZ twins must have dichorionic placentae; by applying Weinberg's rule (1902) it was apparent that more MZ twins should have existed than the number of twins found to have monochorionic placentae. This conclusion was supported by the observation that some twins with dichorionic placentae were physically indistinguishable. Later studies show that between 18.5 and 37.5 per cent of MZ twins do in fact have placentae with two chorions (Corney 1975b).

In contrast it seems unlikely that human DZ twins ever have monochorionic placentae. Six studies of a total of 3452 twin pairs of known zygosity failed to find any (Corney 1975b). Occasional reports of mono-

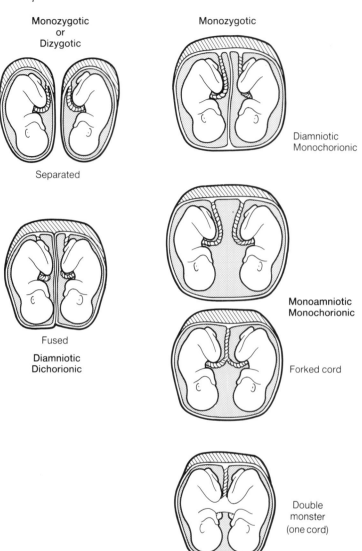

Fig. 6.2   Placentation of twins. From Strong and Corney (1967) by permission of the authors and Pergamon Press.

chorionic placentae in DZ pregnancies lack validity in that essential histological evidence is missing. Nylander and Osunkoya (1970) demonstrated the importance of this in their interesting case of unlike-sexed twins with an apparently monochorionic placenta. Only on histological investigation did they find fragments of chorionic tissue at the base of the septum, from which they concluded that these must be remnants of a dichorionic septum that had disintegrated.

A rare exception to the rule that monochorionicity confirms monozygosity was a case reported by Bieber and his colleagues (1981) where the infants were of unlike sex—a normal XY boy and an (acardiac) female (XXX). These twins were shown to be monovular but not MZ, as two spermatozoa had been involved. It was thought that this was a case of polar body twinning.

Vascular communications

Perhaps the greatest difference between monochorionic and dichorionic twins is that the former share a blood circulation whilst the latter rarely have any blood in common. This can have far-reaching implications. In mono-chorionic twins the most powerful intrauterine influences determining growth are often related to the inter-twin haemodynamics, and this may also apply to malformations (see p. 55). In dichorionic pairs, on the other hand, the sites of implantation of the two placentae are probably of para-mount importance.

Monochorionic placentae

For several centuries it had been known that communicating vessels occur in monochorionic placentae (Smellie 1752) and in 1870 Hyrtl demonstrated all the, now well-recognized, types and combinations of anastomoses—the superficial arterioarterial and venovenous and the deep (parenchymatous) arteriovenous. Schatz (1900) went on to confirm this work and then focussed his attention on the deep arteriovenous anastomoses. He gave much thought to the effects on the fetus of this shared or, as he called it, 'third circulation' (the first two being the fetal circulation of each twin). It was not until the 1960s that interest was revived (Corney 1966; Benirschke and Driscoll 1967; Strong and Corney 1967).

It is now generally accepted that most, if not all, monochorionic placentae have at least one type of anastomosis, of which arterioarterial, often com-bined with arteriovenous, is the most common (Benirschke an Driscoll 1967; Strong and Corney 1967; Cameron 1968; Boyd and Hamilton 1970; Robertson and Neer 1983). Superficial anastomoses can often be seen with the naked eye but the patterns can be determined accurately only by injection studies.

Similar communicating channels exist in monochorionic monoamniotic placentae (Wharton *et al.* 1968; Bhargava 1976), although not invariably (Benirschke and Driscoll 1967; Strong and Corney 1967).

The fetofetal transfusion syndrome

When no superficial anastomoses are present to compensate for the ar-teriovenous blood flow a chronic haemodynamic imbalance may develop between monochorionic twins (Fig. 6.3). This results in the fetofetal transfu-sion syndrome. One fetus transfuses the other via arteriovenous ana-stomoses and causes anaemia to himself and polycythaemia to the recipient (see Fig. 7.2). This is often disastrous for both.

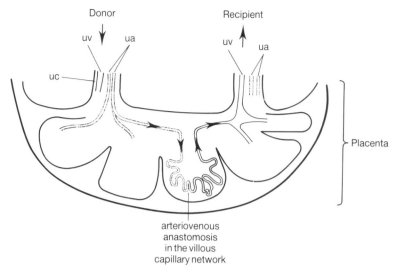

Fig. 6.3 The arteriovenous anastomosis present in the chronic form of fetofetal transfusion syndrome. Uc, umbilical cord; uv, umbilical vein; ua, umbilical artery.

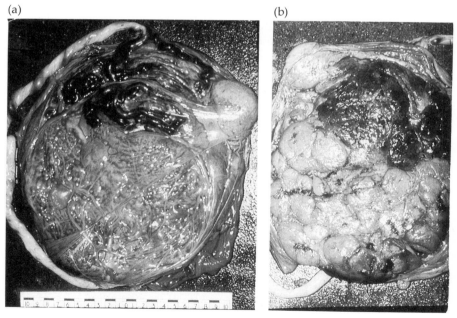

Fig. 6.4 The placenta in the fetofetal transfusion syndrome. (a) Fetal surface; (b) maternal surface. The donor portion is large and pale while the recipient portion is engorged and smaller. By permission of Mr J Erskine.

The appearance of the placenta in this condition is striking and charac-teristic (Fig. 6.4). The recipient's portion is deeply coloured and is often smaller, with dilated engorged blood vessels. The histology, however, is unremarkable and normal for the period of gestation. In contrast, the donor's portion is pale and bulky with high placental:fetal ratio. On micro-scopy the chorionic villi are oedematous and pleomorphic. The two layers of the trophoblast are thicker and well-preserved and syncytial knots are scarce. The fetal capillaries are often filled with nucleated cells (Fig. 6.5). Some authors have compared the appearance with that found in the placentae of Rhesus-sensitized infants (Benirschke and Driscoll 1967) but Aherne *et al.* (1968), in their detailed morphometric studies, found that the characteristic villous hyperplasia did not occur. They showed that both the volume and surface area of the chorionic tissue were much greater in the donor twin. They thought, however, that this was due to oedematous swelling alone. The total volume and surface area of the fetal capillary beds in the two territories were similar but, as the capillary diameter in that of the donor was sometimes only half that of the recipient, these capillaries must be much longer.

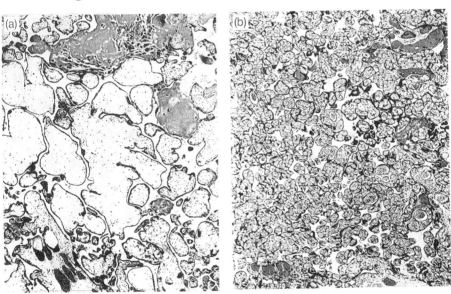

Fig. 6.5 The histology of the placenta in the fetofetal transfusion syndrome. (a) Donor—the chorionic villi are bulky and fetal vessels are scarcely visible; (b) recipient—fetal capillaries are numerous and engorged with blood. From Strong and Corney (1967) by permission of the authors and Pergamon Press.

Little is known about the function of this grossly abnormal placenta but Aherne *et al.* (1968) thought that the donor fetus might well receive less nourishment than his twin. This poor supply could, in part, be due to a reduction in maternofetal transfer across the abnormal placental basement membrane but, Aherne suggested that it may also be due to a sluggish blood flow in the narrow, elongated fetal capillaries of this part of the placenta. The low levels of the maternally derived protein IgG found in newborn donor twins provide further evidence of a disturbance in maternofetal transfer (Bryan 1976; Bryan *et al.* 1976).

The great majority of cases of the transfusion syndrome have diamniotic placentation, but several instances of the syndrome in monoamniotic twins have been reported (Rausen *et al.* 1965; Meyer *et al.* 1970; Pochedly and Musiker 1970).

Dichorionic placentae

Although common in some animals, such as the cow, vascular communications in dichorionic placentae in man are extremely rare (Benirschke and Driscoll 1967; Strong and Corney 1967; Corney 1975b). Many earlier reports are of dubious accuracy. Cameron (1968) however, reported two authentic cases from the Birmingham Twin Study, in both of which the twins were probably MZ. The previously mentioned case of unlike-sex twins with only a remnant of septal chorion had visible vascular communications and blood examination showed chimerism (Nylander and Osunkoya 1970) (see p. 55).

There have been no satisfactorily proven examples of the fetofetal transfusion syndrome in dichorionic placentae. Those cases in which it has been suspected (Michaels 1967; Allen 1972) did not have injection studies. It may well be that the twin was anaemic for other reasons, such as fetomaternal haemorrhage (Strong and Corney 1967; Bryan 1976).

Examination of the placenta

In 1961 Benirschke wrote a paper entitled *Accurate Recording of Twin Placentation. A Plea to the Obstetrician.* His plea has been echoed since to both obstetricians and paediatricians (Strong and Corney 1967; Corney 1975b; Burn and Corney 1988), but by many it remains unheeded. The placenta may receive but a cursory glance; information that may be vital to the immediate care of a sick baby, let alone to twin studies, is all too often consigned to the incinerator. Comments in the medical records frequently give no indication of the placental membranes and remarks such as 'single' and 'binovular' are misleading.

As soon as the first twin is delivered the cord should be labelled according to the hospital practice. This will vary between hospitals but must remain consistent within any particular hospital. Confusion arises if obstetricians adopt individual methods. Probably the most satisfactory and logical practice is to give the first cord a single clamp (or tape) and the second two clamps, on the grounds that only standard (and readily available) equipment need be used.

After delivery of the placenta the site of insertion of the cords should be described and any anomalies or discrepancy in thickness and length noted. A simple sketch diagram in the obstetric notes should be routine practice. If an umbilical artery is missing the paediatrician should be informed.

Samples of cord blood for zygosity determination should be collected (taking care to avoid contamination with maternal blood) into heparinized bottles clearly labelled 'Twin 1' and 'Twin 2'. Clotted blood can also provide useful, although more limited, information. These samples should be stored at 4°C (not frozen) until sent together with similar samples from both parents, if possible, for testing of genetic markers or for DNA analysis (see p. 29). If placental tissue is also required (see p. 29) a full-thickness block of placenta (about 10 g) should be taken from diametrically opposed sites and stored at −20°C (unless immediate facilities for examination are available). If injection studies of the placental vessels (see below) are planned, this specimen should be taken later.

If the placentae are separate or easily separable they should be weighed individually. Fused dichorionic and monochorionic placentae will obviously be weighed as one. If there is a clear demarcation between the two territories, a rough estimation of the relative size of the two portions should be made. Note that the septum is not necessarily an indication of the territorial boundaries as injection studies have shown that often the two do not coincide (Strong and Corney 1967; Fig. 6.6).

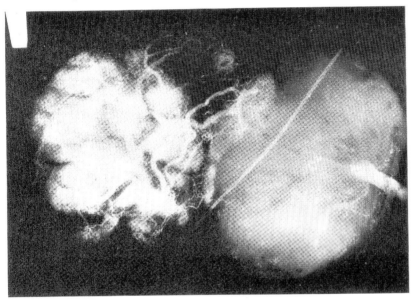

Fig. 6.6 X-ray of fused dichorionic placentae. One placenta has been injected with contrast medium. A catheter lies along the base of the septum showing that the junction of the vascular territories does not correspond to the insertion of the septum. From Strong and Corney (1967) by permission of the authors and Pergamon Press.

The most important part of the twin placenta is the relationships of the membranes; these should be examined gently to avoid tearing. Characteristically, the amnion is more transparent and friable than the chorion and can readily be stripped from the placenta, leaving a smooth surface (of chorion).

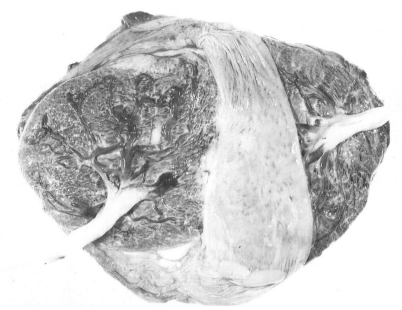

Fig. 6.7   Fused dichorionic diamniotic placenta. From Strong and Corney (1967) by permission of the authors and Pergamon Press.

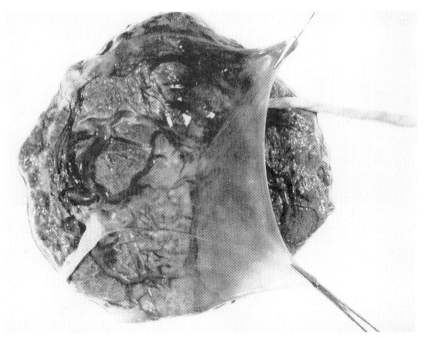

Fig. 6.8   Monochorionic diamniotic placenta. From Strong and Corney (1967) by permission of the authors and Pergamon Press.

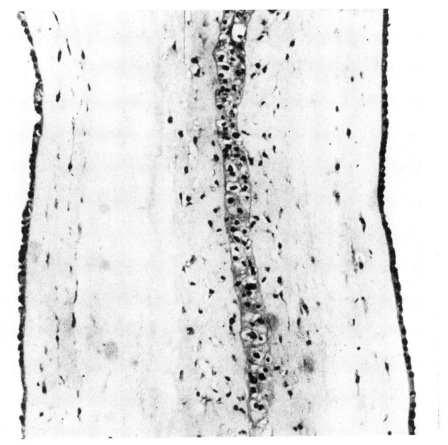

Fig. 6.9 The dividing membrane of a fused dichorionic placenta. The two outer layers are composed of amnion. Between them the two layers of chorion have fused in the mid-line (H&E × 34). From Strong and Corney (1967) by permission of the authors and Pergamon Press.

The amnions should peel right back to the umbilical cords and form a collar at their bases. No septum will then remain in monochorionic placentae whereas in dichorionic a single (fused) or two separate layers of chorion persist. The chorion is more opaque (Figs. 6.7 and 6.8) and cannot be separated from the placenta, except by tearing, as it is an integral part of the placental tissue. The chorionic ridge at the base of the septum is a good clue to a dichorionic placenta (Bleisch 1964). Occasionally, difficulty arises if the septal membranes are fused and this can only be resolved by histology (Fig. 6.9). For full details of histological examination see Bourne (1962). Usually, however, macroscopic examination by an experienced observer is as reliable as histology (Nylander 1970c; Corney 1975b) and the latter needs only to be done in doubtful cases.

Accurate identification of vascular anastomoses will rarely be required for

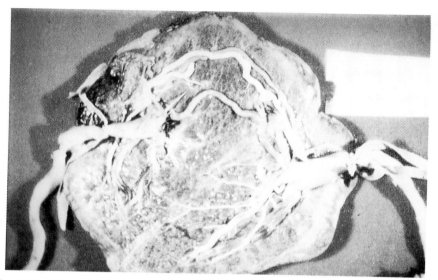

Fig. 6.10 Monochorionic diamniotic placenta. The vessels of twin 2 (right) have been injected and the vessels of the other twin have filled through both arterial and venous anastomoses. From Strong and Corney (1967) by permission of the authors and Pergamon Press.

clinical purposes. Injection studies are usually confined to research projects. However, the techniques are (usually) not difficult to apply and the result can be both informative and decorative (Fig. 6.10). Those interested should gain experience on 'straightforward' specimens before a complicated case presents itself. Many coloured liquids (including red wine) have been injected to demonstrate placental vessels and their communications. Full details are given in Strong and Corney's (1967) beautifully illustrated book *The Twin Placenta* and by others (Benirschke and Driscoll 1967).

The use of radiopaque materials has enabled fascinating X-ray studies to be made (Strong and Corney 1967; Aherne *et al.* 1968; Fig. 6.11). For the practitioner who just wishes to demonstrate the existence and types of communicating channels, milk or coloured saline are the simplest and most readily available media. If the vessels are intact, all the blood can be washed out through catheters inserted into the vessels of the umbilical cords. If they are torn or examination has been delayed, particular areas can be catheterized and examined separately.

Quantitative morphological studies of twin placentae are described by Aherne and his colleagues (Aherne and Dunnill 1966; Aherne *et al.* 1968) but are research procedures and are beyond the scope of this book. More detailed descriptions of the examination of the placenta in general are given elsewhere (Benirschke and Driscoll 1967; Strong and Corney 1967; Boyd and Hamilton 1970; Corney 1975b; Fox 1978).

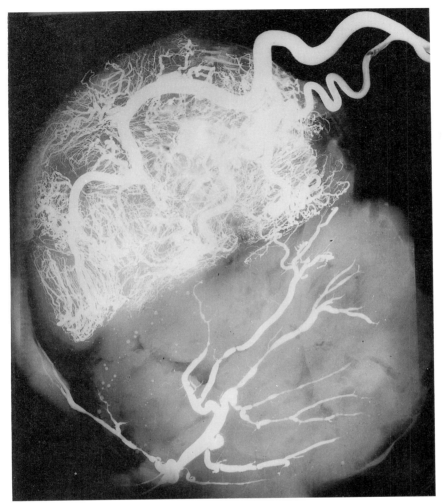

Fig. 6.11   Monochorionic diamniotic placenta. Contrast medium has been injected through the umbilical arteries of twin 2 and flowed through an arterial anastomosis of twin 1. It has just begun to fill its umbilical arteries in retrograde manner. From Strong and Corney (1967) by permission of the authors and Pergamon Press.

Ultrasound

Many couples expecting twins will have no strong preference for either a MZ or a DZ pair but if they are firmly told to expect one or the other they will become adjusted to the idea and feel seriously disconcerted if what they expect to be very different children turn out to be indistinguishable. Many are incorrectly told that because two placentae are visible on ultrasound scan the babies will be DZ. Similarly, because a fused dichorionic placenta is a single organ, some parents have been led to expect MZ children instead of the boy and a girl who were later delivered.

Ultrasound examination can never distinguish between like-sex DZ twins and dichorionic MZ but in skilled hands the chorionicity of the placentae can be accurately determined in most cases (D'Alton and Dudley 1989; Winn *et al.* 1989). Antenatal detection of chorionicity is particularly valuable in supporting the diagnosis of a fetofetal transfusion syndrome (p. 52); when considering selective feticide (see p. 42) and in cases of the death of one twin fetus (p. 71).

7

Newborn twins

The birth of twins always causes excitement in the delivery room but is also bound to cause some anxiety too. The complications that may arise during the labour and delivery of twins have already been discussed (see Chapter 5). Because of the risk of these complications, and of prematurity, two members of the paediatric staff should be present whenever possible and two full sets of equipment for resuscitation must always be available.

Length of gestation

The average length of a twin pregnancy is about 260 days—3 weeks shorter than for singletons (MacGillivray 1975b). About 30 per cent of twins are born before the 37th week and are, therefore, preterm. The reasons for the shorter

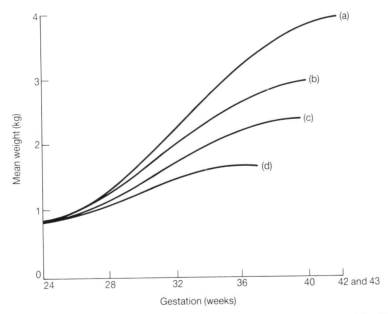

Fig. 7.1 Birth weights of multiple births in relation to gestation. From MacGillivray (1975c) by permission of the author and WB Saunders Co. Ltd. (a) Singletons; (b) twins; (c) triplets; (d) quadruplets.

gestation are still uncertain (see p. 74). In many cases, however, it would be a disadvantage to the twin fetuses to continue intrauterine life to term. Uteroplacental function seems to be suboptimal during the last few weeks in many twin pregnancies. This is suggested by the rapidly increasing discrepancy in weights between twins and singletons as they approach term (Fig. 7.1) and by the rising perinatal mortality rate after 38–39 weeks gestation (Stucki *et al.* 1982).

Poor placental function may also explain why MZ twins tend to have a shorter gestation than DZ (Weekes *et al.* 1977a; MacGillivray 1982). The 'third circulation' may well reduce the efficiency of maternofetal transfer still further.

Assessment of gestational age

The gestational age of the newborn can be assessed by certain neurological and physical criteria. This is well-established practice with singletons (Dubowitz *et al.* 1970). Studies have shown the same criteria to be equally appropriate in twins (Keet *et al.* 1974; Woods and Malan 1977). Twins with only small intrapair differences in weight tend to have more similar scores to their co-twin than those with large weight discrepancies. Although the lighter twin has similar scores on neurological criteria he tends to have a lower score than his twin on physical criteria (Woods and Malan 1977). The pattern shown by the lighter twin is similar to that of an intrauterine growth-retarded singleton.

In his study of 33 pairs of twins Keet *et al.* (1974) found that there was no significant difference in the mean combined neurological and physical score between the heavier and lighter babies. However, in the group with large weight discrepancies (over 15 per cent) only three out of 12 lighter twins had a higher score than their co-twin.

Birth weight

Just over 50 per cent of multiple births in 1982–4 in the UK weighed less than 2500 g, compared to 6 per cent of singletons (Botting *et al.* 1987). As well as being of low birth weight, many of these infants, particularly the more mature, are light for their gestational age when compared with singletons (Fig. 7.1). Indeed, the optimal birth weight for twins appears to be between 2.5 and 3.5 kg, whereas for singletons it is between 3.5 and 4 kg (Butler and Alberman 1969). As in singletons, male twin infants tend to be heavier than females (Parsons 1965; Corey *et al.* 1979).

In twins with large intrapair discrepancies in weight the heavier infant is usually appropriately grown for its gestational age when compared with singletons. The lighter infant, on the other hand, must have suffered from intrauterine growth retardation and runs all the risks of a light-for-dates baby, in particular that of hypoglycaemia (Reisner *et al.* 1965).

The birth weight of twins appears to be unrelated to birth order. Most recent studies have found no significant differences between the mean weight of firstborn and secondborn twins. Earlier studies tended to show that the firstborn was heavier but the difference is removed when macerated stillbirths, which are nearly always both smaller and secondborn, are excluded from the sample.

Bleker and colleagues (1977) found that parity had a greater influence on birth weight in twins than in singletons and suggested that this might be due to the adaptation of the uterine vascular system following a previous pregnancy which then better equips it to cope with the extra demands of a multiple pregnancy.

The problems of low birth weight and of prematurity are many and the reader is referred to textbooks on neonatal medicine for guidance on their management. Mention here will be made of disorders that are either peculiar to twins or have particular expression (e.g. intrapair differences) in twins.

Haemoglobin levels

Neither zygosity nor birth order appear to affect the level of haemoglobin in the cord bloods of twins (Bryan 1976). Intrapair discrepancies, once the cases of fetofetal transfusion syndrome have been excluded, are also similar in DZ and MZ twins (Kauppila *et al*. 1975; Bryan 1976). However, Abraham (1969) suggests that the first of MZ twins may be depleted of blood due to interfetal shunting during delivery. Although he found no difference in haemoglobin levels at birth, by 24 hours of age the firstborn had significantly lower levels.

Clemetson (1956) found that cord haemoglobin levels in dichorionic twins were significantly higher in the lighter twin and suggested that this may be

Table 7.1   Characteristic features of the two forms of fetofetal transfusion syndrome

		Acute	Chronic
Cause	Placenta	Arterior-arterial or venovenous transfusion	Arterio-venous transfusion
Pregnancy	Ultrasound	Normal	Diverging BPD
	Amniotic fluid	Normal volume	Polyhydramnios
Placenta	Appearance	Normal	d—Pale, bulky, oedematous r—Engorged
	Vascular anastomoses	Visible superficial	Invisible arterio-venous
	Histology	Normal	d—Trophoblast immaturity r—Normal
Infants	Birth weight	Similar	r—Heavier than d
	Blood film	Normal	d—Erythroblastosis r—Normal
	Complications	d—Shock++ CCF++ Anaemia+	d—Birth asphyxia+ Anaemia++ CCF± Small-for-dates
		r—CCF++ Polycythaemia+ Jaundice+	r—Polycythaemia++ Jaundice+ CCF±

d, donor; r, recipient; BPD, biparietal diameter; CCF, congestive cardiac failure.

due to relative intrauterine hypoxia. Polycythaemia is well-recognized in association with intrauterine growth retardation in singletons.

In addition to the known causes of anaemia in the newborn, mono-chorionic twins may be anaemic as a result of their shared intrauterine circulation. The donor twin of both the acute (see p. 77) and chronic fetofetal transfusion syndrome (see p. 52 and Table 7.1) and a single survivor with disseminated intravascular coagulation (see p. 71) are two examples of this.

The chronic fetofetal transfusion syndrome

An intrapair discrepancy in cord blood haemoglobin levels of over 5 g/dl has been suggested as the diagnostic criterion for the fetofetal transfusion syndrome. Rausen *et al.* (1965) found no discrepancy of such magnitude in a series of DZ twins, all of whom would be expected to have dichorionic placentation. As haemoglobin concentrations may not be available for infants who die before, or soon after delivery, a combination of other criteria, such as polyhydramnios in one sac, large birthweight discrepancies and characteristic placental histology, will often be needed in making the diagnosis.

Even when they are available, haemoglobin levels should not be used as the only criterion for the diagnosis as they will not distinguish the fetofetal transfusion syndrome from other causes of anaemia in one twin. Intrapartum blood loss or fetomaternal haemorrhage, for instance, could both result in large intrapair discrepancies in haemoglobin level.

Extreme examples of intrapair haematological differences have been described: haemoglobin discrepancies exceeding 20 g/dl (Bosma 1954; Klingberg *et al.* 1955; Sacks 1959), individual haemoglobin levels greater than 30 g/dl (Bosma 1954; Sacks 1959), and alarmingly high haematocrit levels. In Sacks' (1959) case the haematocrit of one twin who survived apparently unscathed was 93 per cent. At the other extreme donor twins have survived haemoglobin levels of less than 4 g/dl (Klingberg *et al.* 1955; Shorland 1971). Even with smaller discrepancies in haemoglobin levels there may be striking differences in the blood films of the two infants—a normoblastaemia being evident in that of the donor (Strong and Corney 1967).

Nutrients are, of course, transfused together with the haemoglobin and it is not surprising that the recipient twin is usually much heavier than the donor (Fig. 7.2). Studies of protein chemistry have shown much higher levels of all proteins in the recipient (Kloosterman 1963; Bryan 1976; Bryan *et al.* 1976). The donor twin may have very low levels of total proteins and albumin and, presumably, colloid osmotic pressure (Bryan 1976). Hydrops fetalis has occasionally been reported in both recipient and donor and it is surprising that this is not more common, particularly in the donor, in view of the profound anaemia and hypoalbuminaemia. However, some infants who are free from oedema at birth may become severely oedematous within a few days (Bryan and Slavin 1974).

Two cases of the fetofetal transfusion syndrome have been described in which the donor twins had 'blueberry muffin' skin lesions, which showed dermal erythropoeisis on histological examination (Schwartz *et al.* 1984).

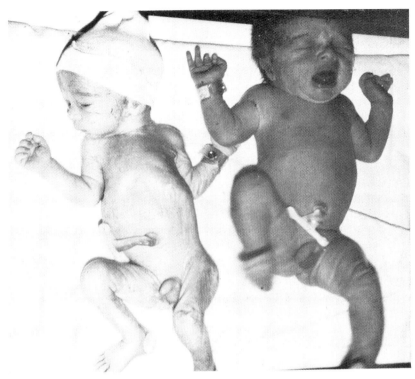

Fig. 7.2 The fetofetal transfusion syndrome showing intrauterine growth retardation and pallor of the donor (weight 1.6 kg; Hb 7.9 g/100 ml) and plethora of recipient (weight 2.7 kg; Hb 21 g/100 ml).

The persistence of cutaneous haematopoeisis was thought to be an unusual response to severe long-standing anaemia.

A recently reported finding in the fetofetal transfusion syndrome was that of abnormal bone mineralization in both recipient and donor (Bishop *et al.* 1990). The donor twin had osteosclerotic bones and this was thought to be due to a reduced availability of macrophages, precursors to the osteoclasts responsible for bone mineral resorption, whereas the osteopenia found in the recipient could be due to overactivity of osteoclasts.

Both intrauterine and neonatal death are common in this condition and Villena *et al.* (1991) found that the size of the fetal weight discordancy was a good prognostic indicator, with a much higher mortality rate amongst those with large weight differences.

Management

The chronic fetofetal transfusion syndrome is not usually diagnosed before delivery, although the presence of polyhydramnios or diverging fetal growth curves in a multiple pregnancy should always raise the suspicion. In mild cases the diagnosis is often missed, or made only because of the result of a routine blood count. Sometimes it is only because of a careful placental examination that the condition is suspected. Many of these infants need no special treatment. Others may be severely distressed. The donor twin, already embarrassed by chronic hypoxia from the anaemia, often suffers from severe birth asphyxia, particularly if he is the secondborn.

A blood transfusion is rarely urgent as the fetuses have usually had time to compensate for their haemodynamic disturbances. Indeed, a rapid transfusing to the donor may precipitate cardiac failure, whereas a sudden withdrawal of blood from the recipient might, by reducing the blood volume, increase the dangers from the hyperviscosity of polycythaemia. Both infants may be in overt or incipient cardiac failure and this should be treated before transfusions are attempted.

To avoid a sudden change in blood volume, exchange transfusions are the best treatment for both babies. Theoretically, an intertwin transfusion should be the method of choice and this has been done successfully (Valaes and Doxiadis 1960). In practice, however, the difficulties of coping with two, often very sick, babies together, either of whom might suddenly need resuscitation, usually precludes this apparently logical practice.

Thus, the donor should be given a slow exchange transfusion with fresh partially packed blood. It is unnecessary and potentially dangerous fully to correct the anaemia immediately; one or more top-up transfusions can always be given later. His iron stores are likely to be severely depleted due to loss of fetal haemoglobin and iron supplements may be necessary for several months.

Blood viscosity rises rapidly when the haematocrit in venous blood reaches 70 per cent (or 75 per cent in capillary blood). An exchange plasma or albumin transfusion should be considered in all recipient twins with levels higher than this.

The donor twin should be treated as a light-for-dates baby and a careful watch kept for complications such as hypoglycaemia and hypothermia. As he often has a deficiency of the maternally derived immunoglobulin G (Bryan 1976; Bryan *et al.* 1976) the donor twin could be particularly vulnerable to infections. Although there have been several case reports of donor twins having severe infections in the first 6 months (Herlitz 1941; Perez and Gallo 1965; Abraham 1967; Bryan and Slavin 1974) no controlled study has been reported.

The recipient, although well-nourished, has no less hazardous a start in life. The consequences of untreated polycythaemia can be disastrous. Sludging of the blood may produce vascular thrombi that will, according to their sites, have serious effects, such as convulsions or neurological damage from cerebral vascular occlusions or renal failure due to renal vessel occlusion.

Hyperbilirubinaemia, often difficult to detect in a plethoric infant, can develop with alarming speed as the large load of haemoglobin is broken down. Frequent checks on serum bilirubin are mandatory.

The acute fetofetal transfusion syndrome (see p. 77)

An exsanguinated donor twin may be one of the most urgent emergencies encountered in the delivery room. In a shocked baby the significance of the pallor is easily missed but other resuscitative measures will be of no avail until the hypovolaemia, sometimes severe, is corrected with a transfusion of blood or other plasma expander. The recipient may need urgent reduction of his increased blood volume if cardiac failure is to be averted, by withdrawal of blood from the umbilical vein.

Cord haemoglobin levels are often misleading in the acute form of fetofetal transfusion syndrome; they may be normal with no intrapair discrepancy. Measurements taken 6–12 hours later, when the intravascular circulation has reached equilibrium with the other fluid compartments of the body, often show much greater intrapair discrepancies than the initial samples.

Distinction between the acute and chronic forms of fetofetal transfusion syndrome is rarely difficult (Klebe and Ingomar 1972; Tan *et al.* 1979; see Table 7.1). In the chronic form infants invariably have discrepancies in body weight, characteristic macroscopic and microscopic changes in the placenta (see p. 89) and an erythroblastotic blood film in the donor.

Disseminated intravascular coagulation

If one monochorionic twin dies *in utero*, thromboplastin may enter the circulation of the surviving fetus and cause disseminated intravascular coagulation, resulting in tissue necrosis and haemorrhage. Severe anaemia may develop in those that survive long enough (see p. 71). It is perhaps surprising that this disorder is not more common in single surviving twins.

Other neonatal problems

Respiratory distress syndrome

Respiratory distress due to hyaline membrane disease is common in twins due to their high incidence of prematurity. It is not surprising to find the disease more commonly occurring in MZ twins in view of their higher rate of prematurity (De La Torre Verduzco *et al.* 1976). Concordance appears to be higher in MZ than DZ twins and it has been suggested that there may be a genetic determinant to the disorder (Myrianthopoulos *et al.* 1971). However, if the babies are of shorter gestation it is not surprising that both are more commonly affected. When one twin alone is affected, it is almost always the second born. Likewise if both are affected the second is more severely so (Potter 1963). Butler and Alberman (1969) found that significantly more secondborn infants died from hyaline membrane disease and the risk was increased further in those with a birth interval of over 30 mins. Perinatal anoxia is almost certainly a contributory factor to the secondborn's increased susceptibility to respiratory distress syndrome.

On the other hand, other influences may give the leading twin a positive advantage. It is well-known that some stresses, such as prolonged rupture of the membranes reduce the risk of respiratory distress syndrome and two such cases have been reported in twins (Rajegowda *et al.* 1975). Chorioamnionitis, without rupture of membranes, is more common in the sac of the first twin (see p. 68). This may cause stress that would promote the production of phospholipids and thereby protect the infant from hyaline membrane disease.

The phospholipid profile of a fetus may determine the management of a preterm labour or the timing of an elective caesarean section. Yet there is still uncertainty as to whether levels differ between the first and second twin. Obladen and Gluck (1977) found that surfactant phospholipids were invariably lower in the affected twin and in the vaginally delivered twins this was always the secondborn. Likewise, Weller *et al.* (1976) found that the firstborn of two sets of triplets had much higher phospholipid levels than the succeeding babies. Jenkins and Baum (1981) in their study of lecithin:sphyngomyelin (L:S) ratios in pharyngeal aspirates, found no general trend to suggest that the lungs of the first twin were more mature than those of the secondborn. However, there was no case in which the first had an immature L:S ratio or developed hyaline membrane disease when the second was mature.

Several workers have found no intrapair differences in phospholipids in amniotic fluid taken before the onset of labour (Sims *et al.* 1976; Spellacy *et al.* 1977; Norman and Joubert 1982) whereas the leading twin had a significantly higher L:S ratio in cases of emergency caesarean section after a period of labour. These findings suggest that as long as the sample is taken before the onset of labour, amniotic fluid from one sac is sufficient to predict the lung maturity of both fetuses.

Necrotizing enterocolitis

Necrotizing enterocolitis (NEC) is a disease of unknown aetiology, but is known to be more common in sick and preterm infants and would therefore be expected to occur more often in twins and, when it did occur, it would be expected in the sicker of the two. Surprisingly, in their study of ten sets of twins with NEC, Samm *et al.* (1986) found that the firstborn was invariably affected and in three pairs both babies were affected. This was despite the secondborn infant being less well and suffering from more of the predisposing factors for NEC, such as birth asphyxia. The authors suggested that the firstborn, because he was healthier, might have received insults to the gut from early oral feeding and thus bacterial colonization, which would not have been inflicted on the twin.

Retinopathy of prematurity

In a report of the Cooperative Study of Retrolental Fibroplasia, Kinsey (1956) noted striking increases in the incidence of retinopathy of prematurity (ROP) in infants of multiple births when compared with singletons. The differences were seen even though the mean birth weight and gestational age were both higher in multiple births and the mean number of days in oxygen was lower than in singletons. Two studies of higher order birth infants have also shown a high incidence of ROP (see p. 204). Kinsey suggests, but without offering an explanation, that multiple birth children have a lower rate of spontaneous regression than singletons. However, a large recently published collaborative study from the US has not confirmed this increase in retinopathy amongst multiple birth children (Palmer *et al*. 1991).

Cost of neonatal care

Because of the difference in birth weight distribution a twin infant is much more likely to require neonatal intensive care than a singleton. Papiernik (1991) estimated that on average a twin infant required 11 times as many bed days in intensive care as a single baby with all the cost to the health service that this entails.

Many multiple birth infants will have to be transferred to another hospital for intensive care and it is recognized that these infants have a less good prognosis than those who are born and remain in the same tertiary care unit (Bowman *et al*. 1988). An increasing problem in the UK is the difficulty in finding tertiary care neonatal units prepared to accept all the children from a multiple birth set. Even those who are actually born in tertiary care units may have to be transferred if the unit cannot take all the babies. There have been instances of triplets where each infant has been sent to a different hospital (each many miles from either of the others) with the mother remaining at the hosptial where she delivered. The emotional strain for both parents of this separation from their critically ill infants is intense. Inevitably there will be times when the babies die without the mother ever seeing them.

Perinatal mortality

Despite improvements in both obstetric and neonatal care the risks to the twin fetus and newborn remain at least three times those of a singleton. In the UK, twins account for about 2 per cent of births but 9 per cent of perinatal deaths (Botting *et al*. 1987). Although there has been a steady fall in their perinatal mortality the difference between multiple births and singletons still remains (Fig. 7.3). Similar differences are found in other parts of the world. In a multiple hospital study in the US the perinatal mortality rate of twins was three times greater than that of singletons (Ellis *et al*. 1979). In Nigeria it was four times greater (Nylander 1979) and in Scotland it was nearly six times greater (Registrar General for Scotland 1983). The main contributor to the high death toll in twins is prematurity and its complications. It is therefore not surprising to find that the neonatal death rate is disproportionately greater than the fetal death rates.

Potter (1963) found that intrauterine death was twice as common in twins as in singletons, whereas deaths in the neonatal period were increased five-fold. Other problems specific to a multiple pregnancy increase the perinatal mortality rate further. These other factors include fetal malpresentation and dystocia, the complications of a shared fetal circulation in monochorionic twins, cord complications in monoamniotic twins and the higher incidence of lethal malformations.

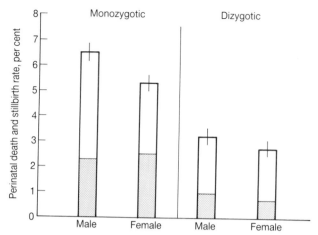

Fig. 7.3   Estimated perinatal mortality (crude figures) for MZ and DZ gestations. Hatched area indicates still births. From Rydhstrom (1990a) with permission of the author and editors of *Acta Geneticae Medicae et Gemellologia*.

Many studies have shown a higher perinatal mortality rate amongst MZ than DZ twins (Potter 1963; Ferguson 1964; Behrman 1965; Benirschke and Driscoll 1967; Myrianthopoulos 1970; Thompson *et al.* 1983; Rydhstrom 1990a) and amongst like-sexed than unlike-sexed twins (Campbell and MacGillivray 1988; Rydhstrom 1990a).

Benirschke and Kim (1973) found a 26 per cent mortality rate in mono-chorionic twins compared with a rate of 9 per cent in dichorionic twins. The higher rate amongst this group of MZ twins is not surprising and the dangers of the 'third circulation' have already been discussed. It might be expected that MZ twins with dichorionic placentation would have the same mortality rate as DZ twins because they are subject to the same environmental influences. However, Corney *et al.* (1972) have shown that MZ dichorionic twins grow less well than their DZ counterparts, so it may well be that all MZ twins are at a disadvantage compared with DZ.

Within each 500 g grouping under 2500 g, multiple births have a significantly lower perinatal mortality, presumably because they tend to be more mature for their birthweight (Patel *et al.* 1984). However, this does not appear to be the case with extremely low birth weight infants, where there will be less difference in weight between twins and singletons at the same gestational age (see p. 47). In a group of infants weighing less than 800 g, twins did less well, with a survival rate of 21 per cent compared with 41 per cent in singletons and a major central nervous handicap rate in survivors of 67 per cent compared with 13 per cent for singletons (Hoffman and Forrest 1990). The combination of high mortality and major handicaps in survivors meant that only 10 per cent of twin infants had a good outcome. Yu *et al.* (1986) had also found a poorer prognosis in twins than singletons who were born between 23 and 28 weeks gestation.

Boys fare worse than girls regardless of zygosity. The highest perinatal mortality rate is amongst male–male pairs (Butler and Alberman 1969;

Fujikura and Froelich 1971; Rydhstrom 1990a). In unlike-sexed pairs Butler and Alberman (1969) found that if the male was firstborn in a pair of unlike-sex than his risk of death was similar to that of his secondborn sister, whereas if the infants were born in the reverse order the boy had twice the mortality rate of the girl. A study of twins in north-east Scotland showed the perinatal mortality rate in boy twins was 61.6 per 1000 compared to 48.8 per 1000 in females (Thompson *et al.* 1983). A later study (Campbell and MacGillivray 1988) found no statistical difference in the perinatal mortality rates for boy and girl twins and it was suggested that this was due to improved standards of care at delivery and in the neonatal period. However, the quality of survival is uncertain and longer-term follow-up studies will be needed to determine the long-term morbidity.

Mother-infant twin relationship

Even if both twins are well and able to be with their mother from the start, their mother will need particular support and understanding. This need will be even greater if one or both babies are ill and separated from her. For most mothers, relating to one baby is a full-time preoccupation both emotionally and physically; relating to two at the same time can be an enormous strain.

It is recognized that mothers find it more difficult to relate to babies from whom they have been separated during the first days following delivery than to babies who have been with them from the start. Klaus and Kennell (1970) have shown the importance of early physical contact between a mother and her baby. With twins the firstborn baby, usually stronger, is often handed straight to the mother. She may, however, get only a glimpse of the second baby before it is whisked away to an incubator. If this happens it is easy for the mother to 'forget' that she has another baby. She should therefore be encouraged to handle the other baby and see as much of him as his condition can possibly allow. If necessary, arrangements should be made for the mother to visit this baby in the special care baby unit as soon as she is ready to leave the delivery room. In many cases it may be wise to send both babies to the unit together (preferably with the mother as well) to reduce the problems of separation.

Mothers of twins will often notice marked differences in the personalities of their babies within a few days of birth and it has been observed that within 3 weeks most mothers talk and behave differently to each infant (Minde *et al.* 1982, 1984). These differences are often shown first in differing feeding patterns. One baby may attack the teat or nipple with gusto and gulp the whole feed down in a few minutes whereas the other may choose to take it slowly over half an hour, with breaks to rest and look around. One may demand frequent small feeds; the other may remain content for many hours.

All mothers aim to give their babies equal attention and to love them equally. They often feel guilty when this does not work out. Particularly in the early weeks, one baby may be more attractive, more responsive and more loveable, than the other. Sometimes the mother is influenced initially by superficial appearances. A mother may have a definite dislike of red-heads and therefore more attached to the one with black hair.

For others the relative sizes of the babies may affect their feelings. Spillman (1984) found that mothers were much more likely to have a preference for one of their babies when there was a weight discrepancy, and that when this occurred it tended to be the larger baby that was favoured.

Different temperaments may make equal love even more difficult. If one baby is an easy feeder and contented and the other is an unhappy crying baby who is difficult to feed, the mother may resent the extra time she has to spend on the unrewarding baby at the expense of the one whom she enjoys much more.

If one baby is much more demanding, his mother may feel guilty about being unable to give the other baby as much attention. She should be reassured that sometimes one baby may *need* more attention and that difficulties of this kind are not uncommon.

Eye-to-eye contact is also vital to the relationship between a mother and her infant. Robson and Moss (1970) have demonstrated how the baby initiates or releases care-taking responses in the mother. If one twin is visually more responsive than the other he may, without the mother realizing, receive more of her attention. Even if she responds to both twins equally she is bound to find it harder to give her concentration to each when there will often be simultaneous demands for her attention. The possible longer-term significance of these early preferences will be discussed later (p. 129).

Many more mothers of twins than of singletons have to cope with the acute emotional crisis caused by the birth of a premature baby. This seems to be unavoidable, even when every effort is made to reduce the separation of the baby from the mother (Blake *et al.* 1975). The very fact of producing a premature baby, even a healthy one, is for most mothers an extremely distressing experience and Minde and his colleagues (1982) found that if one of the babies was notably more ill than the other mothers were much more likely to relate to the healthier infant. A mother of twins is likely to find it particularly difficult to handle her (mixed) feelings if one baby is thriving and the other is critically ill. She may be torn between celebration of the one and anxiety for the other. Once again she and her partner should be reassured that some emotional ambivalence is almost inevitable in these circumstances.

Many mothers easily tell their twins apart; others find it much more difficult. Some may be distressed by the confusion and this must impede their ability to relate to each individual baby.

The parents (and the nursing staff) should therefore be encouraged to identify the babies at all times and to call them by their names. Each cot should be easily recognizable at a distance either from the different covers or by a conspicuous toy—a teddy bear for one and a rabbit for the other. The babies themselves should also be easily distinguishable by, for instance, different coloured clothes.

It is essential that all staff realize that a major problem in raising twins is developing their individuality. This is especially true of MZ twins but also applies to DZ. For this reason parents and friends should not be inadvertently encouraged to emphasize the twinship and where possible the babies' names should be used rather than expressions like 'the twins'. Obviously, staff have no right to interfere with parents who, for example, ask for identical clothes. However, they can at least avoid encouraging the natural but unfortunate tendency to emphasize the twinship rather than the arrival of two babies who will become distinct, even if very similar, persons.

Naming twins

The choosing of names for a baby is clearly a deeply personal matter for the parents. Approval or otherwise is not the responsibility of the medical or nursing staff. Nevertheless, the implications for a child or adult of being landed with a 'twin' name can be tactfully pointed out. Even today, when most parents are aware of the importance of encouraging twins to develop as individuals, the temptation to give rhyming names, such as Sita and Gita, or like-sounding names such as Jean and Jane, Dean and Darren or Kristy and Kirsty seems hard to resist. Similar names for opposite sexes, such as Robert and Roberta, or Dellis and Dennis, even Max(im) and Max(ine), cause added confusion. Even the same initial can cause confusion and embarrassment to teenagers, not least with personal correspondence. However, names of different length can also be a problem. A five-year-old called Christopher may resent the ease with which his brother Sam learns to write his name!

Going home

In hospital the mother of twins is the centre of attention and tends to be the successful applicant for any extra help and support that becomes available. She is often told how lucky she is to have two babies and usually feels this to be true. Rarely is she given any cautions about the physical, emotional and financial problems nor constructive preparation for the tasks that lie ahead.

In the UK, unlike many European countries, a family with twins does not automatically qualify for extra practical assistance, for example, a home help. Thus, everything possible should be done to help the family prepare realistically for the months to come; to organize in advance the help that is available; to invest from the start in any time-saving devices that can be afforded and to ensure that the family doctor and health visitor are alerted to the family's need for support (Linney 1983).

Many mothers are ill-advised on equipment for twins and have no ready access to sources of secondhand articles. Many waste money by automatically buying everything in duplicate. Maternity units should keep close contact with some families with twins in the area, usually through the local Twins Club. Should the new mother wish it, a member is always happy to visit and advise on types and sources of equipment. The mother of undiagnosed twins particularly benefits from this service.

Some Twins Clubs actually store their equipment and first-size clothes at the hospital. Parents then have a wide range readily available. Mothers expecting twins are best encouraged to book, rather than buy, the pram. Selling a twin pram, if one baby dies, can be highly distressing.

As the father has, of necessity, a more important role to play in the care of twins, the earlier he can be encouraged to help the better (see p. 127). Even the most supportive father may be apprehensive about handling a very small baby. His confidence will be greatly increased with practice under supervision in the hospital. Moreover he, like the mother, will find his emotional attachment to the babies will be much enhanced by early physical contact.

Often one baby is ready to go home before the other. If the discharge of the second baby has to be delayed for several weeks its separation from both mother and the other baby will be hard to avoid. Where at all possible, however, it is best for both to be kept together. The notion that it is easier to start with one baby alone seems to be ill-founded; it is harder to adapt to two babies if a routine with one has already been established. Furthermore if the mother is busy at home with one baby she will find it difficult to visit the other. She becomes increasingly attached to the baby that is with her and finds it hard to accept the second baby. The baby who is left in hospital may suffer in his relationship with his mother and in the development of his self-esteem (p. 134; Hay and O'Brien 1987).

One single mother of a 3 kg girl and a 1.5 kg boy went home after 10 days with her daughter. She rarely visited the little boy, who had many neonatal problems. When he finally went home after 2 months she admitted to great difficulty in feeling any affection for him. It was over a year before she even began to accept him as she did her daughter.

Another baby whose discharge had been delayed much longer than her twin brother's was admitted later suffering from non-accidental injury. Such rejection of one baby by the mother may raise the difficult question as to whether one child alone should be placed for adoption (see below).

When temporary separation of the babies is unavoidable, the mother should be strongly encouraged to visit the one remaining in hospital. Transport may be needed and a nursery and feeds for the twin must be available so that he can always be brought too. This allows the mother to spend long periods in the hospital without worrying about the other baby.

Older siblings will also need special consideration. They may well have been separated from their mother for several weeks if she was in hospital before delivering the twins. After the birth the twins are often the over-whelming focus of attention. The sibling will therefore feel all the more rejected and insecure. These children should be with their mothers and the babies and given the opportunity to play an active part in their care whenever they want to.

Adoption

In the past twins who were being adopted were often separated in the process. Fortunately most, if not all, adoption agencies now place twins together. This is at least the practice with healthy twins and few would dispute that this is a right and necessary policy.

Despite the difficulties of mothering twins and the disadvantages associ-ated with twinship itself, it seems wrong to separate children who have developed so closely before birth. A single surviving twin often appears to miss his partner, even if that baby dies at birth. Furthermore, a sadness for many adopted children is that of having no true (blood) relations. A twin or other sibling can greatly enhance their sense of security.

There is more disagreement about what should be done if one baby is ill or handicapped. A number of questions are bound to arise. Should the chances of a successful placement for the healthy baby be jeopardized or delayed? Should a child be burdened with a handicapped sibling when this can be avoided? Although there is no shortage of adoptive parents for a single baby, or even for a healthy pair of twins, handicapped babies are much harder to place. Despite these obvious problems, however, many people— particularly parents of twins—feel that the babies should remain together. Apart from other considerations the healthy twin may sooner or later feel a heavy guilt for having 'deserted' his needy sibling. Nor need there be any delay in placing the normal baby with the intended adopting parents, as the other twin can follow as soon as he is fit enough.

A dilemma arises if the parents of the twins wish to have only one child. Should they be allowed to place one for adoption or should they have to choose between keeping both or giving both away? If only one child is placed for adoption that child will not only feel that he has been rejected by his parents but that his twin was chosen in preference to him. Moreover, the twin who stays with the parents may respond with anger because he may feel it was sheer chance that he was kept and not rejected. The favoured twin may also, of course, feel intense guilt towards his lost twin.

In other circumstances the Social Services department may suggest separating the twins. If the mother is clearly not relating to, or is even abusing, one child it may indeed be necessary to take that child into care. If, despite support and help with rehabilitation, the mother remains unable to accept the child, adoption may be the only long-term option. In these circumstances it is unlikely that it would be right for the other twin to be taken from his home so that the twins could be placed together. Separation may therefore become inevitable. If this occurs, it is essential that the twins should be allowed regular contact with each other. The profound loss experienced by twins who have lost their twin and the lengths to which they will go to trace them has been seen repeatedly by Professor Tom Bouchard from the Minnesota Center for Twin and Adoption Research and in the UK by the late John Stroud, who did so much to enable them to be reunited in later life.

Parents who are considering adopting twins need special counselling. They must have realistic guidance as to the emotional and physical demands of two babies. In addition it is obviously important that they clarify their own motives for adopting two babies and make sure that the attractiveness of twins as such is not a significant consideration.

Adoption agencies provide information and many arrange group meetings for prospective parents. The Twins and Multiple Births Association (Appendix 2) has a register of families with adopted twins and many of the parents are happy to talk to prospective parents, as well as to social workers and other professionals involved with the adoption.

8

Feeding twins

For many mothers of older twins the blurred memory of the first 6 months of the babies' lives is one of an endless round of feeding. Establishing the easiest and most satisfactory feeding routine for both the mother and her twins is of enormous importance, so this whole chapter is devoted to it.

Breast-feeding

Many pairs of twins have been fully breast-fed and have thrived. Some have known no milk other than their mother's until after their first birthday (Addy 1975; Brewster 1979; Linney 1980; Stables 1980; Noble 1990). It is well known that supply rises to equal demand and a healthy mother has a remarkable capacity to produce the required volume of milk. It has been shown that milk production in mothers of twins is approximately double that of mothers who are breastfeeding singletons (Saint et al. 1986). Saint et al. (1986) found that the milk yield of three mothers who were fully breast-feeding their twins at 6 months ranged from 0.84 to 2.16 kg per 24 hours, and similar yields were reported by Deem (1931). These figures should reassure professionals that there is no reason whatever to discourage expectant mothers of twins from breast-feeding on the grounds that they may have difficulty in producing enough milk.

Despite this, many mothers of twins are still discouraged, even dissuaded, from breast-feeding on the mistaken assumption that they will be unlikely to have enough milk or that they will find the breast-feeding too tiring (Leonard 1982). In Addy's study of 173 mothers of twins, 12 were positively advised against breast-feeding and a further 15 assumed that it was not possible and were not enlightened until it was too late (Addy 1975).

A few mothers have produced enough milk to satisfy three babies (Saint et al. 1986; Noble 1990 and two personal reports). A mother of triplets produced 3.08 kg of milk per 24 hours at 2½ months. She fed each baby nine times per day, eighteen sessions in total as she fed two together and then one on their own (Saint et al. 1986).

There have, unfortunately, been few studies on feeding patterns in twins. In particular, none have monitored the growth of those who were fed with breast milk. It is of practical importance to know how their growth compares with that of bottle-fed twins and with both breast- and bottle-fed singletons. The largest study is that of Addy (1975), in which 173 Californian mothers replied to written questionnaires. Forty-one of these mothers breast-fed their twins for varying lengths of time up to 10 months. The growth of these babies was said to be satisfactory but no measurements were taken.

Measurements of lactose, protein and mixed fat in the milk of mothers fully breast-feeding at 6 months were studied by Saint and colleagues (1986). They found that the concentration of lactose was rather higher than normal but that the total energy intake was similar to that of singletons.

Advantages

The advantages of breast-feeding are well documented (Gunther 1973; Jelliffe and Jelliffe 1978). They include nutritional, immunological, psychological, practical and economic advantages; for twin babies the benefits are even greater.

As many twins are born prematurely they are likely to be particularly vulnerable to infections. The immunological properties of breast milk give some protection against both bacterial and viral invasion (Howie *et al*. 1990). Furthermore, mothers have more difficulty in relating to premature infants, partly because of the inevitable separation if the baby has to be nursed on the special care baby unit. Studies have shown that mothers have fewer problems in relating to their infants if they breast-feed them. This may go some way to compensate for the separation.

Breast-feeding is also the only way a mother can feed and nurse both

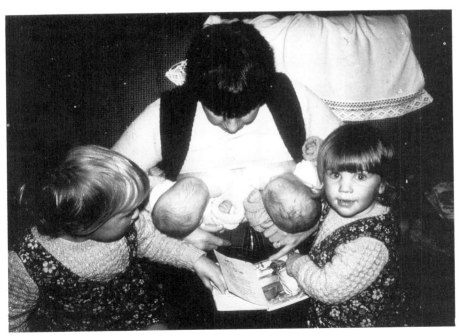

Fig. 8.1   Mother breastfeeding 6-month-old twin girls and entertaining the 2- and 3-year-old sisters at the same time.

babies at the same time. As time is at a premium for her, and opportunities for cuddling much reduced, any means of providing the mother of twins with more nursing time should be welcomed (Fig. 8.1).

Finally the cost of powdered milks for two babies is considerable, particularly to a family budget that is already likely to be under strain. The estimated daily food supplementation to the lactating mother's diet for each baby is 450–600 kcal (Department of Health 1991) (in practice many mothers require less than this). This extra nutrition needed for breast-feeding can be provided by relatively cheap foods. It has been calculated that the cost of supplementary foods need be no more than one-third of that of powdered milk (Jelliffe and Jelliffe 1975). In developing countries the additional hazards of overdilution and bacterial contamination of bottle feeds have been well documented (Muller 1976).

Disadvantages

The most obvious disadvantage of breast-feeding to the mother is that she can have no respite during the early months, when she will often be very tired. However, a mother can sometimes get a full night's sleep or an outing during the day without resorting to a feed of formula milk. If she expresses her milk between feeds a bottle can be stored in the fridge or freezer, to be given later by another helper. Breast-feeding two babies is also much more difficult to do discretely in public. Some mothers find this a further major curtailment to a social life that is already much reduced. This particular disadvantage will be removed if social acceptance of breast-feeding in public spreads.

Preparation

The question of feeding should be discussed with the couple as soon as a multiple pregnancy is diagnosed and the advantages of breast-feeding pointed out. Although a mother may have seen singletons being breast-fed, it is most unusual for her to have seen breast-feeding of twins. Indeed, some assume it is not possible and do not even consider the idea. Arrangements should therefore be made for the mother to visit another mother of twins at feed time (Fig. 8.2). Such a visit will always result in many queries being answered that might never even have been voiced in the antenatal clinic. Sometimes a lasting and supportive friendship will develop between the two mothers.

If the mother has already been admitted to hospital when the twins are diagnosed a visit to a mother feeding twins in the postnatal ward will be much better than nothing. It will at least demonstrate the technique. However, the memory of someone still feeding when the twins are several months old is much more likely to give effective encouragement during the first, often difficult, weeks. Even a videotape, film (or at least photographs) of a mother breast-feeding twins can be both instructive and encouraging to an expectant mother if for some reason a personal visit is not possible.

The rate of successful breast-feeding of twins can be substantially eased with such antenatal education followed by support and encouragement

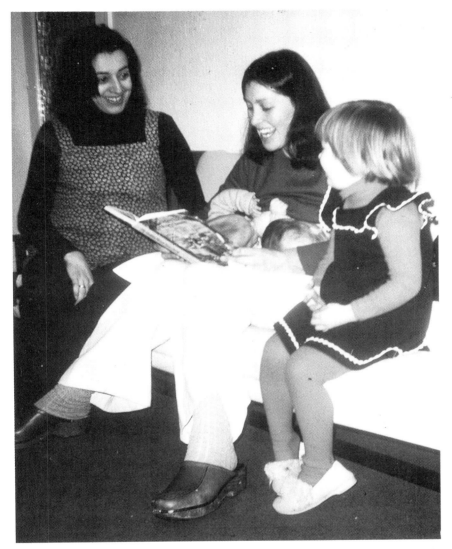

Fig. 8.2 Expectant mother of twins receiving advice on breast-feeding from mother of 5-month-old boys.

when the babies arrive. In one maternity unit it was found that of 12 mothers who had planned to breast-feed their twins only one was successfully doing so after 6 weeks. Following the introduction of these more positive and supportive measures the number of mothers continuing to breast-feed after 6 weeks rose the following year to 11 out of 12 (Bryan 1977a).

Several studies have shown the importance in singletons of early suckling both for the establishment and for the continuation of breast-feeding (Kennell *et al.* 1976; Salariya *et al.* 1978). Although this is just as important, if not more so, in twins it is rare for both babies, or even one, to be put to the breast in the delivery room. The mother is more likely to have had a tiring and difficult delivery or the babies may be premature or suffer from birth asphyxia. All these factors make it more difficult to arrange for the twin infant to suckle early. Nevertheless, far more twins could be safely put to the breast in the delivery room than is now the practice.

Techniques

The mother's first decision is whether to feed the babies together or separately. There are advantages to both and a mother soon discovers which suits her best.

There appears to have been little work on the relative physiological advantages of the two methods. Tyson (1976) reports a higher prolactin response in mothers who suckle their twins simultaneously. It appears that the amount of prolactin released is a function both of the intensity of sucking and of the number of breasts stimulated. This suggests that (at least in the early days, when a full milk supply is still to be achieved) there are advantages in feeding both babies together if the mother is concerned about her milk supply.

If the babies are fed separately the mother can give her full concentration to each and she may find she is generally more comfortable. However, feeding times will then take up a large portion of the day and she may also be distressed by the cries of the second hungry baby. Theoretically it is better to alternate the order of feeds. In practice the same baby often demands the food first. Either way a baby should be offered one breast only at a feed. Otherwise the first baby, by taking the fore-milk from both breasts, will receive milk with a much lower fat content than his twin.

The main advantage of feeding the babies together is the time saved, and time is a precious commodity. Some mothers find that it is actually more comfortable if both their breasts are emptying at the same time rather than having the feeling of tension in the overflowing unsucked breast.

The positioning of the babies during a feed is obviously a matter of personal preference. An astonishing number of different positions have been devised and some of these are illustrated here (Fig. 8.3). Most mothers tend to stick to one position but some alternate.

The place preferred for feeding is equally variable. Some mothers like to feed from their bed whenever feasible. The sofa with supportive cushions for the mother's back and pillows for the babies is popular, so is a large armchair. A triangular cushion, originally designed for patients sitting in bed, is an excellent support when reversed (i.e. in front of the mother), for both babies (Fig. 8.4).

Most mothers prefer to change the babies' sides at each feed and have various ingenious methods of remembering who's due for which breast. A safety pin attached to a bra strap is a particular favourite, others keep daily charts and others trust to intuition and don't worry too much.

Some mothers find that the babies are happier on the same side each time and it has been claimed that the babies then regulate their own milk supply.

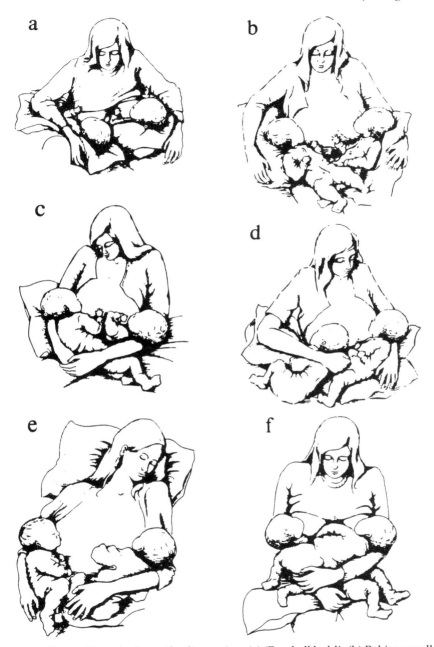

Fig. 8.3 Six positions for breastfeeding twins. (a) 'Football hold'. (b) Babies parallel to mother's body. (c) Babies criss-crossed and supported by pillows and mother's arms. (d) Babies facing same direction. (e) Mother in almost lying position and babies parallel to her body. (f) Babies are criss-crossed but supported only by mother's arms—suitable for 'emergency' feeds only. Drawn by Joan Moore.

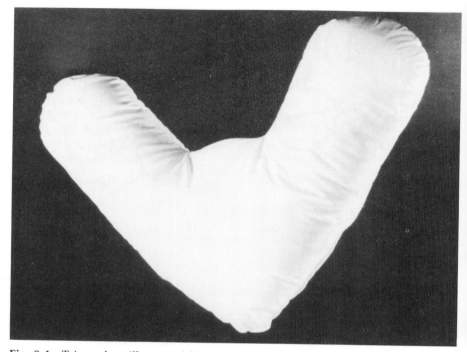

Fig. 8.4 Triangular pillow used for supporting twin babies during breast-feeding. By permission of J.D. Williams and Co. Ltd., The Dale St Warehouses, Manchester.

Lopsidideness of the breasts is said to be a disadvantage of this method but I have yet to hear of this actually happening. In theory, one-sided visual stimulation for such a large portion of a baby's waking hours could be detrimental to his development but as yet there is nothing to substantiate this idea.

An increasing number of mothers of twins are choosing to feed their babies on demand as the advantages of this, rather than scheduled feeding to the clock, become more appreciated. In Addy's (1975) study 78 per cent of the babies were so fed. Any disturbance to the mother's routine seems to be offset by the advantages of having more contented babies.

A number of mothers find the most practical method is to feed both babies when one has indicated that he is hungry. This is particularly important at night, so that the mother can avoid being woken again shortly after feeding one baby, by the other.

Establishing breast-feeding

Many mothers with just one baby have some difficulties with breast-feeding during the first few days. For mothers of twins the problems are proportionately greater and many find the first week a frustrating struggle.

The mother can be helped in many ways. In particular she should have the opportunity to suckle the babies in the delivery room and as often as she wishes to thereafter. Rest and minimum tension are essential. Both are difficult to provide for a mother with two babies to care for. The more help she can have with looking after the babies, the better. The father should be made aware of the problems and encouraged to help from the start and other friends and relatives should be enlisted whenever possible to help with the household tasks.

Many mothers become frustrated and tearful if left to feed the two babies simultaneously on their own. In the early days it is often difficult to keep both babies attached to the breast. If one falls off the second may also be lost as the mother struggles to retrieve the first. If she resorts to feeding them separately her milk supply may be reduced. She may then become frustrated because the feeding round seems endless and a lactation crisis can set in (Fig. 8.5).

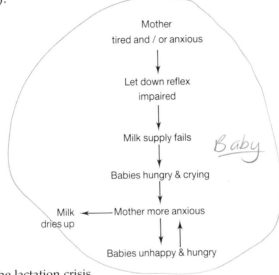

Fig. 8.5   The lactation crisis.

It is most important that all mothers with twins should have someone by their side throughout the feed until they are entirely confident and choose to be left on their own. This need not be a highly qualified midwife. The father or an understanding friend can perform the task perfectly well.

In some pairs of twins, particularly if there are large differences in weight between the two babies, one twin has a much stronger suck than the other. This can be a positive advantage to the weaker baby as his twin's stronger suck will invoke a let-down reflex in both breasts, thereby supplying extra milk for both. Alternating breasts at each feed allows the smaller baby to have the benefits of the larger milk supply that the larger twin has stimulated.

Breast-feeding counsellors, some of whom have particular expertise in advising mothers of twins, can give invaluable emotional support as well as practical suggestions.

For a mother to maintain her milk supply it is essential that she has a good, well-balanced diet as well as adequate rest (Leonard 1982). Too often she cannot find time to take proper meals in an unrushed way.

Problems

Lack of encouragement

Many mothers complain not only of lack of information about breast-feeding twins but also of the negative approach of doctors, midwives and health visitors. In many centres this attitude is changing but there is still need for more teaching about the breast-feeding of twins so that midwives can give more informed advice.

Many mothers find the postnatal ward, with its inflexible timetable, a harassing environment and because breast-feeding takes longer initially, as the babies may take time to get positioned, they may resort to bottle-feeding to conform more easily to the rules of the ward. This is a most unfortunate outcome and should not be allowed to happen.

Lack of milk

Although supply should normally rise to meet demand the equilibrium is only too often disturbed by the extraneous factors already mentioned. The babies may be premature and have an inadequate suck, the mother's anxiety may have reduced her let-down response and the lactation crisis may intervene (see Fig. 8.5).

It is often difficult to decide if and when to give complementary feeds with cow's milk. As many twins are small-for-dates, and therefore at risk of hypoglycaemia, these may be necessary sooner than would otherwise have been wished. Some mothers continue to give combined breast- and bottle-feeds for many months. Others alternate each feed, offering one baby the breast and the other the bottle. Full breast-feeding can usually be achieved by giving the babies increasing feeding time at the breast.

Occasionally, a mother chooses to breast-feed one baby entirely, usually the frailer, and bottle-feed the other. No doubt it is better to breast-feed one baby than neither but the mother will inevitably develop a much closer relationship with that baby and may need to compensate with special attention to the other one. Sometimes the decision will be made by the babies themselves. One may reject the breast, and feed well from the bottle, whereas the other may clearly enjoy the breast-feed. Although emotionally and practically awkward it would seem a pity to deprive the breast-fed baby of a nutritionally and emotionally good experience, if at all possible.

An innovation that may prove a great help to some mothers of twins is the Lact-Aid Nursing Supplementer (Avery 1972). This provides additional milk to the baby without interfering with sucking. The milk is supplied through a narrow tube leading from a plastic bag of milk that hangs round the mother's neck. The tube is strapped to the breast and the baby sucks the nipple and tube together. Using this method adoptive parents have managed to estab-lish full breast-feeding of their single babies. Although no case has yet been reported, there is no reason why adopted twins should not be breast-fed in this way, especially if started early.

There have been occasional reports of a mother who has given one of her twins to another lactating mother to feed (Mead 1957).

Bottle-feeding

The obvious advantage of bottle-feeding twins is that the task can be shared. In particular, the father is able to play a larger role in the care of his babies. The disadvantages include the increased cost, the greater amount of work in sterilizing bottles, making up feeds, etc. and, most important, the inability to nurse and feed both babies simultaneously. It is possible to nurse one baby by propping the other in a cushion but many mothers resort to propping both. This means that the babies have no direct contact with the mother. A few ingenious mothers devise ways of nursing one baby in their crossed legs and the other in their arms.

Many mothers are tempted to leave one or both babies feeding unattended (for example with the bottle supported by a cushion). The consequent dangers of choking should be obvious but may not always appear so to a harassed mother.

Preparation of the feeds

Any safe short-cuts to this time-consuming chore should be welcomed. One of these is, of course, to make up the whole 24 h milk supply at the same time. A large plastic bucket or small dustbin will allow all bottles, jugs and teats to be sterilized together. The milk can be made up in large jugs but it should be transferred at once to the bottles and immediately refrigerated. If left in jugs and not thoroughly stirred at each serving the first feeds will be too dilute and the later ones dangerously concentrated.

Weaning

If mother and babies are content there is no hurry for the babies to be weaned from the breast. Extended breast-feeding is particularly valuable for twins as it ensures a continuing physical closeness with the mother. Ideally, the twins should wean in their own time. One may well choose to do so several weeks before the other.

Solid foods

Introducing solids to twin babies is an added chore for the already busy mother. It is therefore wise to postpone this as long as possible. There is rarely a need to consider solids before 4 months of age and many babies, especially the breast-fed, will not want solids until 6 months. Even then one baby may well be ready to start before the other. In the same way the children will have different tastes and appetites and these should be respected. Because one child asks for a drink or a snack it should not automatically be assumed that the other wants or needs the same.

Many mothers start with the firm intention of having a separate spoon and dish for each baby; few keep it. When feeding them together it is much easier to use the same spoon and dish. Dishes, divided into two by a partition, are useful for gauging the approximate quantity eaten by each child.

Many twins are slow in learning to feed themselves as they lack opportunity. Mothers fear the mess and find it quicker to feed the children themselves. In extreme cases healthy twins may approach their second birthday with little idea of how to use a spoon (personal observation). This practice should be strongly discouraged. Exploration with food and the process of feeding is an important part of a child's development and should not be suppressed. Two high chairs, two large plastic bibs and an extremely large plastic mat are essential equipment and the children should then be given the freedom to experiment.

9

The first year

To be the mother of twins is the dream of many pregnant women. And for those 'doubly blessed' the happy expectations are reinforced by the general public view, which tends to see only the positive aspects of having twins. Social pressures allow few mothers to think of the possible difficulties (Leonard 1982)—the difficulties of looking after two babies, each of whom is likely to be more frail, more difficult to feed and more vulnerable to infection than the average single baby. And then there are the difficulties of responding emotionally to two babies at once and, perhaps hardest of all, of developing a distinct relationship with both at the same time. Few mothers are prepared for these problems. Many therefore suffer a painful shattering of happy expectations (Bryan 1977a).

Inevitably, a mother of twins spends less time with each baby than she would if she only had one. This was clearly shown in Goshen-Gottstein's (1980) study from Israel of mothers of young twins. She found that these spent 35–37 per cent of their time on activities related to the care of the twins, whereas the average mother of a singleton spent as much as 22–29 per cent of her time on that one baby.

Nearly all mothers regret the lack of time for simply enjoying their babies. Costello (1978) found that mothers of 6-month-old singletons spent on average over twice as much time playing with one child as mothers of twins did with both.

Many mothers find that their reserves of both physical and emotional energy are expended before the end of each day, let alone the end of the first year. Many feel guilty that their previous domestic standards cannot be upheld and that they can give so little attention to their husband. Marriages are often put under great strain during this time. Mothers deeply regret that they have so little time just to nurse and enjoy each baby (Bryan 1977a).

This frustration over the need to identify with one baby is particularly keenly felt by mothers whose twins are their firstborn. This is partly because the normal caretaking activities are bound to take longer in inexperienced hands, but also because the mother feels cheated of a unique relationship. The main reason many mothers of twins want a third, single child is to have the experience of which they have been deprived—that of giving their undivided attention and love to one baby (Leonard 1982).

Over the last few years there has been increasing concern about the prevalence of depression amongst mothers of young children. Incidences as high as 40 per cent have been reported amongst working-class mothers at home with young children (Wolkind 1981) and it is now recognized that maternal depression constitutes a psychological risk factor for the children (Rutter *et al.* 1990). The most important precipitation factors for depression in the early months are stress and social isolation. Mothers of twins are thus especially vulnerable.

Recent studies have confirmed an increase in both depression and anxiety in mothers of twins (Powell 1981, Haigh and Wilkinson 1989, Hay *et al.* 1990, Thorpe *et al.* 1991). In a study from Australia, Hay and his colleagues (1990) found that depression was five times and anxiety three times as common amongst mothers of twins than in mothers of singletons. Taylor and Emery (1988) did not find a higher incidence of depression in general in mothers of twins during the first 6 months but they did note a small but significant group with very high anxiety scores, which did not occur amongst the control groups.

But many of the symptoms of depression are also those associated with fatigue; most mothers of young twins become extremely tired. In the Australian study, 76.2 per cent of mothers of twins reported being constantly exhausted during the first year compared with 7.9 per cent of mothers with single babies (Hay *et al.* 1990). Taylor and Emery (1988) found that 50 per cent of mothers of twins had less than 6 hours rest at 3 weeks and that throughout the first year they had less sleep than mothers with single children. Mothers of twins tend to perceive their children as more difficult than singletons (Groothius *et al.* 1982; Taylor and Emery 1988; Hay *et al.* 1990). However, this so-called difficult behaviour may sometimes be less to do with the children than with their mother's depression and their consequent reaction to their children's behaviour.

A worrying finding is that depression may well continue long after the time of acute fatigue. Thorpe *et al.* (1991) found that mothers of 5-year-old twins had a higher malaise score, indicating depression, than mothers of singletons, even when the singleton mothers had two closely spaced children.

Management

Any saving of energy by reducing the physical burden of twins makes a mother better able to face the inevitable emotional strain. Too many mothers could have saved many exhausting hours had they been given more advice on the practical care of two babies and perhaps if they had been more ready to accept outside help (Bryan 1977a). Divorce amongst parents of twins was found to be more common in those who had had poor support during the first year (Hay *et al.* 1990). Too many mothers learn by trial and error when parents from the local twins club, for example, could have given useful guidance. Many mothers are too proud to accept help with domestic chores and continue doing these whilst allowing friends to feed and play with the babies. It needs to be emphasized that offers of help should usually be diverted to other tasks, so that the mother can spend more time with the babies.

There will, of course, be times when the mother welcomes a break from her babies. Indeed, her mothering may be enhanced by the feeling that she can escape from that role occasionally and give opportunity and space to her own needs, and of course to those of her partner.

Practical aspects of feeding have been discussed in Chapter 8. Washing (and drying) is also time-consuming and fuss-free clothes are invaluable. Those needing ironing should be avoided. A tumble-dryer is money well spent, for those who can afford one. Most families now choose to use disposable nappies. Mothers often struggle to bath their babies daily, believing this vital to health. There is plainly no need for this and most cannot easily bath two babies without a second pair of hands. It may well be advisable to limit bathing to times when father's help is available, or to bath each child separately on alternate days.

Many mothers complain of the isolation they feel during the first year. Often family and friends rally round for the first 2 or 3 months. Help may then suddenly dwindle, leaving the mothers alone during a period of great stress and fatigue.

One of the most common complaints of mothers is of immobility leading to isolation. Broadbent (1985) found that mothers of twins left the house much less often than those with a single baby. Mothers saw less of their friends and therefore got little encouragement and little feedback on how well they were coping. They felt out of touch with their former life and had little chance of outside entertainment. Their partners often had to take time off work (and often used up their remaining annual leave) to accompany them, for instance, to the clinic or hospital appointment.

Because they are confined to home or the immediate vicinity, mothers become increasingly reliant on their partner; which can reduce their self-esteem or strain the relationship.

Parents who would have regularly taken one baby on a visit to friends often find the performance of taking two babies is just too much. Getting two babies ready, getting them there and then anxiously keeping an eye on two crawlers in someone else's precious home is not worth the strain.

The large majority of mothers lack a car in the daytime and for them transport is a major problem. Public transport with two babies in arms (plus pushchair and shopping) is almost impossible. In one group of 23 mothers only one took a bus alone with the twins during the first year; she returned by taxi!

Another mother boldly took twins together with an older brother on extra seats attached to an adult tricycle. Most mothers stick to their feet with a twin pram, pushchair or buggy. Two single buggies clipped together have the advantage that they can be separated at weekends or at other times when a second pair of hands is available. Likewise, a single buggy can be clipped on to a twin buggy if three children need transporting. Sometimes a mother prefers to have one baby in a sling and the other in a pushchair. Some may carry both babies in slings one in front and one on her back.

Some mothers find outings an ordeal because of the attention the twins attract. Many relatively private people find it difficult becoming a constant focus of interest to strangers, which is the inevitable fate of a mother pushing a pram containing a pair of young twins. The public appear to think they have a right to stare, ask extremely personal questions and even touch the babies.

Visits to a Baby Clinic are dreaded by many parents of twins and are therefore often avoided (Taylor and Emery 1988). Few clinics have the facilities to cater for a double pram. Many mothers end up holding two crying babies and being quite unable to talk or listen to either the health visitor or the doctor. No mother of twins should be expected to come to the clinic or the doctor's surgery alone. Home visits for weighing and immunizations are greatly appreciated by parents but, unfortunately, are rarely offered. Taylor and Emery (1988) found that not only were twins taken to see their Family Doctor far less often than singletons, they also received fewer visits to their home from the doctor. The twins were therefore receiving less medical supervision. Yet, if anything, twin infants would be expected to be more prone to illness than singletons. However, mothers of twins reported fewer symptoms in their twins than did mothers of singletons. This is likely to be a reflection of the mothers reduced powers of observation due to fatigue and workload rather than a true indication of the health of the babies. All these factors point to the need for *increased* supervision of these families.

Special Twins Clinics provide a more relaxed atmosphere where a mother is more likely to feel able to discuss all the problems that are arising. At these clinics there are always spare hands to hold the babies, which allows the mother to see the doctor on her own, before the children are seen. The volunteers are all mothers of twins so they can give emotional as well as practical advice and support. Unfortunately, at present, there are only four such clinics in the UK (see Appendix 1).

Sleep

The endurance of a mother, let alone the happiness of the family, can ultimately depend on whether or not the twins allow the family a good night's sleep. One wakeful baby can be disruptive enough but not only can two take turns to disturb the household, one of them can set the other going and then each reinforce the other's distress.

There is obviously no simple answer to sleep problems, nor a single arrangement that suits every family. The number of rooms available, their ambient temperature and the sleeping patterns of the babies all have to be considered. However, many parents have blamed themselves in retrospect for allowing unnecessarily troublesome sleep patterns to develop in their twins.

During the early months a cot divided by a partition across the middle so that one baby sleeps at either end is satisfactory. Later, when they are in separate cots, some babies are comforted by being close enough to touch each other. If they do wake they may then resettle on their own. On the other hand, many disturb each other, so that if one wakes, the second is woken unnecessarily. The cots should then be well separated and, when practicable, perhaps even put in different rooms.

Mothers often reinforce bad sleeping habits. For instance, a mother may rush, at the first whimper, to comfort one so as to prevent the other being disturbed. The children may welcome this easily won attention and demand it more and more. When they are sleeping separately, the wakeful child may be left longer and a vicious circle may be avoided.

It is often assumed that if there are several children in the family the twins should always sleep together. However, some families find that it is much better to separate the twins, so that one or both sleeps with another sibling.

The father's role

Clearly a mother with twins will turn to her partner for help very much more than she would do for a single child. Most fathers seem to respond well to this call (Bryan 1977a). The notable feature about those mothers who cope well in the first year is that they have a good and secure relationship with their partner (Hay *et al*. 1990).

The father's role has changed greatly in the last 10 or 20 years. They were already involved in many domestic tasks and the social climate now encourages men to take a more active interest and practical part in the care of the children. Economic circumstances have pointed in the same direction. Women are sometimes now the main wage earners and, with the additional expenses, it may be essential for a mother of twins to continue earning. Thus, in some families the father may be responsible for a substantial amount of the twins' care.

Although twins tend to have less contact than singletons with both their mother and their father, the proportionate amount of time spent with their father is likely to be greater. It is not surprising therefore that Lytton (1980) found that more 2-year-old boy twins than singletons chose their father as their primary figure of attachment. This is one of the few bonuses for the father.

Nevertheless, he may find the first year, in particular, a severe strain. He is almost bound to lose some of his wife's attention and care. He may become jealous of the demanding twins. Because of the added financial strain of a larger family he may also have to work longer hours or, more likely, cut down on luxuries. On top of all this he is then expected, and rightly, to help with the children and domestic tasks to an entirely unaccustomed degree. Because of all this the position and feelings of fathers of twins deserve more attention than they often receive, and contact made possible through the Twins and Multiple Births Association can be valuable.

Identification

Despite increasing awareness of the importance of twins being encouraged to develop their own individuality from the start, many parents find it difficult in practice during the first year. Social pressures and attitudes militate against it. Friends, relatives and particularly grandparents want to celebrate a twinship and like to see the children dressed alike. Few take the trouble to call the babies by their names. Indeed many parents fail to do so and just call them 'the twins'. In the case of MZ twins some parents even forget which name they originally gave to each child. Zazzo (1960) found that 10 per cent of the parents of MZ twins did not remember to which child they had originally given which name.

And yet patterns set in the first year are difficult to change. Many parents, both for simplicity and for their own satisfaction, initially dress the babies alike with the firm intention of changing later. But then the babies get used to looking alike and resent a change. Many parents who leave the change until the second or third year meet with vehement opposition. One pair as young as 10 months old, when given different clothes for the first time, refused to be consoled until they were allowed to be dressed alike again.

Outfits in similar styles but different colours seem to be a good compromise. The attraction of the twinship is retained whilst allowing people, at least for that day, to remember who is who. Colour coding may even extend to names, one pair being christened Jasmine and Emerald. In retrospect, parents may feel they have been too rigid on colour coding. One pair were so attached to their own blue or red coding that biscuits wrapped in green paper were refused and, more seriously, the 'red' child was miserable on starting at a school with a compulsory blue uniform.

Obviously, clothes should not be the only way of recognizing a child and any distinctive feature such as a different hairstyle should be pointed out. There may be a place for initialled clothes for MZ twins and people should then be encouraged to use the names.

Photography is another context in which parents tend to treat their children as a unit. Significantly, some families have no photographs of either child on his own. Worse still, parents sometimes cannot remember who is who on a photograph. A note should be made on the back each time. Twins are even more difficult to distinguish in photographs than in real life. A poignant example arose with 2½-year-old MZ boys. The children had been photographed many times but always together. One twin suddenly died of meningitis. The father, in particular, could not bear to see photographs of the dead son. This meant that all the early pictures of the survivor had to be hidden away.

Intrapair relationships

From the start, the emotional environment of a twin baby differs radically from that of a singleton for he must develop two strong emotional ties simultaneously; to the mother and to the co-twin. His most constant companion is his twin rather than his mother and he is often further confused by many changes of caretaker (Robin *et al*. 1988). Not only will the father handle the babies more often but others, including relatives and neighbours, are more likely to be involved in caretaking activities, particularly feeding.

The age at which twins seem to become distinctly aware of each other appears to vary greatly. At this stage, when most babies are beginning to explore their own bodies, twins may spend quite as much time in discovering the body of their twin. Initially, indeed, they make no distinction. It is not uncommon to see twins peacefully sucking each other's thumb. It may be a painful stimulus such as having his finger bitten that first tells an infant the limits of his own body in relation to that of the other.

The effect and degree of the intrauterine relationship of twins is unknown. Studies of fetal activity on ultrasound film have shown the varied and distinct interactions that twins may have with each other. One fetus may be the more active or aggressive while the other is calm and soothing. Follow-up of the infants showed that these characteristics tended to persist at least through the first year (Piontelli 1989).

Certainly, by 5 or 6 months, twins are sufficiently comforted by each other's presence for it to have a quieting effect (Leonard 1959). Too often parents, busy with household chores, take advantage of this, and assume that the mother's attention has become less necessary, whereas for twins, just as for single children, one-to-one communication from an adult is essential to their language development (see p. 139).

The quality of the attachment of a twin infant to his mother and to his co-twin was closely explored by Vandell *et al.* (1988). It might be expected that a twin with an especially strong attachment to his twin would have a less strong link with his mother and vice versa—the reverse was found. Twins who had a strong attachment to their mother during the first 2 years also related strongly to each other. Thus, the argument that a secure attachment to their mother is needed to free infants to make other relationships appears to apply to their twin as well as to unfamiliar people.

Maternal attitudes

Most mothers want to treat their twin babies equally and plan to give them the same amount of time and attention. In practice this is not easy as one baby, often the smaller, can be much more demanding. Few mothers can give their full attention to a placid, seemingly contented, baby whilst the other baby is crying. Too often she is unable to concentrate fully on either baby. She may, for instance, be feeding one whilst soothing the other.

The physical similarity of the babies, particularly of MZ twins, can obstruct the formation of a close relationship. If a parent cannot readily tell their babies apart, it is inevitably more difficult to relate to them as individuals with their different temperaments and needs.

Mothers may continue to feel a preference for one baby (see p. 108) and demonstrate this in the way they talk of their children or by the quality of their responses to them. Nevertheless, most mothers are remarkably fair in the time and care they give to each and indeed a mother may actually compensate the less favoured twin by spending more time with him or her.

As discussed earlier, a mother's relationship may be affected by the size of the baby. The mother's attitude to the smaller of a pair varies. She may reject it with the feeling that it is in some way imperfect. The rejection may be promoted by inadequate bonding in the neonatal period (see p. 108). On the other hand its very smallness and weakness may inspire special care and protection. Several studies have shown the latter reaction to be the more common, at least during the first year (Allen *et al.* 1971; 1976). This extra attention to the weaker baby may to some extent compensate for its initial deficit and facilitate its development in relation to its co-twin (Field and Widmayer 1980).

Some parents have unjustifiably higher expectations of the larger twin, even if the smaller one has been fit and well from the start. They assume for instance, that the larger one will walk first and expect other skills, even those unrelated to strength such as speech, to be more advanced (personal observation).

Siblings

The effect of twins on other siblings has only recently begun to attract attention. Many of these children are deeply affected, even damaged, by the presence of an inseparable pair within the family. This is particularly so where there is only one single child: he may feel very isolated. He will have been the sole focus of attention but is now suddenly relegated. Furthermore, his parents are a pair, so are the twins. Both pairs seem to exclude him and very often the twins do. The isolation is intensified if the twins have their own language or other communication.

Bernstein (1980) goes as far as to say that older siblings may feel incomplete and 'search' for their own twin using doll or animal substitutes. They may have developed a special fear of being alone, particularly at nights. The toddler who has been used to the relatively straightforward relationship with two parents may be agonizingly confused by the sudden influx not only of twins but of the many new relationships they bring about.

He is inevitably now deprived of much of his mother's time and attention. She, at least, will be aware of the problem but not so the many well-meaning but thoughtless friends and acquaintances who focus all attention and admiration on the twins and do not see the unhappiness of the older child (Fig. 9.1). One mother was so concerned by this phenomenon that she had a seat especially arranged on the pushchair pram so that the twins could not be seen until the toddler had been acknowledged.

Not surprisingly, the older sibling may react to this stressful situation with difficult behaviour. In Australia 64 per cent of families with young twins reported problems with the older child during the first 6 months after the twins' arrival and, in many cases, this persisted. In this same study siblings were found to have 'lower self-concept' and less emotional involvement with the younger children in the family (Hay *et al.* 1988).

Lytton (1980) described the older sibling of twins as 'the classical difficult child', either diverting his parents' attention from the twins by negative attention-seeking or by showing aggression towards the twins. There is always the danger that such behaviour will provoke parental child abuse. In the US Groothius *et al.* (1982) found a nine-fold increase in abuse in multiple birth families and in half of the families it was the sibling rather than one or both of the twins who was abused.

Some older children on the other hand may become silently hostile and withdrawn (Collier 1972) or take the opposite and more worrying route, striving for attention by being extra good at home and at school.

Single children, especially those close in age to the twins, may need more

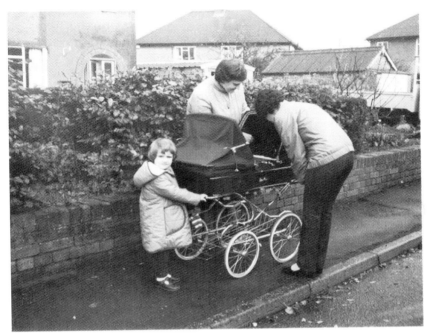

Fig. 9.1 Attention focussed on young twins while elder sister is ignored.

help and support than the twins themselves. This is rarely appreciated and we need to learn more about this neglected group.

Similarly, little is known about the younger sibling of twins. At least they are not displaced from the focus of attention, but they may well suffer from being thought of and known as 'the twins' sister' with no regard for their own identity.

On the whole the twins themselves benefit from having siblings. The more there are, the looser their own bond is likely to become. In this respect DZ twins have some advantage over MZ in that they tend to come from larger families (Phillips and Watkinson 1981).

Sudden infant death syndrome

The sudden unexpected death of an infant during the first year is a tragedy that can hit any family. However, some infants are known to be at particular risk and twins are amongst these. The incidence of the 'sudden infant death syndrome' (SIDS) or 'cot death' in twins appears to be about twice that of infants in general (Carpenter 1965; Kraus and Borhani 1972; Imaizumi *et al.* 1981; Beal 1983); amongst triplets the risk is higher still (Kraus and Borhani 1972). Like- and unlike-sexed pairs appear to be equally affected, as do both males and females (Carpenter 1965; Froggatt *et al.* 1971). The results of a large study in Australia (Beal 1983) suggest that the higher risk to twins is limited to infants weighing less than 2000 g at birth and that in this group there is a five-fold increase in risk compared to singletons of similar birth weight. Where there was a substantial intrapair discordancy in birth weight, it was the smaller twin who died in all seven cases.

A further finding in the Australian study was that three of the 20 twins who died were single survivors whose twins had been stillborn. This is at least three times the incidence expected amongst twins in general.

SIDS is known to be more common amongst prematurely born infants and those who have been separated from their mothers at birth. Thus it is not surprising that twins are more vulnerable. However, it would seem that at least amongst low birth weight twins the twinship in itself adds a further risk factor and the reason for this is not clear (Carpenter *et al.* 1979; McCarthy *et al.* 1981; McMullen 1986).

In families where one infant has died unexpectedly subsequent children have a five- to ten-fold greater risk of themselves dying unexpectedly (Carpenter *et al.* 1979). Amongst twins the risk is higher still. There have now been many reports of both twins dying either at the same time or within a few days of each other (Cooke and Welch 1964; Carpenter 1965; Froggatt *et al.* 1971; Kraus and Borhani 1972; Beal 1983; Bass 1989). Occasionally both babies are found dead in the cot together. However, Bass (1989) challenges the idea of simultaneous infant death and suggests that the majority of cases, if not all, can be explained by avoidable injuries. In all thirteen cases of unexplained simultaneous death he considered that the deaths had been due to some form of insult, such as overheating, noxious gases or, in two cases, homicide.

One study found that the concordance rate for SIDS was 8.6 per cent in like-sexed twins and 7.6 per cent in unlike-sexed twins (Spiers 1974). In another series of 112 cases of SIDS in twins over half the co-twins had some abnormal signs around the time of the death of their twin and two died on the same day. On the other hand in 39 per cent of pairs the parents had recognized no abnormal signs in either the dead twin or the survivor (Carpenter 1965). It appears that the excessive risk to the co-twin lasts only for 1 month, and that much the most critical period is the first few days. For this reason immediate and very close supervision should be given to the surviving twin, if not several days of observation in hospital (Emery 1979).

The effects on the family and, in particular, on the surviving twin of an unexpected death in infancy can be severe and complex. They are discussed in Chapter 13.

10

The preschool twin

The preschool period is especially critical for twin children. It is important enough for singletons in that problems in these early years can have a lasting effect on their adult personality. In twin children, however, the considerable extra complication is whether each of them will become properly independent or for ever function as half of a duo, unable to cope without the constant support of his co-twin.

Intrapair relationship

Despite some inevitable sibling rivalries and jealousies, twins are usually strongly interdependent. They have always had each other and therefore been less dependent on others. Parents often say that their twin children appear to have less need of parental approval and are consequently less responsive to parental guidance and discipline (see p. 137) although, interestingly, the attachment of twins to their mother was found in one study to be similar to that found in the singleton population (Vandell *et al*. 1988).

When disappointed in their parents, however, they can always turn to each other for consolation. This powerful intrapair relationship must be a significant factor in the development of a twin child and has been described by Zazzo (1960) as 'the couple effect'.

This very interdependence and companionship may indeed be vital to the emotional survival of some twins. Koluchova (1972) describes a pair of MZ boys who were isolated from the outside world from the age of 18 months to 7 years. They were deprived of any stimulation, spent many hours each day in the cellar and their only toys were a few bricks. They were frequently beaten by their stepmother. Their remarkable progress when removed from this environment and their apparent lack of long-term damage has been attributed to their close attachment to each other (Koluchova 1976; British Medical Journal 1976).

For an MZ twin the differentiation of his own ego and body from those of his partner must be a complicated process. If dressed alike the process may well be delayed still further. DZ twins learn to identify their mirror images several months before MZ twins (Burlingham 1952) and the majority of twins recognize their co-twin's reflection in a mirror before their own (Bernabei and Levi 1976) (Fig. 10.1). The characteristic confusion was exemplified by a 5-year-old MZ girl, who when trying on a new dress, told

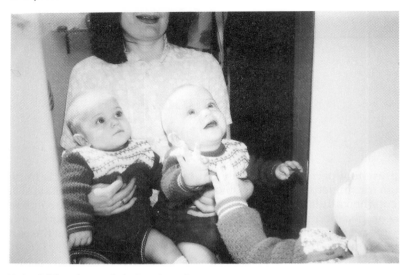

Fig. 10.1   MZ twins and their mirror images.

her twin to stand in front of her, 'So that I can see what I look like' (Mittler 1971).

Many twins respond to the name of the other twin as well as their own and often call themselves by their twin's name. For instance in a pair of MZ twins, Bert referred to his brother, Bill, as 'other-one-Bert' (Burlingham 1952). Leonard (1959) found that 60 per cent of 2-year-old single children gave their own name on request whereas only 40 per cent of twins did so.

Behaviour

Most twins do not seem to mind which of them was born first; nor, of course, should they. It is however surprising and unfortunate how often this information interests other people and in turn may have a lasting effect on the twins. A firstborn twin often attaches undue importance to his rank and Hay and O'Brien (1987) have found that it is one of the factors that later determines a twin's self-esteem. If a firstborn child boasts of his superiority a parent might tell the story of the African tribe where the second born is considered senior. They say it is only after the firstborn has checked that the world is ready to receive him is the second twin delivered.

Matheny and Brown (1971) found that birth order was not an important influence on behaviour, although Hay and O'Brien (1987) did find some effect and leadership and aggression, traits characteristic of the eldest child in the family, were also more commonly found in the firstborn of twins (Very and Van Hine 1969).

Birth weight is another factor affecting the self-esteem of a twin child but the strongest influence appears to be coming home first from hospital (Hay and O'Brien 1987). Birth weight discordance, however, was associated with other differences. Of 18 weight-concordant pairs only two showed markedly discrepant behaviour, whereas in ten out of 18 weight-discordant pairs behaviour significantly differed. The lighter twin tended to have more 'problem' behaviours and was less proficient in various aspects of cognitive behaviour.

Gifford *et al.* (1966) vividly illustrate these points in describing the progress of a pair of birth-weight-discordant MZ girls from birth to 6 years. The larger was always the more contented, placid and serious whereas the smaller was more active, impetuous and charming. Their IQ scores at 14 years were almost identical but the children's approach to the test was entirely different.

In the Louisville Twin Study over 200 mothers were interviewed periodically about the behaviour of their twins. At 1 year the differences were mainly in temper and attention span whereas by 4 years the main difference was in the degree of sociability (Wilson *et al.* 1971).

Not surprisingly, there was a higher degree of concordance in behaviour between MZ twins than DZ. However, this effect of zygosity does not necessarily apply equally to interests and activities. In young children, at least, it appears that their activities are more a result of parental influence than any particular personality trait. Lytton (1980) found that 2- to 3-year-old MZ boys were no more similar in their choice of toys or forms of play than DZ twins. Later, however, the pattern changes. By 6 years, Loehlin and Nichols (1976) found a significantly greater similarity in the activities of MZ than DZ twins. MZ twins also tend to cooperate more effectively in a joint task than DZ (Segal 1984), presumably because their approach to the task is more likely to coincide.

Twins should always be encouraged to develop their own interests. If one asks to go to a football match there is no reason to assume his brother will also want to go. If one is tired or hungry, why should the other automatically be so?

Separate outings should be arranged from an early age. Not only do they increase the twin child's independence but most children (and adults) find it easier to build relationships one-to-one than one-to-two. These periods also give a parent some precious time alone with one child.

Several workers have shown that there is no correlation between similarity of appearance and similarity of behaviour within a twin pair (Cohen *et al.* 1975; Matheny *et al.* 1976; Plomin *et al.* 1976). This is perhaps not surprising as the more physically alike the two children, the greater may be their need to differ in behaviour.

Wilson and colleagues (1971) found a surprising degree of age-to-age stability in intrapair behavioural differences. But this is by no means invariable. Many parents report a switching, particularly in leadership, from time to time. Which twin dominates may vary both over time and with the situation (Lytton 1980).

A group of children who were defined by their parents as being the dominant of a pair of twins were compared with their co-twins. The main differentiating factor was that the dominant twin tended to talk more than his partner. There was no intrapair difference in their verbal IQ, in their size or in their degree of parental attachment (Lytton 1980).

I have already suggested that the natural individuality of twins—as of all children—should be respected, indeed encouraged (see p. 127). There is, however, a danger of some parents artificially accentuating differences of personality or behaviour. It is inevitable that parents should constantly compare and contrast the behaviours of two children of the same age and hence look out for differences. But this process often leads to the exaggeration of character traits that in fact lie well within the normal range. Parents may therefore speak of one of their twins as the 'placid' or 'lively' one and relatives and friends soon learn these stereotypes and, perhaps unconsciously, respond to the two children accordingly. More serious, however, is the fact that children tend to live up to parental expectations of being the one who is 'good' or 'naughty', 'quiet' or 'noisy', 'untidy' or 'tidy'. Parents should be helped to realize that a balance has to be struck between encouraging and exaggerating differences between their children. They need to acknowledge that the range of 'normal' behaviour is wide and that children vary greatly in their sociability, for instance, or in their degree of attentiveness.

Parents usually believe themselves to be equally fond of each twin but this is not necessarily shown in their behaviour towards them. One child may be blamed for more misdemeanours than he deserves whereas the same actions in the other may pass apparently unnoticed. If parents expect certain behaviour they tend only to notice when the expectation is fulfilled. Goshen-Gottstein (1980) describes a pair of twins whom the mother had 'labelled' as early as 7 months. Ruben, the boy, was labelled as naughty and wild and Ruby, the girl as sweet and easier. Regular observation of the children did not confirm these differences yet at the age of two the mother still treated them according to this pattern. She often wrongly suspected Ruben of aggression towards a baby brother but was blind to the several occasions on which Ruby pulled the baby's hair.

On the other hand, some parents do recognize that they feel closer to one baby than the other. They may well feel unhappy and ashamed about these feelings and many do not admit to them until months or years later. Such parents might have been greatly relieved to learn at the time that these unequal affections are not at all unusual and that most of these difficulties resolve themselves over time. Indeed, Minde *et al.* (1990) have actually suggested that there can be beneficial aspects to a parental preference between twins. They found that differential, and even preferential, treatment of twins, instead of being harmful to development, actually benefited both children. They suggested that the differences in the twins' experiences might further their sense of self and autonomy. There was no doubt, however, that the more favoured child did better. Whether it was the favouring that stimulated the development or whether it was the brighter child that evoked the preference was not elucidated.

Young twins may have greater difficulty with social interaction than singletons. Infant twins as young as 6 and 9 months are less sociable than singletons in that they show less interest in and interact less with unfamiliar peers (Vandell *et al.* 1988). This may, of course, be because there is much less novelty for twins in being offered another child to whom to relate. Kim *et al.* (1969) found that 3½-year-old twins in a nursery were more solitary, less affectionate and less aggressive. This may well be due to the relative isolation of a twin unit because, by the age of 5½, after 2 years in the nursery, these twins had overcome their inhibitions and their behaviour was not significantly different from singletons of the same age.

A marked difference between twins and singletons is that of distractability. Twins tend to have more difficulty in concentrating and this is likely to be due to the constant distraction caused by their twin throughout the early years. Rarely do they have a peaceful time alone. The parents, because of the situation they find themselves in, may reinforce the problem. Clark and Dickman (1984) found that parents show frequent shifts of attention from one child to another, whereas parents of singletons are more likely to have prolonged uninterrupted interactions. Similarly, Betton and Loester (1983) found that when one twin was alone with the mother he received more encouragement and positive reinforcement; when she was interacting with two at the same time much of her time was spent keeping order.

Winnicott (1958) urges consideration of the positive aspects of the capacity to be alone, through which a child can discover himself and become aware of his feelings. With twins the practical difficulty of providing two children with the experience of safe yet rewarding solitude is very considerable. The parent can rarely find time to devote any kind of concentrated attention to one twin without the other twin calling either out of real need or out of jealousy. It is unlikely that the parent of twins will be unflurried and composed enough to create the atmosphere needed for a gently creative 'alone together' solitude to emerge. No child is likely to spend less time on his own than a twin. Twinship and solitude are virtually antithetical. Perhaps more attention should be given to the pyschological consequences of this unique kind of childhood. Arranging for each twin to attend play-group on his own for one session a week is a good way for the parent to have regular uninterrupted periods alone with each child.

Discipline

By 36 months almost twice as many twins as singletons were described by their mother as 'difficult' (Hay and O'Brien 1984).

The discipline of preschool twins poses a unique challenge. Three- and 4-year-old MZ boys seem to be the most problematic of all. Even experienced parents can be disconcerted to find how ineffective are the forms of control they had used successfully with their older children.

The difficulties probably have several origins. A child responds to discipline because he wants the love or respect of the person giving it. If the person he most minds about is a twin who encourages him on, he is naturally less likely to respond to parental pressures. Furthermore, the ingenuity of two minds together with combined effort and joint perseverance can be much more devastating than the effects of a single child.

Care must be taken not to punish both children for the misdemeanor of one. This can be difficult when neither will confess to the act but whenever possible reprimands and other punishments should be given individually and in private, away from the twin.

Biting

Biting 2-year-olds are some of the most regular visitors to the Twins Clinic. Biting appears to be at once more common and more extreme in twins than single children. This is not surprising, as there are few better ways of ensuring a parent's attention than drawing blood from another child! One mother resorted to carrying her 2-year-old son constantly in order to prevent him biting the other two triplets. He therefore gained exactly the attention he wanted.

There was no easy remedy in this case; nor for biting in general. Essentially, however, the less issue made of it the better and any necessary actions should be accompanied by quiet but firm handling without signs of parental agitation. If the biting fails to elicit special attention, let alone excitement, it is much more likely to be abandoned.

If one twin is behaving badly he should be quietly reprimanded but the most effective deterrent is often to give lots of positive attention to the other twin. In this way the offending child may learn that he will get more attention for good behaviour than bad!

Toilet training

Twins tend to toilet train at a later age than singletons. Toilet training of twins is best delayed until one child is interested and actually showing signs that he is ready to be trained. Too often parents struggle to train both at once. It is usually much easier to concentrate on the child who is showing most promise and the other will usually follow his twin's example when he sees the advantages, not least parental praise, in acquiring such skills.

Laterality

Over no aspect of twinning has there been more disagreement than laterality. The reported frequency of left-handedness in twins has varied from 5 per cent to as much as 31 per cent and even the effect of zygosity is a source of contention. One study showed that left-handedness was three times more common in MZ than DZ twins. Another found the incidence in MZ twins to be half that of DZ. In only 11 out of 18 studies was left-handedness found to be more common amongst MZ twins (McManus 1980).

Many earlier studies suggested a higher incidence of left-handedness in twins. More recently these conclusions have been challenged (McManus 1980). McManus anlaysed 19 studies of laterality in twins and found that none of them was satisfactory. Criteria had varied and twins and singletons were rarely seen by the same investigators. Most of the studies had been made before the advent of reliable zygosity determinations and some had actually (and wrongly) assumed that symmetry reversal was pathognomonic of monozygosity (Newman 1928).

Several workers agree with McManus that there is no significantly higher incidence of left-handedness amongst twins (Husen 1959; Zazzo 1960; Koch 1966). Phillips (1981) points out that to use the writing hand as a measure of laterality may be misleading, as this is subject to cultural pressures. In the

Birmingham study he found that 86 per cent of twin children had consistent laterality for writing and for manual skills and that 14 per cent of these were left-handed. Six per cent differed in the hand they used for writing from that used for manual skills. The remaining 14 per cent had mixed laterality. This last group was nearly twice as large as that found amongst singletons. The overall incidence of left-handedness in twins was higher than that in singletons but significant only at the 10 per cent level. However, intrapair concordancy for left-handedness was five times the expected figure.

There may well be two separate populations of left-handed children. One of these groups would be genetically determined and hence no more common amongst twins than singletons. The second 'pathological' group would be that of children whose left-handedness is a result of an insult to the normally dominant left cerebral hemisphere during the intrauterine or perinatal periods. This group is certainly likely to be disproportionately represented amongst twins.

Mirror imaging

MZ twins can be mirror images of each other, which means that they have lateral asymmetry, including the reversal of superficial features such as hair whorls and tooth eruption, the reversal of internal organs (*situs inversus*) and opposite handedness. This lateral asymmetry probably arises from the late division of the embryo when the left and right sides had already been determined (Burn 1991).

However, such a complete lateral asymmetry is rare and, of the internal organs the heart is the most commonly affected (see p. 64 and Burn 1991).

Language

It was first recognized in the 1930s that twins were slower in their language development than singletons (Day 1932; Davis 1937) and this has been confirmed in many subsequent studies (Alm 1953; Koch 1966; Mittler 1976; Conway *et al.* 1980; Watts & Lytton 1980; Hay *et al.* 1987). Many twin children, particularly boys, whose overall intelligence is normal show significant deficits in their verbal performance (Alm 1953). Alm found that, by 4 years, twin children were, on average, 6 months behind singletons and, by defining language delay as a failure to use a sentence at 30 months of age, Zazzo (1979) found that 44 per cent of MZ and 43 per cent of DZ twins were retarded.

In her study of 5–6-year-old firstborn North American boys Koch (1966) found that twins were less talkative than singletons. Watts and Lytton (1980) found that by 9 years the verbal performance of twin boys was still delayed.

The most comprehensive large study of speech development in twins was that by Mittler (1976). He studied 200 4-year-old twins—30 per cent MZ and 70 per cent DZ—and applied the Illinois Test of Psycholinguistic Abilities, which includes subtests for nine different aspects of speech development. He found that twins had an overall score 6 months behind that of singletons and that performance was influenced neither by zygosity nor birth order. Twins performed less well than singletons in all except one subtest, the exception being speed of reaction to speech. Perhaps the constant presence of another competing recipient for communications from parents stimulates the development of this particular skill.

A particularly interesting finding in Mittler's study was that of the much greater effect of social class on language development in singletons than twins. In singletons there were 12 points (53 versus 41) difference in scores between social classes I and II and social classes IV and V, whereas the difference between the same groups in twins was only five points (44 versus 39). Possibly twins are less able to take advantage of their otherwise linguistically favourable environment. It may well be that some mothers from social classes I and II, who would normally have looked after a single child on their own, employ help (generally less educated than themselves) when there are two children.

However, even with twins, the education of the mother does to some degree affect the speech development of the children. Lytton *et al.* (1977) found that 2½-year-old MZ boys had significantly inferior verbal skills than DZ twins, and that this could be entirely accounted for by the difference in the education of the mothers in the two groups.

Savic (1980) has studied the pattern of communication between twins and their mothers in detail. As a result of her close observation of three pairs of twins over a 2-year period from 1 to 3 years of age, she concluded that twins pass through the stages of speech development in a different way to singletons. Twins have to develop a much more complicated form of interaction. They must learn earlier than most how to communicate within a triad and when to engage and disengage in discourse. Concentration on this essential skill may mean that other aspects of speech development are postponed.

Speech delay in twins is neither inevitable nor irremediable and it has been demonstrated that twins can make conspicuous progress with appropriate teaching (Koluchova 1972, 1976; Douglas and Sutton 1978). Mittler (1971) tells a remarkable story about 4-year-old twin boys. The mother sought help because the boys had no speech, were overactive and wild; she was at her wits' end. Assessment showed that their intellectual function was subnormal and they both had IQs in the low 60s. The mother was advised to treat them and talk to them individually, to dress them differently and in every way to try to prevent them acting, or being thought of, as a single unit. One year later they were transformed. Their speech was fluent and an IQ assessment gave them each a score of 120. It is plainly vital that more is learnt about detrimental factors in the early environment of twins and that remedial efforts are not delayed.

Too often parents of twins are given unhelpful and misleading reassurance that 'They will grow out of it', which is not true, or that 'It's because they are twins', which may be true but is not helpful in remedying a condition that may have bad long-term consequences.

Earlier studies suggested that the language delay was entirely due to the difference in environment experienced by twins and singletons (Mittler 1970; Lytton *et al.* 1977). Indeed, the findings of Record *et al.* (1970) pointed strongly away from biological factors in that they showed that single surviving twins whose twins had died in the neonatal period did better in their language development than twins brought up together. Yet these single twins were likely to have had perinatal experiences that were at least as traumatic as members of surviving pairs.

Findings by Myrianthopoulos *et al.* 1976 and from a more recent large study from Australia (Hay *et al.* 1987) suggest that the delay may be related to both biological and environmental factors in about equal proportions. Previous studies tended to look at each perinatal factor individually. When the various factors were studied cumulatively a strong association between perinatal problems and language delay was found. The finding of an association between language delay and problems with fine motor but not gross motor performance is consistent with biological influences related to perinatal events. As more very preterm infants survive from multiple pregnancies the proportion affected by perinatal complications is likely to increase. A stronger association between early language problems and later reading difficulties in twins has also been found (see p. 160).

The environmental factors affecting twin development are likely to be many and these have been usefully reviewed by Mogford (1988) and Redshaw and Rutter (1991).

Lytton and his colleagues in Canada have shed much light on the differences between the environment in which a twin is brought up and that of a singleton. Many of these differences could be expected to militate against optimal language development. It has also been suggested that twins have less need to use the conventional form of communication—language—as they have so many other means of relating to each other (Zazzo 1960).

Twins have problems with communication from the very start. There is the almost constant presence of three potential participants in any act of communication, so there are always two recipients and two responders to any message within the triad.

It is not surprising that verbal interaction of all kinds appears to be lower in families with twins. Not only do twins talk less than singletons but parents of twins communicate less with their children. When they do talk they tend to use shorter and grammatically less complex utterances (Lytton *et al.* 1977). In his study on mother–child interaction, Lytton (1980) found that this may in part be because the mother has less time and is under more strain, but many mothers also believe, mistakenly, that twins have less need of maternal attention because they entertain or comfort each other.

Lytton found mothers to be less responsive to the distress or demands of twin children. They also give fewer commands, suggestions and, in particular, explanations. Often, the mother does not have the time to wait for the response of one child before her attention is demanded by the other. Rules are less consistently carried through. Mothers also demonstrate less affectionate behaviour and give less praise and approval (Lytton 1980).

Tomasello *et al.* (1986) suggested that it was not that mothers of twins talked less to their children but that responding to two children meant that each child received less speech specifically directed to him personally and participated in fewer and shorter individual conversations.

Acquisition of speech is a highly complex process that is heavily dependent on personal interaction. Children learn to speak through learning, imitation and stimulation. The main models for singletons are parents or older siblings. For the twin the main model is the co-twin. Thus, speech is likely to be immature and deviations from normal will be reinforced. Some observers have gone so far as to assume that twins communicate with each other in preference to their mother. Savic (1980) found that this was not so. Twins are often forced into communicating mainly with each other but, given the choice, they prefer relating to their mother. In addressing the adult they will more often choose the diadic than triadic forms of communication (Table 10.1). Savic found that twin children directed speech to their mother over twice as often as to their co-twin.

Table 10.1   Communication between 1- to 3-year-old twins and their mother

Direction of communication	% Time
Mother ⇄ Twin	20.33
Twin ⇄ Mother	18.41
Twin ⇄ Twin	13.88
Twin → Mother	29.65
Mother → Twin	0.91
Non-directed	9.73
Triadic	6.49

Source: Savic (1980).

Single mothers of twins appear to compensate for the absence of the father by providing sterner discipline and criticism. Although they reassured their children even less than married mothers of twins they gave them greater stimulation and these children tended to have greater verbal comprehension than other twins (Lytton 1980). These findings are the results of a study of only five families, so no firm conclusions can be drawn. Nevertheless it shows that at least some compensation can be made for the lack of a second parent.

Cryptophasia

Much has been made of the 'secret language' of twins. There is no doubt that this cryptophasia, idioglossia or autonomous speech does exist—a language quite incomprehensible to others. Occasional instances of isolated pairs with exclusive cryptophasia have been reported. Scobie (1979) described a pair of MZ girls who had little contact with anyone but each other during their first 5 years. They had developed their own relatively elaborate language but to others had no recognizable language at all.

Exclusive cryptophasia is, however, extremely rare and there is little evidence that the use of a special intertwin language is in itself harmful to normal speech development. Incidences quoted will vary according to definition. About 40 per cent of twins have been reported to have cryptophasia by several workers (Mittler 1970). Some have found it to be more common amongst MZ twins (Alm 1953; Zazzo 1979). Zazzo (1979) considered that 48 per cent of the 2½-year-old MZ twins he examined had cryptophasia and only 27 per cent of DZ. Others have found no difference in the incidence in MZ and DZ twins.

Stuttering

Stuttering has been little studied in twins. Koch (1966) found that 11 per cent of twins stuttered at one stage but only 6 per cent were still doing so by the time they started school. The problem was more common amongst boy twins than girls. Rife (1940) found a slightly higher incidence amongst twins than singletons and like Koch (1966) found it to be equally common among MZ and DZ. Concordance, although low in both groups, was over twice as common amongst MZ twins.

Illness in twins

Apart from a vulnerability to infections in the early months due to prematurity, twins are, in general, neither more nor less prone to most physical illnesses than singletons. Malignant disease may, however, be an exception. It appears that some cancers may be less common in twin children. Hewitt and Stewart (1970) found that there were fewer cases of non-radiogenic cancers than would be expected amongst like-sexed twins who died before their tenth birthday and they suggested that this was due to the elimination of those fetuses whose later neoplasms would have resulted from cell damage incurred at, or shortly after, conception.

Twins under school age also appear to be less prone to leukaemia, which is surprising as twins are, if anything, more likely to be exposed to radiation in intrauterine life. Leukaemia, when it does occur, was found to be more common in pairs of disparate birth weight. The larger infant was the one more commonly affected (Jackson *et al.* 1969).

Staying in hospital

If one twin has to go into hospital during the early years the effect on both children may be shattering. Not only are they separated from each other, often for the first time, but one will also be separated from his parents. If the admission is unexpected there will not even be the chance to prepare the children for separation. Yet many hospitals will not allow admission to the healthy twin and, unfortunately, few positively recommend it. In one study of 139 twins admitted to hospital before the age of 7 years only one was accompanied by his twin for non-medical reasons (Griffiths 1981).

Every effort should be made to admit both children and the mother especially, of course, if the babies are being breast-fed. In the rare instances where this is impossible then the healthy child should at least be allowed to stay with his twin throughout the day.

Accidents

No figures are available on the accident rate in twins but it would be surprising if it was not relatively high. It is often difficult to keep a simultaneous eye on two active crawlers or toddlers who have no sense of danger.

Worse than this, however, is the terrifying daring of a bold child encouraged by another. Siblings, let alone single children, rarely get into the same predicaments. In most pairs of siblings there is either an older child with some sense of reality or a younger one who is physically unable to tackle the project. With twins the combination of mutual encouragement and physical cooperation results in more reckless feats—or attempts at them.

There is an added danger for MZ twins. If they are dressed alike particularly in outdoor clothes, many parents cannot distinguish between their twins at a distance. But if a child is about to chase a ball across a busy road a failure to call the correct name may cost a young life (Fig. 10.2).

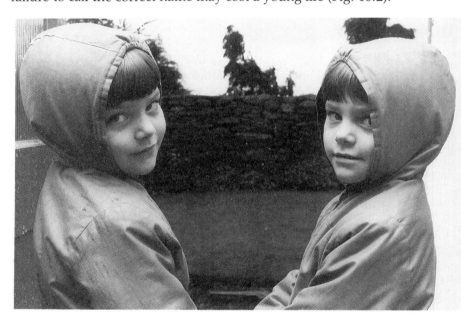

Fig. 10.2   MZ twins indistinguishable when dressed in outdoor clothes.

Some children are undoubtedly accident-prone but it is difficult to know whether an initial accident results in behaviour conducive to further disasters or whether such behaviour is inherent in particular children. Using twins from the Louisville Twin Study, Matheny *et al.* (1971) went some way to answering this question. They reviewed all pairs of twins in which at least one child had had an accident resulting in hospital admission. By referring to their previous records they found there were certain types of behaviour that were more common in the injured children than in their less accident-prone twins.

Child abuse

The non-accidental injury (NAI) of a child by his parent is known to be more common in families under emotional or financial stress and amongst children who were premature or separated from their mother during the first days after birth. It would therefore be reasonable to expect that twins would be at exceptionally high risk of abuse. The mother of DZ twin boys who were born at 28 weeks' gestation weighing 1 kg each was just such a case. After a very stormy neonatal period these much-wanted babies were finally taken home at the age of 3 months with much rejoicing to join their 18-month-old sister. They cried almost incessantly for the next 2 months, by which time the poor mother, despite the excellent support of her husband, was so exhausted and desperate that she begged not to be left alone as she feared that she might harm the babies. Fortunately she admitted to these feelings of aggression. She was given round-the-clock support and within a few months things were much better and the much-loved little boys have thrived. The mother has since given great understanding and support to other mothers living through similar crises.

Accurate data on the frequency of NAI in twins is difficult to find. However, a study from Japan found a much higher incidence of child abuse amongst families with twins (Tanimura *et al.* 1990). This nationwide survey found that 10 per cent of child abuse victims were products of multiple births, almost ten times the rate found in the general population. In 81 per cent of cases only one child was abused. In the cases where both children were abused it was much more likely that the twins were normal babies and that the mother had severe psychosocial problems.

In the far more common cases where only one child was abused, the abused child tended to be the disadvantaged one either because of disability or because he had suffered more neonatal complications, been separated from his mother or been more difficult to care for. A difference in development or responsiveness in the twins was a key factor in provoking abuse of the disadvantaged child.

A significant increase in abuse in families with twins, even when they were full-term, was found in a smaller study by Groothius *et al.* (1982). They also found that siblings of twins were at risk (see p. 130).

Child abuse can, of course, take many forms. One of the most worrying forms that is often missed is the so-called Munchausen syndrome by proxy (Meadow 1977). In these cases the mother deliberately creates symptoms and abnormalities in the child by various means, including drugs and physical insults. This syndrome has been reported in a pair of MZ twins, who presented with recurrent unexplained bleeding (Lee 1979).

It is not uncommon for one child, particularly in pairs of different sex or size, to become the scapegoat and hence the target for parental aggression. If the situation becomes so serious that the abused child must be removed from his parents a dilemma arises. Must he also be separated from his twin or should his twin join him in care at the cost of the second twin being 'unnecessarily' separated from his parents? There is no easy answer. But whatever happens the twins should continue to see as much of each other as possible. They are likely to remain extremely important to each other.

11

Starting school

Starting school is an important milestone for any child. Both parents and children think about it a lot before the big day comes. When the children are twins there are additional aspects to consider. The parents must decide whether the children should be in the same class, or even in the same school. Perhaps the twins should start together and be separated later. But if so, at what stage?

There are no simple or universal answers to these questions. The advantages and disadvantages will need to be weighed for each individual pair and each individual child.

Until recently the little guidance available was based on personal impressions and anecdotal evidence. Now, however, a large study from Australia has provided useful data on the current situation including the perceptions of both teachers and parents in relation to school-age twins. Gleeson and her colleagues (1990) found that in Australia 30 per cent of twins were separated in their first year and that the number increased to nearly 65 per cent by the fourth year. For a substantial minority (23.5 per cent) the separation was not permanent, varying from year to year.

Contrary to what has been generally assumed, the study found no convincing evidence that separation led to a better development of a twin child's individuality, although over 90 per cent of teachers saw this as the main reason for separating twins.

Together or apart?

The gradual loosening of the bond with his parents is a normal stage in a child's development. Starting school has an important part in this process. Twins have a second bond to loosen, often equally strong—that with their co-twin. Most parents expect their twin children to be in separate classes by the time they reach secondary school but careful thought is needed by teachers and parents in deciding whether to separate them earlier. Clearly any decision by the Education Authority about an individual child should be made in close consultation with the parents. Yet in the Australian study it was disturbing to read that 75 per cent of parents felt they had been inadequately consulted about whether or not the children should be separated. Parental reports on the childrens' reactions at home were often not taken into account and the twins themselves were rarely asked about their views.

Very few teachers had received any training about the special needs that twins, particularly boy twins, may have, such as reading difficulties and distractability. Too often they drew extensively from single and, therefore inevitably, non-representative experiences. In 10 per cent of schools there was said to be a fixed policy as to the separation, or non-separation, of twins. Although in no case was this found to be a statutory rule, such rigidity of approach is worrying. More recently, Queensland has actually issued a directive from the Department of Education recognizing that not all twins are the same and that schools should not have a fixed policy on their management.

Teachers would benefit from reading leaflets produced by TAMBA in the UK and the La Trobe Twin Study and AMBA in Australia (see Appendix 2).

Advantages of separation

When separated from his twin a child need no longer be compared with his twin, nor will he be so likely to have particular personality traits emphasized just because they are different from those of his twin (see p. 136).

Some twins like to perform exactly equally with each other and they may contrive to achieve similar results at school. The brighter child may therefore tend to underachieve whereas the slower may be put under undue stress to keep up. Other pairs are conscious of differing abilities, real or imagined, and accept the varying roles expected of them. Either way the children would be better separated.

Parents themselves may become unnecessarily anxious about the childrens' progress if, being in the same class, their differences are readily seen. Children vary not only in their rates of progress but also in the timing of periods of acceleration and periods of assimilation. Parents may be worried by these differences in performance. Just because one child is racing through the reading books and the other is taking them more slowly, there is no reason to assume that the second is failing. Parents need reassurance, but if the children themselves are very conscious of their differing progress they may be happier in separate classes where the differences become less obvious.

Sometimes if one twin is obviously more talented in a particular direction the other will opt out completely. For instance, if one is a star cricketer and the other only average the second may not wish to play at all. Had they been in different classes or schools the second twin would probably have been happy to join in with the others. In this way there may be many kinds of school activities in which the less talented twin may not allow himself the chance to develop as well as he could.

A problem arises if one twin is not only less able than his twin, but also less able than the rest of the class. In this situation a single child would, in some schools, be held back a year. With twins the decision may be more difficult and teachers and parents may not agree on the best strategy (Gleeson *et al.* 1990). Parents were found to be much more reluctant than the teachers for the twins to be in different years. Once held back it is most unlikely that a child will catch up that year and join his twin. To be in a lower class may be particularly difficult through the adolescent years. For this reason it may be worth giving the less-able twin the benefit of the doubt for a little extra time to see if their progress improves. If separation becomes inevitable, different schools may be the best answer, so that their different abilities become less obvious to others as well as to themselves.

However, no child can be protected for ever from recognizing that he is less talented in particular areas than other children, and so it is with twins. We are not all equally endowed and sooner or later twins, like everyone else, have to accept that life is not always fair. Although it may be harder for a twin child, the earlier he can accept the differences the easier will he find it and the happier his relationship with his twin will become.

Girls tend to develop faster in the early school years and this can be a problem in mixed-sex pairs. The girl often tends to 'mother' the boy. At the time he may be quite happy to accept this but in the long-term it may harm his relationship with other children, particularly boys.

Some twins are highly dependent on each other. Obviously some mutual support, particularly in the early days, can be beneficial and twins may settle more quickly if they start in the same class. However, if the dependence is either so intense that it excludes other relationships, or is so unbalanced that one twin performs on behalf of both, it must become harmful. It is not uncommon to find pairs of 5-year-old twins in which one twin answers every time, regardless of who is asked the question.

An extreme example was seen in a pair of MZ boy twins who had changed schools many times due to their father's frequent changes of post in the armed forces. One twin had always been the leader and had answered all questions addressed to his brother as well as to himself. It was only when they reached their first school medical examination at the age of 8 years that the retiring twin was found to have a severe degree of hearing loss. This had never been noticed because of the co-twin's constant intervention on his behalf.

School gives the child, often for the first time, a part of life that is independent of his parents. Some of this life he may want to keep to himself and not necessarily share with the family. If one twin repeatedly reports all that has happened to the other (whether it be good or bad) the second may be distressed, and he is being denied his important right to privacy.

Twins together can make a powerful unit. If they combine forces to be disruptive they can cause chaos in a class, just as they can in a family, and they are then better separated. They should also be separated if one tends to distract the other. Distractability has been found to be a common problem with twins (Gleeson *et al.* 1990), probably because of their much reduced opportunity for periods of uninterrupted activity in the early years.

Many twins use their 'twinship' to confuse teachers and entertain other children. This is harmless fun in small doses but can become a destructive and attention-seeking habit. Phillips and Watkinson (1981) found that 24 per cent of twins played tricks of identity with teachers.

Disadvantages of separation

When kept together twins seem to have less problems settling into school than single children (Koch 1966; J. Stevenson, personal communication).

This is no doubt because they feel less vulnerable. Although they have lost their mother they still have the security of their twin. Most people would agree that if the twins like being together then they should start school in the same class, at least for the first term. If twins are so dependent on each other that they pine and do not join in school activities when parted, there is no point in enforcing separation until they have help to reduce their dependence on each other.

This problem usually arises only with twins who have had no previous experience of acting independently. In these cases separation must be planned as a very gradual process. For instance, the first stage may be for children to sit at different tables within the same class, or at mealtimes, and then generally progress from there.

Although some twins compete excessively, others benefit from the mutual help and mild rivalry. This has been described as the combined pacer and runner effect, with twins alternating in response to each other.

Timing of separation

If twins start school together the timing of the separation must be carefully planned. It is usually better if they separate when a change is due anyway. Otherwise one will remain in the same room with the same teacher and friends and the other may feel rejected as he sets off alone into the unknown.

Some schools may be flexible enough to allow the children to move whenever it seems in their best interests. Others may have a more rigid policy and insist that changes only take place at certain stages in their school career or at the beginning of the academic year. It is important that parents should discover the policy (if any) of their particular school at the outset as it may influence their initial choice of school.

Choice of school

In the UK it seems that most twins go to the same school as each other. In the Birmingham Twin Study out of 201 pairs of twins of primary school age, 199 were at the same school. One child went to a special school (for the disabled) and his twin was at the normal primary school. Only one pair was separated from choice (Phillips and Watkinson 1981).

In the same study, 13 per cent were in different classes by the age of 7 years but only 2 per cent were separated at 5 years. In her study of North American children, Koch found that many more were separated, particularly amongst the boys. At the age of 6 years, half the boys were in different classes and just under a quarter of the girls (Koch 1966).

In rural areas there will probably be only one local school and this is unlikely to have more than one class per year, so the children must necessarily remain together. In towns, where there are more primary schools and most of them will be larger, parents have a choice. Secondary schools appear less sensitive to the needs of twins than primary schools and parents may have to emphasize the importance of respecting the individuality of each child.

Teachers' attitudes

Many teachers welcome the arrival of twins and are eager to accept advice from the parents as how best to help them cope with their twinship in school. Others will have set and often false ideas about twins. They may expect them to be slower than other children, to look alike and to like being treated alike. Many teachers assume that they will not be able to tell the twins apart and therefore make little effort to do so; they see them as a pair with no distinguishing differences in personality or aptitudes. Some twins have even been given shared projects when all the other members of the class have individual ones.

Some teachers, however, may be too keen to compare and contrast the behaviour and abilities of the twins. Care must be taken not to prejudice or otherwise influence teachers by describing particular characteristics of the twins, except, of course, where this is medically or otherwise essential. While each child needs to be recognized and treated as an individual, teachers should be discouraged from comparing them.

It may be helpful to actually arrange separate appointments with a teacher when discussing the progress of each child. Similarly, when messages are being taken by the children from teachers to parents or vice versa, separate messages should be given to each child whenever appropriate.

If twins are in different classes parents will inevitably be faced with the different attitudes and approaches of two teachers. To cope successfully with this it is important that the activities of each child are discussed independently and that, wherever possible, any help with homework is given separately.

Other people's attitudes

As in the rest of their lives twins, particularly MZ, always cause interest at school. Indeed they may attract friends through this without needing to make the social effort otherwise required to develop friendships. They may therefore find it quite difficult when they are first separated and are no longer recognized as part of an interesting pair—losing their so-called prima donna effect; this particularly applies to girl twins.

As with teachers, other parents and children must be encouraged to think of the children as individuals and to make every effort to distinguish them, always calling each by his name. Too often the problems encountered by twins are actually created by other people's attitudes.

Preparation for school

Twins, like any children, need long and careful preparation for school. They need particular help in learning to be independent of each other and the more each has been used to doing things on his own the easier the transition will be. Some parents find it helpful if each attends some playgroup or nursery sessions on his own. Some send the twins together for one morning and on the other two mornings send one or the other on his own. This increases their independence and also allows each of them a period of the parent's undivided attention.

If twins are used to being dressed alike it is important that they get used to looking different. Initially twins, particularly MZ, find this disconcerting and it is helpful if this phase can be worked through before they start school.

Starting school

For those in separate classes it is often helpful if a friend or relative can come to school with the mother until the children have settled. Otherwise a mother may feel torn if both children are tearful and needing her and she has to leave one comfortless.

For twins who are not used to being separated from each other the first few weeks are bound to be stressful. The teachers should be made aware of this. They should ensure that the twins see each other at intervals through the day and are allowed, for instance, to sit together at meals.

If the twins are in the same class it is important that the teacher and the other children should be able easily to tell who is who. In MZ twins different hairstyles are helpful and, of course, different clothes. Even with school uniforms there is usually some opportunity for differences with, say, jumpers and cardigans, skirts and pinafores. Initials on badges can be helpful until everyone is sure they can tell them apart. Names should be avoided because of the danger of attracting strangers. It may be necessary specifically to ask the teacher—and hence the class—not to refer to them as 'the twins'.

Unfortunately, it is not only the teachers' attitudes that may be misguided. The parents themselves may insist on the children looking alike. One teacher had this problem with a pair of 11-year-old MZ twin girls who neither she nor the class could tell apart. The twins always dressed alike but their abilities were quite different. One was intelligent and confident and the other was shy and found school work difficult. The teacher's approach to each child should have been very different but she found the constant confusion of identity a severe handicap to her relationship with them. She asked the mother if they could have some form of identification even if it was only a coloured hair slide. The mother adamantly refused.

On the whole, twin children are popular, although they may be less gregarious (Koch 1966). They usually have no trouble in making friends. They are used to cooperative games and are usually better at these than with individual activities. Phillips and Watkinson (1981) found that most twins made some separate friends; only one-third of 7-year-olds always shared the same friends. Occasionally, one twin may be much more outgoing than the other and have a much larger circle of friends, but this is not necessarily harmful. Each may be finding his own natural inclinations and allowing twins to develop their own individual relationships is vital to their adolescent development.

Finally, it must be remembered that many twins have no problems at school and are as happy and successful as single children. However, by being aware of the possible problems and, where necessary, taking preventive or remedial action, teachers will help a far greater number of children to enjoy and benefit fully from their time at school.

12

Growth and development of twins

Twins are at a disadvantage from the moment of conception. The problems facing them both in intrauterine life and in early childhood have been described in earlier chapters. But what of their long-term mental and physical development? Is this affected by these earlier problems, or indeed by the 'twin situation'?

Physical growth

In view of the relatively high proportion of twins who suffer from intra-uterine growth retardation it is not surprising to find that on the average adult twins are smaller than singletons. Male twins in Sweden, at the time of their 'call-up' for military service, were 1.3 cm smaller than their singleton counterparts (Husen 1959). More surprising, perhaps, is the relatively small discrepancy in adulthood considering the marked difference in size between twins and singletons at birth (see p. 98). Several studies have shown a remarkable catch-up, particularly in the case of the smaller of a size-discrepant pair, during the first year (see below).

The most comprehensive data on growth in twins have come from the Louisville Twin Study (Wilson 1983), in which 900 white North American twins were studied from birth. By 1979 over 400 had been followed beyond their eighth birthday and, as a result, Wilson (1979) has produced the centile charts for height, weight and occipitofrontal circumference (Figs. 12.1 and 12.2).

By 4 years twins had almost caught up with singletons in height but not in weight. Similarly, Buckler and Buckler (1987) found that twin children were taller than they were heavy, which is the pattern often found in intrauterine growth-retarded single children. Wilson suggests that this may be because the normal rate of replication of adipose cells during fetal life was reduced because of the greater nutritional demands imposed by a twin pregnancy. On the other hand, Chamberlain and Simpson (1977), in a random sample of nearly 200 British 3½-year-old twins, found that the twins were similarly proportioned to singletons but were significantly lighter and shorter.

None of these studies has made allowances for prematurity and Elliman and her colleagues (1986) have shown that even at 3 years correction for prematurity may make a significant difference to the relative values for height and weight.

Wilson (1974a) found that the boys grew relatively faster during the first 6

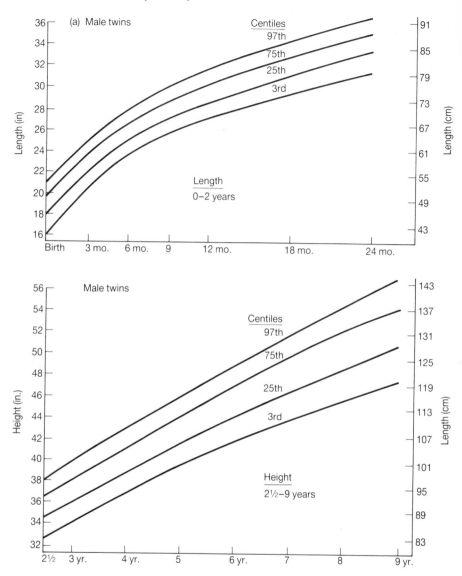

Fig. 12.1   Centile charts for height in twins from 0–9 years. (a) Boys; (b) girls. From Wilson (1979) by permission of the author and the editors of *Annals of Human Biology.*

months whereas girls accelerated during the third year. The catch-up of both sexes in relation to singletons continued and by 8 years of age there were no significant differences in either height or weight between twins and singletons.

However, Buckler and Buckler (1987) found that, although their heights

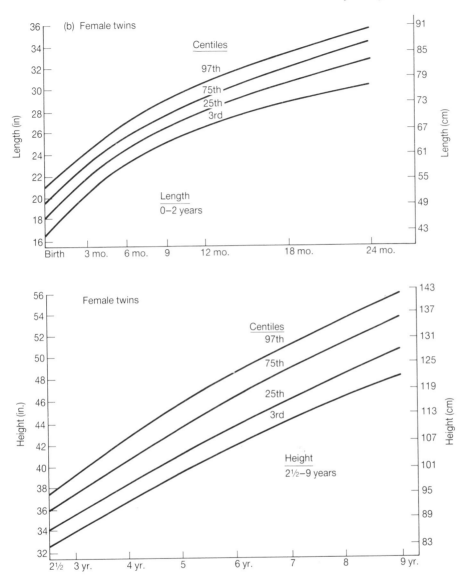

were the same as the general population, twins were shorter and lighter than their siblings, although the deficit in height was limited to the group who had been very light for dates (below 5th centile) at birth. When this group was excluded there was no significant difference in height between the twins and their siblings.

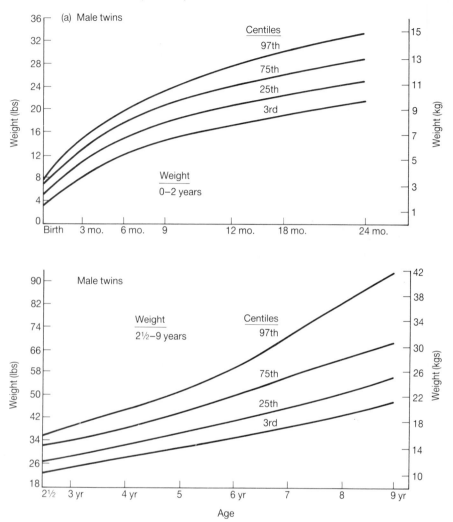

Fig. 12.2 Centile charts for weight in twins from 0–9 years. (a) boys; (b) girls. From Wilson (1979) by permission of the author and the editors of *Annals of Human Biology*.

The Louisville Twin Study did not show growth rates in relation to birth weight. It may well be that larger pairs do better than smaller. Drillien (1964) found that, even with good home conditions, twins who weighed less than 2.5 kg at birth never made up their initial growth deficit. But a contemporary study is needed to confirm this point, as the children in Drillien's study were born during an era when it was the practice to restrict the food intake of low birth-weight babies.

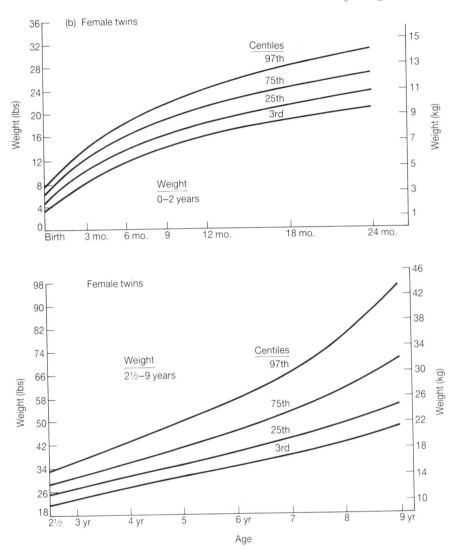

A longitudinal study of growth patterns in older twins has been reported by Ljung *et al.* (1977), who followed over 300 twin pairs from 10 to 18 years. In boys they found that the differences in height, weight and peak growth velocity between twins and singletons were all small and much less than the differences between twin and singleton girls. The girls showed a significant deficit particularly during puberty—their peak height velocity, peak weight velocity and menarche all came later than in singleton girls. It was suggested that this relatively better performance by twin boys might be due to selective survival, as there is a higher early mortality amongst twin boys than twin girls (Figs. 12.3 and 12.4).

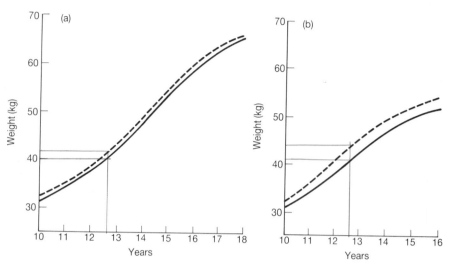

Fig. 12.3   Weight charts in twins 10–18 years compared with singletons. (a) boys; (b) girls. From Ljung *et al.* (1977) by permission of the authors and editors of *Annals of Human Biology.* —Twins; --- controls.

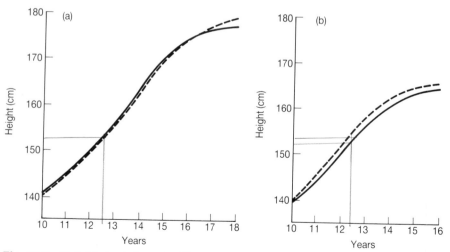

Fig. 12.4   Height charts in twins 10–18 years compared with singletons. (a) boys; (b) girls. From Ljung *et al.* (1977) by permission of the authors and editors of *Annals of Human Biology.* —Twins; --- controls.

Zygosity

Over the years the growth of MZ twins becomes progressively more concordant and that of DZ less concordant (Wilson 1979); this is to be expected. As extrauterine environmental influences are likely to be similar for both members of a twin pair then the genetic influence will dictate any differences in growth pattern from birth onwards. In intrauterine life, however, the environment of one fetus may be very different from that of the co-twin, particularly in MZ pairs.

Genetic influences take time to counteract the effects of prenatal experience and it may be several years before long-term growth patterns are established. Tanner *et al.* (1956) showed that the 'genetic target curve' in singletons is not reached until the age of 2 or 3 years. Vandenberg and Falkner (1966) found the same tendency in twins. The concordance for growth was very similar for MZ and like-sexed DZ twins during the first few months but thereafter the DZ twins became increasingly discordant. Not surprisingly, as they are dictated to by the same 'gene-action system', MZ twins also tend to have similar patterns of growth, making their periods of growth spurt or latency coincidental (Fig. 12.5).

The effect of other intrauterine influences was considered by Falkner (1978). He found that postnatal growth in MZ twins can depend in part on

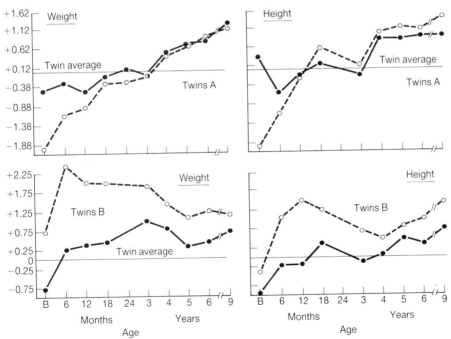

Fig. 12.5 Growth charts in two pairs of MZ twins of discrepant birth weight showing later similarity of intrapair growth. From Wilson (1979) by permission of the author and editors of *Annals of Human Biology*.

types of placentation. MZ monochorionic pairs became progressively more similar in weight between birth and 4 years, their initial intrapair difference of 14.4 per cent falling over the period to 2.9 per cent, whereas MZ dichorionic pairs maintained a remarkably similar intrapair discrepancy (9.5–10.7 per cent) throughout.

Although intrapair comparisons of growth have been made in relation to zygosity, most studies have not distinguished between MZ and DZ twins in comparing twins with singletons. It is possible that MZ twins have a reduced growth potential due to their loss of size in early embryonic life. This early zygote division has been proposed as an explanation for the lower birth weight of MZ twins (see p. 48). Husen (1959) did find that adult male MZ twins were significantly (even if only 0.85 cm) shorter than DZ twins. However, genetic factors could also explain the DZ twins' greater height. Mothers of DZ twins are on average taller than MZ (see p. 22).

Intrapair discrepancies in birth weight

There is disagreement in the literature as to how the smaller of a pair of twins fares physically and mentally in the long-term.

Several workers have found that when there were large intrapair differences in birth weight in MZ twins, some discrepancy persists (Babson and Phillips 1973; Wilson 1979; Henrichsen *et al.* 1986). In a group of ten MZ pairs with intrapair weight differences of over 750 g, Wilson (1979) found that, at 6 years, the smaller twin was still significantly lighter and marginally shorter, but had no significant reduction in IQ.

The degrees of intrauterine growth retardation in the smaller twin is probably more important than the size of the intrapair weight discordancy. In a group of MZ twins with large birth weight discrepancies (25 per cent or more) Keet *et al.* (1986) found that where the smaller twin was above the 10th centile for weight at birth the catch-up growth was good. For those below the 10th centile the prognosis had to be more guarded, particularly, as with singletons (Holmes *et al.* 1977; Walthers and Ramaekers 1982), for those with a normal ponderal index. Those with a low ponderal index, even if their weight was below the 10th centile, had more chance of catching up.

However, there have been several case reports of astonishing catch-ups (Buckler and Robinson 1974; Falkner 1978). Just occasionally the growth of the smaller-born twin will actually overtake the larger one. This may be due to a chronic debilitating disease or disability in the larger-born twin. Sometimes, however, there is no apparent explanation. For example, at birth one MZ twin, the donor in a fetofetal transfusion syndrome (see p. 52), weighed 1560 g and his co-twin weighed 2700 g. By 18 months there was only 180 g difference in weight and by their ninth birthday the smaller was actually 1 cm taller than his brother. He then went into puberty over a year ahead of his brother and, at the age of 14 years, his radiological bone age was 11 months ahead of his brother. At one stage he was 8 cm taller.

Why some smaller MZ twins should show such a remarkable ability to catch up whilst others remain permanently smaller is uncertain. It may well be that there are two distinct groups of intrauterine growth-retarded twins. One, the catchers-up, would be those who probably suffered from malnutrition only in the latter part of pregnancy, and thus they had acquired their full cellular complement and, therefore, potential for growth. The other—the laggards—would be those whose differential growth was established early in pregnancy, thereby reducing their long-term growth potential.

Mental development

It is popularly said that twins are less clever than single children. Some parents worry that this reduced intelligence will be a serious handicap to their children. It is true that most, although not all, studies have shown that the mean IQ of twins is somewhat lower than that of singletons (Mehrotra and Maxwell 1949; Scottish Council for Research in Education 1953; Husen 1961; Drillien 1964; Record *et al.* 1970; Kranitz and Welcher 1971; Churchill and Henderson 1974; Myrianthopoulos *et al.* 1976; Zazzo 1979). However, the great majority of twins will be well within the normal range for singletons. Indeed, there have been many examples of brilliant pairs of twins, as well as individual twins, in all walks of life (Scheinfeld 1973; Bryan 1992).

Husen (1961, 1963) reported a large study of Danish school-age twins of 11–15 years. He found that the mean IQ of twins was between one-quarter and one-third of a standard deviation below that of singletons. This was not just due to a large number of low scorers. The overall distribution of scores was similar to that found in singletons but with the curve shifted to the left. Zazzo (1979) found that this was true throughout the socio-economic groups, suggesting that, even in the most favourable conditions, twins were at a disadvantage.

Drillien (1964) found that at all ages between 6 months and 4 years the developmental quotients (DQ) of twins were lower than singletons. She divided both her singletons and twins into four groups according to birth weight. There was a positive correlation between birth weight and DQ in both twins and singletons at all ages, and twins scored consistently lower than singletons.

In the Louisville Study, however, it was found that although twins were relatively retarded at 18 months, they had caught up by their sixth birthday and by this age there was no significant difference between twins and singletons (Wilson 1974b).

There is plainly scope for more research in this area. In considering the inferior performance of twins the detrimental effect of close sibling spacing in itself must not be forgotten. Singletons born close together are known to be at a disadvantage and twinship is the extreme example of close spacing. Zazzo (1960) demonstrated this. Whereas singletons in general scored seven points higher in IQ testing than twins, siblings born close together were superior to twins by only 2.25 points.

Reading

Reading problems have been shown to be more common in twins than singletons (Bakwin 1973; Watts and Lytton 1980; Johnston *et al.* 1984; Ghodsein 1989) and there is a stronger connection with early language problems and later reading problems than in singletons (Johnston *et al.* 1984). Eight- to 9-year-old boy twins had reading difficulties of a different type to single children. Together with delayed reading they tended to have a cluster of problems including spelling, letter reversal and numeracy difficulties.

Children frustrated by their inability to read may develop antisocial and attention-seeking behaviour. Hay *et al.* (1987) found that conduct disorders were more common amongst twins than single children. However, Ghodsein (1989), in analysing the British National Child Development Study data on behaviour at 7, 11 and 16 years, found only a slight increase in overall behavioural difficulties in twins, and these tended to be conduct disorders in boys.

Zygosity

Again, few studies have differentiated between MZ and DZ but, where they do, MZ twins are more alike in their mental development than DZ (Husen 1963; Wilson 1974b). MZ become increasingly concordant with age and parallel each other for spurts and lags (Fig. 12.6). DZ twins become progressively less concordant and eventually match singleton siblings as closely as they do each other (Wilson 1978, 1981).

Placentation

It has been suggested that differences in placentation might in themselves affect the long-term development of twins. Melnick and Myrianthopoulos (1979) found significantly less variability in the intrapair scores of MZ monochorionic 7-year-old twins than MZ dichorionic. Indeed, they found that intrapair differences in MZ dichorionic twins were surprisingly similar to those in DZ twins. It is difficult to explain this finding and others have not confirmed it (Brown 1977; Welch *et al.* 1978). If anything, MZ dichorionic twins could be expected to be more alike as they have smaller intrapair birth weight discrepancies and they are not at risk from the potentially long-term effects of the fetofetal transfusion syndrome.

Birth weight

It is well known that light-for-dates singletons tend to have lower IQ scores than those who are appropriately grown at birth. It is not surprising, therefore, to find that within a pair of MZ twins the heavier born is likely to be more intelligent than his lighter co-twin (Scarr 1969; Munsinger 1977; Henrichsen *et al.* 1986) and this applies throughout the socio-economic groups (Willerman and Churchill 1967). Most studies have shown this trend, although some have not found that the difference reached levels of significance (Fujikura and Froehlich 1974).

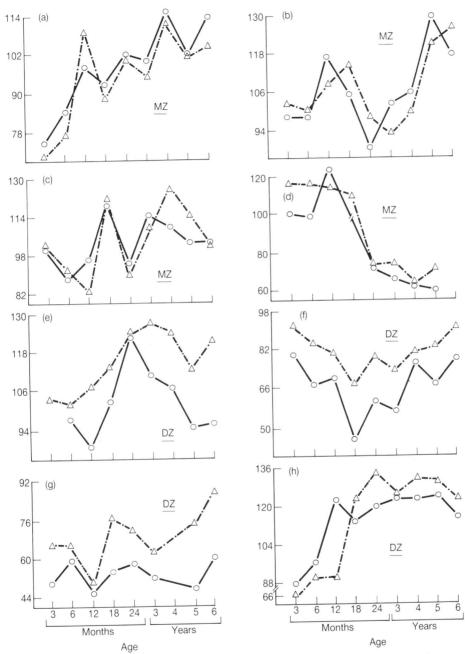

Fig. 12.6   Mental development of eight pairs of twins showing greater concordance in pattern in MZ pairs than in DZ. From Wilson (1978) by permission of the author and editors of *Science*. Copyright 1978 by the American Association for the Advancement of Science.

Kaelber and Pugh (1969) compared a group of MZ twins who differed in birth weight by less than 300 g from their co-twin with a second group whose intrapair discrepancies were over 300 g. The average IQ difference between the heavier and lighter twins in the first group was 0.48, whereas in the second it was 5.76. Scarr (1969) reported similar findings in a group of 52 MZ pairs.

Babson and Phillips (1973), in their serial observations of nine MZ pairs with an average birth weight difference of 36 per cent, found that the lighter twin remained smaller and less intelligent into adulthood. However, there was less intrapair discrepancy in school performances than would have been expected from the results of the test scores, which suggests that the smaller twin had made an extra effort to compensate for his deficit.

A study of the neurological outcome for twins with large birth weight discrepancies (Ylitalo *et al.* 1988) found a higher incidence of problems in fine motor performance, coordination and visuomotor perception in the smaller twin.

Those who find that the smaller twin does less well blame the prenatal environment for his handicap, whereas those who find that the little one does almost as well as his twin consider that the strength of the common genetic influence over-rides other factors.

A common postnatal environment may blur the effects of birth weight discrepancies on mental development, particularly if the smaller twin has the constant stimulus of a more intelligent twin and, probably, extra encouragement and help from parents. To eliminate these postnatal influences Munsinger (1977) studied 23 pairs of twins who were separated at birth and who appeared, from the literature, to have been of obviously differing size at birth. He surmised that, in most cases, if not all, the fetofetal transfusion syndrome had been responsible for the differences. In this group the heavier twin had a higher IQ in 19 instances and the average discrepancy was 11.4 points, with an overall average IQ of 93.5. In contrast, 26 pairs of separated twins of similar birth weight had a discrepancy of only 3.9 and an overall average IQ of 99.9. From these results he concluded that any estimates of heritability in behavioural genetics would be biased if MZ twins of discrepant birth weight were included and that the strength of genetic influences would be underestimated.

13

The disabled twin

The parents of twins face not only the double risk of having a child with a disability but, because the children are twins, the risk is further increased because many forms of disability are more common amongst twins. The high incidence of congenital malformations has already been discussed (see p. 55). Some twins are left with scars such as mental retardation or cerebral palsy from an intrauterine insult. Others may be damaged as a direct result of their intrauterine twin relationship (see below). A number, although fewer than was previously believed, suffer lasting damage from perinatal hazards.

Mental retardation

It is generally agreed that mental retardation is more common in twins than singletons (Berg and Kirman 1960; Illingworth and Woods 1960; Allen and Kallmann 1962). The only form that actually appears to be less common is that due to trisomy 21—Down syndrome.

Exact figures are difficult to obtain as most data are derived from institutionalized patients amongst whom there may be a selective bias. For instance, a family might cope at home with one retarded child but be defeated by two. On the other hand, if one of a pair of twins is disabled the parents may feel less inclined to separate the two by sending one away. This also applies, of course, to other disabling conditions, such as cerebral palsy.

Severely disabled individuals are often not included in studies of the general population, for instance in groups of schoolchildren or, as in Husen's study of those undergoing routine medical examination for military enrolment. Nevertheless, Husen (1959) found that the number of young adult twins with an IQ of less than 75 was twice that in the general population.

The secondborn twin and the smaller of a pair appear to be at greater risk than their co-twins (Berg and Kirman 1960). This would suggest that pre- as well as perinatal insults are the important aetiological factors. Likewise, MZ twins are more commonly affected, probably due to their more hazardous intrauterine existence.

Cerebral palsy

Depending on differences in definitions and standards of data collection, cerebral palsy occurs in from 2 to 4 per 1000 of all births. For twins the only report from a total population is of 79 multiple births (74 twins and 5 triplets) in Western Australia from 1956 to 1985, where the incidence of cerebral palsy in twins was 6.3 per 1000 live births and in triplets was 32 per 1000 live births, compared with 2.4 in single live births (Petterson *et al.* 1990).

Many authors have found that twins are over-represented amongst children with cerebral palsy (Asher and Schonell 1950; Benda 1952; Greenspan and Deaver 1953; Yue 1955; Russell 1961; Eastman *et al.* 1962; Alberman 1964; Durkin *et al.* 1976; Stanley 1979). Incidences vary from 5.4 to 10.4 per cent (Asher and Schonnell 1950; Alberman 1964) amongst groups of cerebral palsied children, which is three to five times the incidence of twin individuals in the general population. Within a pair, the smaller of the two at birth is at greater risk (Russell 1961).

Griffiths (1967), in her study of 78 twin pairs in which one or both twins had cerebral palsy, found only four instances of concordance but 16 of the children were single surviving twins, their co-twin having been stillborn or having died in the neonatal period. Of those whose twins had died 80 per cent were thought to be MZ. Petterson *et al.* (1990) found six out of nine MZ pairs were concordant for cerebral palsy whereas amongst the 21 pairs of DZ pairs there were no instances in which both twins were affected. In 24 cases the co-twin had died in the perinatal period.

Earlier studies found that the highest incidence of cerebral palsy was amongst secondborn and breech-delivered infants. When the first twin was affected, the mean delivery interval was 25 min, compared with 228 min when the second twin was affected (Griffiths 1967). There were two distinct neurological pictures amongst the children, depending on their birth order. The firstborn infant who developed cerebral palsy was more likely to have been premature and vertex-delivered, and characteristically suffered from spastic diplegia. Affected secondborn twins tended to be more mature and to have a more severe form of cerebral palsy, such as quadriplegia and/or athetosis. In these cases the damage was thought to be related to malpresentation and birth asphyxia but in many instances these factors are simply indices of an already abnormal fetus. More recent studies, however, have found no significant effect of birth order on outcome (McCarthy *et al.* 1981, Petterson *et al.* 1990). Petterson's study also revealed an increasing sex ratio with increasing plurality. In affected twins the ratio was 2.1 compared to 1.3 for singletons and all five affected triplets were boys.

Alberman (1964) also found a bimodal distribution to cerebral palsy in twins and suggested that there may be two separate aetiological groups. The first group were babies of less than 32 weeks gestation and the incidence of cerebral palsy in the group was no higher amongst twins than singletons of the same gestational period. However, in the second group, whose incidence peaked at 37 weeks gestational age, the occurence of cerebral palsy was greatly in excess of that expected in babies of such maturity.

Another aetiological factor in cerebral palsy peculiar to twinning has been emphasized by Durkin *et al.* (1976). Of 19 twins with cerebral palsy and severe mental retardation, nine had a stillborn co-twin. The author suggests that the cerebral damage could have been caused by intrauterine disseminated intravascular coagulation, as a result of the surviving monochorionic fetus sharing a placental circulation with a macerated dead fetus (see p. 71).

Many of the studies on cerebral palsy in twins were reported in the 1960s. The pattern is likely now to be changing as obstetric care improves and more very preterm infants are surviving.

Studies in the general population have shown that improvements in obstetric care over the past 30 years have been associated with a fall in perinatal mortality but not with any change in the prevalence of cerebral palsy (Edmond *et al.* 1989).

This may be due to the increasing numbers of low birth-weight survivors who are more liable than normal birth weight babies to suffer from cerebral palsy. It is possible that any fall in the numbers due to birth trauma or asphyxia is balanced by an increase in the numbers of low birth-weight survivors.

As yet there are no data available to show whether there has been any change in the distribution of the different types of cerebral palsy in twins, although from recent research it appears that the number of firstborn twins with cerebral palsy is now rising. (MacGillivray 1990).

Any deviation from normal in the development of a twin child will often be detected earlier than in a single child because the mother is made more aware of the defects of one child as she watches the progress of the other. This early detection can be very valuable in ensuring early investigation and, where necessary, intervention.

Parental reactions

The response of a parent to a disabled child, especially if the disability is recognized at or soon after birth, may be very similar to that of bereavement. Denial, anger, guilt and grief are all reactions common to both. The parents mourn for the healthy child that 'might have been' and parents with one normal twin have no difficulty in imagining this—the image of the healthy child is constantly there alongside the disabled one. Rather than rejoicing in the normality of the one child the parents may, often unconsciously, blame the healthy child for the disability of the other. There are other yet more complex dangers. For example, parents may not only overpraise the achievements of the disabled twin but fail sufficiently to celebrate those of his healthy sister or brother. The parents may feel guilty about feeling unqualified joy about these or fear such enthusiasm would hurt the disadvantaged child. Joy can be 'denied' as well as pain or loss. Many parental attitudes may be similar to those towards a single surviving twin (see Chapter 14).

Furthermore, the mother has the additional 'bereavement' of effectively losing her motherhood of twins. Many mothers find it difficult to relinquish the image of the twinship, even when the two children have very different physical and mental ages. It is not unusual to see twins dressed alike, even when one is severely disabled. One mother refused initially to allow a surgical boot for her 4-year-old daughter as it would mean that, for the first time, these MZ girls would not be identically dressed.

Responding appropriately to both children may be a genuine problem, particularly in the preschool period when the healthy child may still not understand the implications of his twin's disability. Appropriate encouragement for the two children can be difficult. A healthy 3-year-old whose own physical feats appeared to go unnoticed, resented the praise showered on his diplegic brother who had just learnt to crawl. Another child noticed that his disabled brother received a hug every time he fell down and was disconcerted to find that he did not receive one himself when he contrived assorted accidents.

The fact that the disabled child's achievements receive exaggerated praise may irritate him as much as it does his non-disabled twin. Well-meaning people often overcompensate in praising a disabled child, even where no special tribute is appropriate. The child may indeed often enjoy it being accepted without comment that he can perform entirely adequately in some areas.

It is not uncommon for a healthy twin sibling to regress in their development and imitate their disabled sibling during times of stress. It may be helpful at such times to attempt to compensate for the extra attention given to the disabled child by helping the healthy child acquire his own special friends and to have more separate outings with his parents.

Visits to doctors and therapists may often be time-consuming and the problems of taking (or leaving) the healthy twin may, at times, be insurmountable. Plainly, every consideration should be given to such families. Arrangements for the care of the healthy twin should be as much the concern of the paediatric team as for their patient. It is often quite practicable for the twin to join in the activities of the therapy groups. The mother will then be more relaxed and more able to concentrate on the disabled child.

Reactions of the twins

It has been found that siblings of disabled children are more prone to conduct disorders, aggressive behaviour and to depression (Breslau and Prabucki 1987). There have been no such studies on the twin of a disabled child but it would be surprising if the emotional stress were not at least as great as for an ordinary sibling. Indeed, there are likely to be additional and more complex emotions experienced by these children—the healthy twin may feel both guilt and jealousy. He may well feel jealous of all the time spent on his twin. The mother will often feel that she alone is capable of feeding and caring for the disabled child, whereas any passing friend or neighbour can feed the healthy one. The disabled child may have to be carried by his mother for many years, whereas the other one has to trudge behind as soon as he is able to walk.

Similarly, far more attention from parents, professionals and visitors may be focussed on the disabled twin. Numerous therapists and helpers become 'special friends' to the disabled child, often ignoring the healthy one. It is the more important that he too should have his special visitors.

Some children will show their jealousy in aggression, others in more complex behavioural patterns. One bright 8-year-old twin became so jealous of all the extra attention and 'treats', such as taxi journeys and riding (for the disabled) that her sister enjoyed that she became increasingly withdrawn and hostile and finally reached a crisis when she developed a hysterical hemiplegia.

Inevitably, some of the normal family activities, such as hiking or museum-visiting, may have to be curtailed. Some school-age children find it difficult to cope with the embarrassment of having a twin who does not look normal or behave in expected ways. This may make them reluctant to have friends to the house.

Some healthy twins come to feel guilty in later years that they have been spared their twin's affliction particularly, for instance, if they received more intrauterine nourishment. Some may strive to make amends. One MZ boy of 13 was referred to me because of his refusal to participate in any extracurricular activities at school. He was a bright child who was doing well at school but would hurry home as soon as obligatory classes were over to play with his severely mentally disabled twin. Such concern on behalf of the disadvantaged twin is very welcome—and helpful—but it can go too far. In cases like this some careful counselling, both for the twin and his parents, may be needed, and possibly also arrangements that relieve some of the healthy twin's burden. For example, someone else to entertain the disabled twin on certain evenings.

It can be very hard for both twins when one of identical twins is disabled. Each can see what he might have been like. One MZ twin described the sight of his disabled brother as 'like looking in the mirror at a caricature of myself'. Even in pairs who are close friends it must inevitably be difficult to watch the accomplishments of your twin sister or brother when you know that you can never achieve the same. For the parents the joy in the success of one child is bound to evoke sadness for the other.

Clearly, as they grow beyond babyhood the intellectual and physical needs of the two children will increasingly diverge. To balance the needs of the disabled child with those of his siblings is always a problem for parents. With twins there is danger that by emphasizing the twinship the development of the more advanced child may be held back. The needs, and particularly the feelings, of the healthy twin are often just as complex and a family may need skilled counselling in coping with them (Bernabei and Levi 1976).

There are, of course, positive aspects. The disabled child has a constant source of stimulation (Fig. 13.1) and the opportunity for regular contact with normal children through his twin's friends. The potentially therapeutic influence of normal siblings on children with disabilities has been clearly demonstrated (Craft *et al.* 1990). A child may be more effective in motivating his disabled twin than the parents. For various reasons, not least pressure of twins on the parents, the disabled twin may be less overprotected than a similarly disabled singleton.

The self-confidence of the healthy twin may also be increased if he feels he has an important role. He may acquire valuable understanding and sensitivity towards disability. The caring attitude developed by many twins is clearly very rewarding but it may sometimes be difficult for parents to strike the right balance between encouraging this caring and avoiding imposing objective burdens, an exaggerated sense of obligation and also thereby feed possible later resentment.

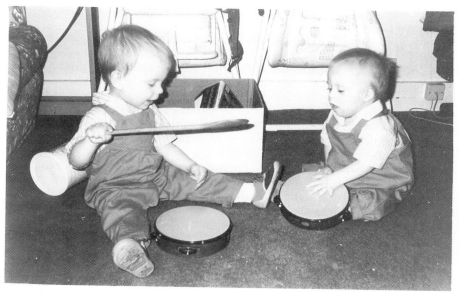

Fig. 13.1 3-year-old child with Down syndrome playing with his twin brother.

This chapter has concentrated on twins discordant for disability. Clearly, if both children are disabled, the physical and emotional burden on the parents can be enormous, not least the (irrational) guilt they may themselves feel. However, such problems are dealt with thoroughly in many general or specialized books on disabled children. The complexities of caring for a healthy and disabled child of the same age are less well understood.

14

Death of a twin

All too many parents of twins have to face the death of one or both their twins. Not only do they have twice the risk of a child dying but from the moment of conception the mortality rate of twins is relatively high.

An unknown, but certainly large, number of single twins are lost in early pregnancy (see p. 34). In later pregnancy the risk of intrauterine death is higher than for singletons; higher still is the neonatal mortality rate (see p. 105). This increased risk of death persists, although at a lower level, at least throughout the first year of life.

For parents of twins the loss of both babies is a tragedy that, for some, is heightened by the shattering of the extraordinary social prestige that attaches to having twins. But, just as the parents once gained the admiring attention of relatives, friends and the medical profession, so also will they now gain the sympathy.

Not so the parents who lose one twin; particularly a twin who was stillborn or died within the first few days. Consciously or not, society forgets the dead baby. Attention and feelings are focussed on the surviving child and the parents are encouraged to do the same. This is understandable, often well-intentioned, and wrong. It deprives the parents of fully mourning, which can often mean that the repercussions of loss are more severe and long-lasting than they need to be (Lewis and Bryan 1988).

With a single bereavement there is the additional difficulty of having a constant reminder in the survivor of the child that might have been; this is enhanced further in MZ twins. Later the parents will have to come to cope with the, often complex, feelings of a child deprived of its close partner.

Abortion and fetus papyraceus

The spontaneous abortion of twins is little, if any, more common than that of singletons. The loss of one of the two fetuses during the first trimester is not, however, unusual (see p. 32). Before the introduction of ultrasound these twin pregnancies were unrecognized, except when a fetus papyraceus was noticed when the single baby was delivered. The only other abnormality might have been a vaginal bleed in the early months.

There are other occasions when a twin pregnancy is missed. Some 'premature' babies, thought to have been conceived immediately after an early spontaneous abortion, are surprisingly large and mature for their length of gestation. It is likely that at least some of these babies are single survivors of the original (twin) pregnancy.

A fetus papyraceus can give rise to considerable anxiety. It is often insufficiently explained to the parents. The surviving twin may feel a sense of something odd or hidden and distressing about their birth.

It is not known how much the early loss of a twin fetus may affect the mother or the single survivor. At least some twins have personality problems related to the loss of their partner. This may be so even when the survivor is not conscious of having been a twin. It may be more important than is yet generally realized that both mother and child should be aware of the twinship (Lewis 1983).

Birth and death before 28 weeks gestation

In the UK, birth occurring before 28 completed weeks of the pregnancy used to be defined as a miscarriage. If a twin was born dead before 28 weeks and a sibling was liveborn and either survived or died later, the legal paradox and ambiguity added to the confusion and distress accompanying any perinatal bereavement and may have further impeded mourning. This experience is movingly described in a personal paper (Gabrielczyk 1987). The legal limit of viability has now been reduced to 24 weeks, which will avoid the problem of ambiguity in almost all cases.

Selective feticide

The intrauterine killing of an abnormal fetus in a multiple pregnancy where the other is normal is now an option available to parents who would otherwise have to choose between terminating the whole pregnancy, despite the sacrifice of a normal baby, or continuing the pregnancy while knowingly carrying an abnormal child (see p. 42).

Although, for many, selective feticide may be the least unacceptable option in this situation, the bereavement of the mother may be profound and the experience itself very distressing. The thought of a live baby lying for many weeks by the side of his dead twin can be very disturbing. Because the baby has not been aborted the process of mourning may be delayed. For many parents the full impact of the bereavement is not felt until the delivery, many weeks later, of a solitary live baby—the undeniable evidence that they will not become the parents of twins. By this time, however, the carers may have 'forgotten' the twin and this failure to acknowledge and respect the dead baby may add to the mother's distress (Bryan 1989). A photograph of the ultrasound scan showing both babies may be a precious and unique proof to parents that they were ever expecting more than one child.

Unlike a straightforward termination of pregnancy, memory of the lost baby will be preserved by the presence of the survivor.

Stillbirth and neonatal death

After months of expectation and anticipation of a life-to-be there is no bigger anticlimax than the birth of a dead baby. Society shuns it. Even the medical profession tends to turn away. It wraps it up and buries it as soon as possible. It tries its best to forget the baby ever was (Bourne 1968). People manage to do this distressingly soon (for the parents) even with a single baby.

With twins this reality avoidance can be accomplished with dangerously greater ease. Attention to the surviving twin provides an escape route. Once out of the delivery room, by concentrating on the live baby, it is quite possible never to mention the dead baby again. Some mothers have found that midwives whom they have known well during their pregnancy did not—perhaps could not—even refer to the baby who died.

In fact the mother, and often the father too, wants to talk about the stillborn baby. They naturally want to ask questions about how and why it happened, to vent anger, to attribute blame, just to share their feelings, rational or not, about the baby they have lost and what he or she might have been.

Mothers invariably feel shame and to some extent guilt about the baby's death. Somehow they feel responsible, even that they have actually 'killed' their baby. The mother's guilt may be increased by misguided remarks such as, 'How lucky you still have a healthy one' or 'Two babies would have been such a handful'.

This concentration by other people on the healthy baby to the exclusion of the stillbirth that the mother is longing to talk about may induce her to idealize the dead baby (her 'angel baby') and positively alienate her from the survivor. Its 'normal' crying, feeding habits and restlessness may irritate her quite unreasonably, so much so that she may come to feel it is punishing her. Child abuse would not be unexpected in situations of this kind and has been reported in a surviving twin of a 'cot death' (Bluglass 1980).

It is known that pregnancy and the arrival of a new baby inhibits mourning (Lewis 1979). A pregnancy following too soon after a stillbirth may have disastrous consequences. If the mother has not adequately mourned her dead baby she is likely to have serious misidentifications of the new child with its dead sibling (Lewis and Page 1978). Twins are an extreme example of this. The mother experiences the joy of the new life and the tragedy of death simultaneously. She is therefore likely to attempt to suppress her grief; those around her encourage her to do so. She may appear to do this successfully for some time but later, sometimes after many years, she may well suffer from severe psychiatric disorders.

Maternity hospital staff should do all they can to facilitate rather than impede, the normal process of mourning (Lewis 1983). Suppressing this natural process of grieving and lament is likely to delay acceptance and have damaging results for each parent, for their marriage and not least for the surviving twin.

In their study of mothers a year after the perinatal death of a baby Rowe and her colleagues (1978) found that mothers who had lost one of their twins tended to suffer from more psychiatric morbidity than those who had lost their only child. A recent study of over 13 000 families with 5-year-olds in the UK similarly found that the highest malaise scores, indicating depression, were amongst the few mothers who had lost one of their twins (Thorpe *et al.* 1991). The group was too small to reach statistical significance and the subject is clearly in need of further study.

It is important that a mother is able clearly to distinguish the two babies in her mind. One mother, who had never seen her stillborn baby, felt that the surviving twin was 'only half a baby' (Lewis 1983). If she had some substantive memories of the dead baby she would have found it easier to avoid the confusion. All parents should be given the opportunity, and be encouraged, to see the dead baby and indeed to handle it.

Naming the dead baby can be particularly important in twins. It becomes much easier for the parent to distinguish the babies in their mind and when they talk about them. For the survivor it is obviously easier if he can refer to his sibling by name.

A photograph should always be taken. Photographs should be as natural a part of death as they are of life. Many parents treasure photographs of their dead baby, which can help to reinforce memories and sort out the emotional confusion between the live and the dead twin. Several types of photographs need to be made of the twins separately and together, dressed and naked, to give as complete an aid to memory as possible, both of the baby and of the multiple birth. If the dead twin is sensitively dressed, the mother and father can hold the two babies, together with any siblings, and the photograph of the family group may be very precious. Black and white photographs may

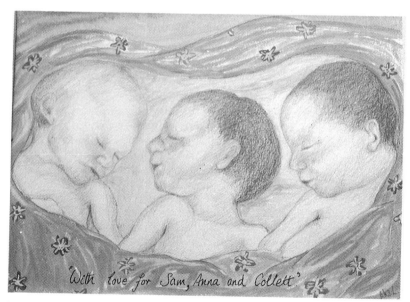

Fig. 14.1 Sketch of triplets who were miscarried at 23 weeks gestation. With permission from Alison Little and the parents.

be easier to show to siblings, relatives and friends, when a baby is grossly discoloured. Similarly, a sketch taken from a photograph can provide an image that can be displayed and seen by others without embarrassment (Fig. 14.1). This is also a way in which the two babies can be shown together, even if they were originally on two photographs (Fig. 14.2). There are a number of artists who are prepared to make such sketches from photographs of dead babies.

Parents have been known to ask for a photograph years later. Spare photographs should always be kept with Medical Records. Some parents who initially refuse photographs (or even destroy them) may later desperately want one. When this is not available an X-ray or a photograph of an ultrasound scan can be a great comfort, if only to confirm that what may seem a nebulous baby did exist.

The value of a photograph of the twinship is strongly felt by many mothers. Even those who have had a stillborn twin would often like to have had a photograph of the live and dead twin together. Some doctors and nurses are clearly disturbed by this idea but it is important that, whatever their own feelings, medical staff should do their best to reassure the parents that no reaction to the death is abnormal or illegitimate.

Blood samples should always be taken for zygosity determination. Even if one or both babies die, parents nearly always want to know whether or not their twins were 'identical'. The zygosity may also be essential for reliable

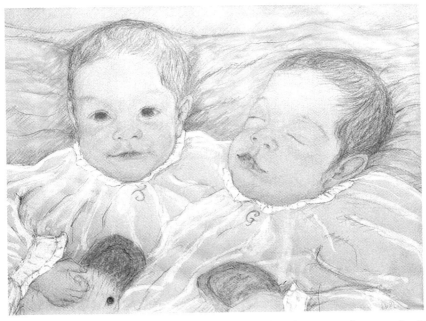

Fig. 14.2   Sketch of liveborn and stillborn twins taken from two photographs. With permission from Alison Little and the parents.

genetic counselling, particularly if either baby was malformed. Furthermore, those with dizygotic twins may like to know that they have a greatly increased risk of conceiving twins again.

Too often the funeral arrangements are taken over by well-meaning hospital staff and the event minimized in the hope that the whole sad episode will be quickly forgotten. Many people, however, need to have a memorable funeral and an individual grave or memorial.

One mother's feelings about her lost baby were so complex and ran so deep that she found herself unable to arrange the christening for her surviving baby that she would normally have wanted. It was only when it was suggested, 4 years later, that the christening might be combined with a memorial service for the stillborn twin that she felt able to face, indeed welcome, the service.

One mother who had lost her twin daughters during the 22nd week of her only pregnancy was still distraught 3 years later and quite unable to continue her work as a writer. She had only seen the babies at a distance through the placental membranes. A memorial service was held where the babies were baptized 'by intent'. The baptism certificates provided the first substantive mementoes and were treasured by the parents.

Similar considerations are relevant when both babies are born alive but one is likely to die soon from, say, gross malformations or severe birth anoxia. In these cases parents are often encouraged to focus their attention on the healthier baby, but this they may later regret. A mother wants to do as much for any baby of hers as possible. If his life is to be short there is all the more reason to give him as much love and care while she can, and she then at least has some experiences to remember. Similarly, if one twin is on the special care baby unit and the other at her bedside, the mother should always be encouraged to visit and think about the one separated from her. She should never be allowed to feel that her frequent visits or requests for information are in any way a nuisance to the hospital staff.

The need for a mother to talk about her dead baby may be intense during the first weeks. It can be trying for those with her and some may feel critical of her apparent lack of interest in the healthy baby. It may, however, be necessary for her to come to terms with the death of her other baby before she can really bond to the survivor. Her needs should be respected. It is only by allowing, indeed encouraging her to think and talk about the baby that the normal mourning process can take place.

Most mothers continue to welcome opportunities to reminisce about the baby who died, particularly with those who were with her at the time of her bereavement, sometimes for many years. Paediatricians, family doctors and clinical medical officers should make clear to the mother that she is welcome to do so. It is good practice for the paediatrician to see the mother and, if possible the father too, with the surviving twin on at least one occasion in his follow-up clinic, even if it is not medically necessary. He will then be able to make sure that she is happy with the baby's progress and it will also give her the chance to ask any questions about the dead twin, or just to talk about him and about her feelings of loss.

Higher order births

The loss of one or more babies in a higher multiple set can be particularly difficult. After many years of infertility the arrival of quadruplets may result in tragedy. They may miscarry before they are viable. They may die one by one over many months, or some may die, others become disabled and a healthy child may have to suffer from the parents' bereavement as well as being the sibling of a disabled child (see p. 199).

If a couple is left with two or more babies it is unlikely they will receive much sympathy. Logically they have enough children. Yet to the parents each child is equally precious. Any implication that the death or deaths might have been for the best, even if objectively this might be thought true, can be profoundly hurtful to the parents and can produce justified anger.

Many mothers who have a higher order birth deeply resent the labelling of the surviving children, as say, 'twins' when they were born as members of a triplet set.

Sudden infant death syndrome

The sudden unexpected death of a baby is a shattering experience for any parent. Four in every 1000 families in the UK suffer the tragedy of Sudden Infant Death Syndrome (SIDS), otherwise known as a 'cot death'. The incidence amongst twins is higher still (see p. 131).

Parents usually feel extreme guilt about a cot death, however unjustifiably. They often believe that something they did or failed to do must have been responsible for the death. This belief is often reinforced by the bewildered and embarrassed responses of their relatives and neighbours, which the parents can often interpret as criticism of their care and confirmation of their guilt. The mother is determined that the same should not happen to the other baby. For this reason as well as for medical reasons (see p. 132) the twin should be immediately admitted to hospital.

Many parents are so obsessed by the fear of the survivor's demise that they become unable to let him out of their sight. The slightest abnormal sign or symptom results in urgent calls to the doctor or hospital.

The whole family will need support and understanding, often for many months or even years. Easy access to, and frequent visits from, the health visitor are often welcomed. The health visitor will, of course, need sensitivity and tact to ensure that their attentions are seen as being supportive rather than supervisory and hence an apparent confirmation of the mother's failure in child care.

Many surviving babies appear deeply affected by the death of their twin, even when they are only a few months old. In part this must be due to the general family upset and the change in mood and attitude of their parents. Nevertheless, the event itself may be of deeper significance to the co-twin than is yet realized. One mother described the shocked expression and ashen complexion of the healthy twin as she lay in the same cot beside her dead sister. It was the appearance of the first baby that led the mother to look at the dead one.

When so little is known about the causes of SIDS, parents find comfort in the knowledge that many other apparently healthy babies with caring parents die in the same way. They often appreciate introductions to other bereaved parents either locally or through the Foundation for the Study of Infant Deaths.

Death in childhood

Twins are little if any more likely to die in childhood than singletons. But for those who do—be it from accidents, chronic illness or acute infections—the effects on the surviving twin can be devastating (Bernabei and Levi 1976). This is particularly so if the twins had had little experience of being separated or if the one who died was the 'leader'. For these children the beliefs of some African tribes that the spirit of the dead twin must be preserved in order to ensure the wholeness of the survivor may appear frighteningly apt (see Chapter 1).

Many survivors feel guilty that they were the one chosen to live. This guilt, of course, is compounded if they think that they were directly—or even indirectly—responsible for their twin's death.

Young children have great difficulty in understanding the finality of death, that their brother or sister will never return. One 3-year-old, whose brother had died in hospital 6 months earlier, insisted on taking some of his toys to the doctor at Christmas-time so that they could be given to his twin. For all ages it is nearly always helpful for them to be as much involved in the terminal illness and death of their sibling, as well as mourning, as reasonably possible. The unknown and unseen is more frightening and incomprehensible than reality. For a twin this must be particularly important. With the chronically ill child there are advantages both to him and his healthy twin of being together through the final weeks. Janet Goodall and the parents concerned have sensitively and revealing described how a family coped with the terminal illness of a 5-year-old at home rather than in hospital. This clearly enabled the older and younger sisters to accept and come to terms with the death of their brother more easily than they would otherwise have done had they been excluded from the whole experience (Cotton *et al.* 1981).

Children need to say goodbye in their own ways. Some will want to help with the funeral arrangements. They may wish to choose the toys to go in the coffin or the outfit in which their brother is to be dressed.

Many parents, whilst still grieving themselves, find the disturbances in behaviour of the surviving twin particularly distressing. One 2½-year-old suddenly lost his MZ twin brother from bacterial meningitis. Having had normal speech development as well as an elaborate 'twin language' he became silent. Six weeks later his mother took him to the mirror to point out some dirty marks on his face. His expression lit up for a few seconds only to turn to anguish as he realized the reflection was his own, not his twin. He refused to go near a mirror again and became increasingly withdrawn and destructive. Other children may suffer profound psychological injuries that do not show any immediate overt symptoms.

The behaviour of some children at these times can be so difficult as to disrupt family life. Both parents may be anxious to help their unhappy child but may disagree profoundly about the best way of doing so. Marital discord is common. Other siblings may also be very disturbed. It is vital that all families should be offered support and bereavement counselling as soon as possible to prevent or at least reduce both the child's difficulties and the family tensions.

Mother's attitude to the surviving twin

Most mothers have ambivalent feelings towards the surviving twin. Some overprotect the survivor, others reject him; many do both. They are thankful to have this baby (or child) to love yet often feel he is in some way responsible for his twin's death. Perhaps he had an unfair share of intra-uterine nutrition. With an older child the mother may feel that an accident that killed one was the fault of the other. Sometimes, of course, this may be true. The mother's feelings and suspicions may be rational or irrational but they are very real and cannot be thrust aside.

Many parents are haunted by the vision of their dead child in the living twin. One mother dreaded washing her 2-year-old's hair because it was when his hair was wet that he looked most like his dead brother. Another mother described how her 18-month-old daughter acquired a number of mannerisms peculiar to her dead MZ twin, which she herself had never before shown. These ever-present reminders of the lost child can be so painful that the mother, at least temporarily, rejects the twin and may give an unfair amount of attention to the siblings. The same problem may even arise with a stillborn baby. One mother who had never seen the stillborn baby found that each time she looked at his live twin she was unable to stop herself wondering what the dead one looked like.

A mother's guilt in failing to produce a live baby may be increased further by her apparent inability to care for the survivor. Through the projection of her own anxieties the baby becomes increasingly 'difficult'. Her humiliation is complete when the baby calms on being handled by the father or other caretakers. She becomes severely depressed and may abandon the baby altogether (Lewis and Page 1978).

Expert and prolonged psychiatric help is often needed for the whole family.

The father

In general it is believed that mothers feel the loss of a baby or young child more deeply than the father. However, this impression may sometimes be gained because of the father's relative difficulty in expressing what he may fear to be 'unmanly' emotions. Certainly he may feel the death of an older child as deeply as the mother (Bowlby 1980). But whatever his own feelings about the actual bereavement, the father will anyway need a lot of support in coping with the mother's grief and the reactions of the surviving twin.

Society often reinforces his inhibitions about expressing his own grief by concentrating its sympathy on the mother.

Most fathers are extremely proud of having twins and in the early months think of them as a single unit. The destruction of this unit leaves an incomplete child, one whom the father may now reject. After the loss of a 2-year-old twin son one father insisted on the removal of all photographs of the pair. He was able to give his love and attention to the 5-year-old sister but wanted nothing to do with the MZ twin, who was altogether too painful a reminder of the lost son.

For both parents there will always be painful reminders of the twinship. Anniversaries such as birthdays are especially difficult when the happy celebration of the surviving child may conflict with the sad memories of the death day of the twin. Some parents light an extra candle for the dead twin. Others set aside a quiet period on anniversaries when they can specially think about him. Most parents will be grateful if others mention that they remember him.

The surviving twin

The number of single surviving twins in the UK is difficult to determine. National perinatal mortality figures distinguish between singletons and twins but they do not reveal the number of twin pairs in which only one twin died.

On the assumption that the twins who have been brought up on their own have lost their co-twin through death then a figure of 15 per cent for single survivors can be deduced from the study by Record *et al.* (1970) on 2164 twins taking the eleven-plus examination. Another study found that 10 per cent of 5½- to 7½-year-old twin pairs had only one surviving child (Phillips and Watkinson 1981). The lower rates of 5 to 9 per cent have been found in several studies of single twin survivors up to the end of the perinatal period, by which time the great majority of deaths would have occurred (Potter 1963; Ferguson 1964; Hendricks 1966; Myrianthopoulos 1970).

The price of being a single survivor may be very high. In her study of over 200 adult bereaved twins, Woodward (1988) found that many suffered a profound loss. Remarkably, she found that this loss was often felt most deeply by those who had never consciously known their twin—because she or he had died at birth or soon after. Many surviving twins felt, justifiably or not, that their parents either blamed them for the death of their twin or would have preferred the other child to survive, particularly if the dead twin was of a different gender. In moments of anger some parents have greatly distressed the surviving child by claiming that they are somehow responsible for the death of their sibling, for example by 'taking all the food from your twin in the womb'. A surviving twin may have to come to terms with survivor guilt and identity confusions, which may affect the development of his personality.

To be the twin of a stillborn baby may be the worst fate of all. Many survivors appear to carry the guilt of their twin's death right into adulthood. This may well be expressed in their relationships with others: they tend to compensate by looking after or marrying people weaker than themselves and they may have a morbid preoccupation with death.

There seems no doubt that overt psychiatric morbidity is higher in single surviving twins than in either the general population or in twins whose co-twin is still alive. Twenty-six per cent of twin-born patients attending the Maudsley Psychiatric Hospital in London had lost their co-twin, and amongst those with psychotic illness the figure rose to 44 per cent (Reveley *et al.* 1981).

Even those twins who appear psychologically and socially unscathed may suffer profoundly from their bereavement. A 58-year-old head school teacher had lost her MZ twin at the age of 6 weeks yet, despite being a member of a large family, she greatly missed her twin and describes a 'desperate sense of loss and loneliness' throughout childhood, which she then revealed to no one. She also had fantasies that the dead twin was still alive; these continued until adolescence. Even as an adult she continued to dream of her lost twin.

Too often the dead twin is not considered relevant (or is thought of as a merely morbid concern) and is never mentioned. It is rare, for instance, for a teacher at school, or even in a playgroup, to learn about a child's twin who died at birth or soon after. Yet the child's first school drawings may well show his need to express his twinship. Perhaps there is a recurring second figure or the loss may be demonstrated by incomplete bodies or objects with missing parts.

One 3-year-old, whose twin was stillborn, was repeatedly attracted to depleted objects (Lewis 1983)—the toy car without a wheel, the doll with a missing arm. Some have secret fantasies, which can be frightening and indeed dangerous if allowed to develop.

A 5-year-old, whose twin died at the age of 6 months, was severely incapacitated by the fear of his brother's ghost. He would not go upstairs on his own or put his hand out of bed for a drink at night. It was only when he was allowed to talk about the ghost and learnt to accept that it would do him no harm that he overcame these fears.

All single surviving twins should hear about their dead twin from the start and be encouraged to ask questions and express their feelings—rational or not. Many feel angry with their twin for deserting them, for causing such unhappiness in the family and for making them, the survivor, feel guilty. They may also feel anger towards their parents for 'allowing' the twin to die.

For the surviving twins who only learn of their twinship later in life it is often a profound relief. At last they understand their previously unexplained feeling of loneliness and loss.

Support from self-help groups

Most parents who have lost a twin continue to think of themselves as parents of twins and of their single surviving child as a twin even if the co-twin was stillborn, and they like other people to do the same (Bryan 1986). For this reason some parents continue to join in the activities of their local twins club. Others, not surprisingly, find the contact with twins and their parents too painful but welcome a chance sometimes to share their feelings with other bereaved parents, particularly those who had twins.

For many parents the greatest source of support is from others who have shared their experience. Through the TAMBA Bereavement Support Group (see Appendix 2), which has four sections (for the loss of one newborn twin, the loss of both including miscarriages, sudden unexpected infant death and the loss of an older child) parents are put in touch with each other individually and through a newsletter. The Multiple Births Foundation also holds bereavement clinics (Appendix 1) where families can have individual appointments but, more importantly, can meet together over an informal lunch.

In 1989 the Multiple Births Foundation established a Lone Twin Network (Appendix 2) which allows bereaved adult twins to be in touch with each other. Many of the twins on this register lost their twin in infancy.

15

Higher order births I : biology

Although this book is primarily about twins it would plainly be incomplete without consideration of higher multiple births. Families with 'supertwins' have most of the same experiences and share most of the same problems and many of them, of course, with greater intensity.

There is theoretically no limit to the number of infants that a human mother can produce at one delivery. Hoaxers, mythologists and imaginative historians have made the most of this. Mayer (1952 a,b) made a comprehensive review of all reports of sextuplets or more, whether they were authentic or legendary, and found there were at least eight reports of the delivery of ten or more infants. One claim was of 365! Traditionally the delivery of multiple offspring has been seen as a punishment for sexual or other misdemeanours.

Rare but authentic cases of multiple births as high as seven have been reported in the past (Mayer 1952b). The incidence of such high multiples has, however, greatly increased since the introduction of ovulation-stimulating drugs for the treatment of infertility.

A case of nonoplets, none of whom survived, is probably the largest reliably recorded multiple birth (Benirschke and Kim 1973; Carey 1976). Octuplets, of whom seven are said to have survived, were reported to have been born 120 miles from Shanghai. However, the report came indirectly from the father via an Italian newspaper and has not been confirmed (Mayer 1952b). An octuplet abortion has been reliably reported (Prokop and Herrmann 1973). There have been a number of septuplet pregnancies, most of which ended in abortion or neonatal death (Mayer 1952b; Turksoy et al. 1967; Burnell 1974; Hodgkinson 1987); in a few cases some of the infants have survived (Aiken 1969).

The first recorded surviving sextuplets were reported from Sri Lanka in 1947. The second set was reported from South Africa in 1974 (Gutowitz et al. 1974) and the third set—the 'Florentine' sextuplets—was reported in detail by Giovannucci-Uzielli et al. (1981) (Fig. 15.1). However, although not reliably recorded, it seems that all the Bushnell sextuplets, born in Chicago in 1866, were alive at 8 months (Nichols 1954). Amazingly they escaped publicity and the three survivors were only 'discovered' at the age of 72. Apparently one girl and one boy had died at 8 months and a second brother at the age of 68 years. Lachelin et al. (1972) reported sextuplets of whom five survived. The only other two sets of sextuplets were born in the UK, six girls in 1983 (the Walton sextuplets) and three boys and three girls in 1986.

Many surviving quintuplets have now been reported, several of whom

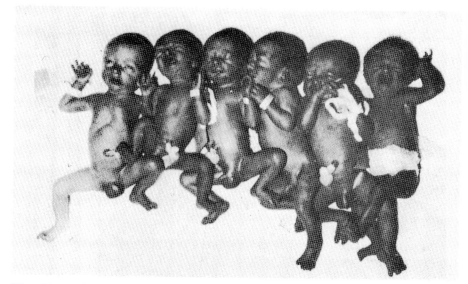

Fig. 15.1 The 'Florentine' sextuplets born at 34 weeks' gestation. Four boys weighing 1430 g, 1520 g, 1540 g, 1700 g and two girls each weighing 1150 g. There were six chorionic membranes in the single placental mass. From Giovannucci-Uzielli *et al.* (1981) by permission of Alan R Liss.

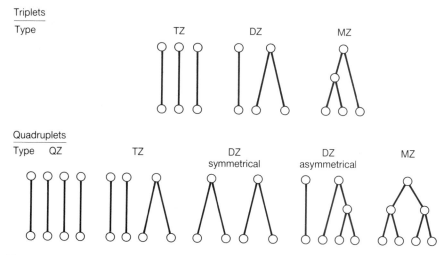

Fig. 15.2 Types of triplets and quadruplets.

are described by Clay in her comprehensive review of higher order children (Clay 1989). Many of the mothers were on treatment for infertility but several had had spontaneous pregnancies. The most famous are the Dionne quintuplets, who were exceptional in being monozygotic (MacArthur 1938). The surviving set reported by Campbell and Dewhurst (1970) had the advantage of close supervision throughout their intrauterine life as they were diagnosed by ultrasound as early as 9 weeks. This early diagnosis is now becoming increasingly common with pregnancies resulting from assisted conception.

'Supertwins', the term used by Scheinfeld (1973) to describe higher multiple births, may be derived from separate zygotes, from a single zygote or from a combination of the two. The possible combinations in a triplet and a quadruplet set are shown in Fig. 15.2. DZ triplets, for example, are derived from two zygotes, one of which later divides into an MZ pair.

Combinations for the higher multiples can be worked out from the basic triplet and quadruplet patterns.

Zygosity

In many higher multiple births the zygosity of the babies has not been accurately determined. There are therefore few data on the relative frequency of the different types. It has been estimated that the ratio of MZ:DZ:TZ triplets amongst Caucasians should be 1:2:3 and details of the calculations are given by Bulmer (1970). Some studies, however, have found higher incidences of DZ triplets than would be expected (Bulmer 1970).

Amongst mongolian racial groups, such as the Japanese, the proportion of MZ triplets, as with twins (see p. 19), is much higher, whereas TZ triplets

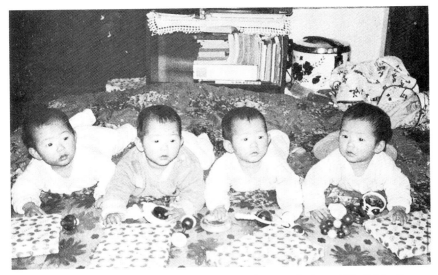

Fig. 15.3   MZ quadruplets from South Korea. By permission of Dr B Martin.

are proportionately more common amongst negroid races. Of 40 sets of triplets born in Ibadan, Western Nigeria, only two were MZ and 24 were TZ (Nylander and Corney 1971).

MZ quadruplets and quintuplets are rare but have been authentically reported (MacArthur 1938; B. Martin, personal communication) (Fig. 15.3). DZ quadruplets may be asymmetrical, with three infants arising from one zygote, or symmetrical when two zygotes split to form MZ pairs. Only occasional examples of the latter have been reported (Nylander and Corney 1971).

Most ovulation-induced pregnancies resulting in higher multiple births are polyzygotic but, interestingly, the numbers that also include an MZ pair appear to be higher than would be expected by chance (Atlay and Pennington 1971, Derom *et al.*). It has been suggested that polyovulation may in itself promote division of the zygote (see p. 18).

Sex

MZ triplets must be the same sex, whereas half DZ sets will be of like sex and only one quarter of TZ.

The sex ratio in triplets is even lower than that found in twins (see p. 14). This higher proportion of females may be due to an increase in abortions of the more vulnerable male (Bulmer 1970).

Incidence

Factors influencing the incidence of higher multiple births are the same as those for twins and are outlined in Chapter 2. There are many reports of triplets occuring in the same family as twins (Miettinen 1954) as well as some instances of two sets in one family (Clay 1989). As would be expected, the incidence of triplets is much higher amongst negroid races and lower amongst Oriental and Caucasian peoples (Little and Thompson 1988). An incidence of 2 per 1000 has been reported from Nigeria (Nylander 1971a). Even so this is not nearly as high as the 6 per 1000 predicted by Hellin's law (see below). A high undetected abortion rate could explain the discrepancy, at least in part.

Hellin (1895) proposed a formula by which the frequency of higher multiple births in a given population could be calculated, this has become known as Hellin's law. If n is the frequency of twins in a population, then n^2 is the frequency of triplets, n^3 of quadruplets and so on. However, Hellin did not take into account the zygosity distributions in different populations. Other models have also been developed to predict multiple births (Peller 1946; Fellman and Eriksson 1990).

In countries like the UK, where the incidence of twins is approximately 1 in 90 deliveries, the deliveries of triplets should be 1 in 9000 and that of quadruplets 1 in 900000. However, the recent introduction of new techniques in the treatment of infertility has transformed the picture with regard to higher order births. In England and Wales, the incidence has almost trebled in the last ten years (Fig. 15.4). A similar picture has been seen in other countries, including Japan (Imaizumi 1990), the US (Allen 1988) and Germany (Grutzner-Konnecke *et al.* 1990). In England and Wales in 1989 figures for multiple births included one set of quintuplets, 11 sets of quadruplets, 183 sets of triplets and 7579 pairs of twins (Registrar General 1989). In the last 10 years there have been three sets of sextuplets and one set of septuplets. The figures on higher order births may, however, be mis-leadingly low in the UK. If a multiple birth infant was delivered before 28 weeks, only those that were born alive were registered. A surviving child may not, therefore, be recorded as belonging to as large a higher order pregnancy as it actually did, or indeed to a multiple pregnancy at all.

New techniques for treatment of infertility, which may cause multiple births, include ovulatory stimulating drugs, *in vitro* fertilization (IVF) and gamete intrafallopian transfer (GIFT). The most commonly used drug is clomiphene citrate (Clomid or Serophene). This drug, and others such as the human menopausal gonadotrophin (Pergonal), have the disadvantage that more than one ovarian follicle may ripen to produce multiple ova, with a resulting higher risk of multiple births. In a study of 2369 pregnancies resulting from treatment with Clomid the incidence of twins was 6.9 per cent, triplets 0.5 per cent, quadruplets 0.3 per cent and quintuplets 0.13 per cent (Merrell Pharmaceuticals Ltd 1981).

With gonadotrophins the estimates were higher still, with an incidence of 15–45 per cent for twins and 5–6 per cent for triplets (Scialli 1986), although more recently better monitoring appears to be reducing the risk (Rein *et al.* 1990). Sextuplets have been born and survived as a result of drug treatment for infertility (Marlow *et al.* 1990). Septuplets were delivered, six alive, but all

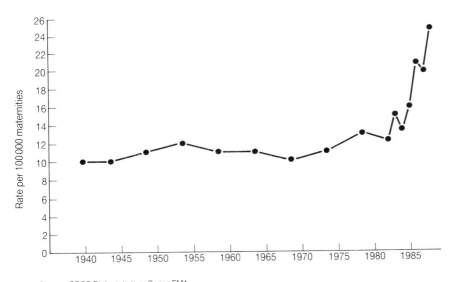

Source: OPCS Birth statistics, Series FM1

Fig. 15.4 Proportion of all maternities which resulted in a triplet or higher order birth, England and Wales, 1939–1989.

died within a fortnight (Hodgkinson 1987). The outcome of other forms of assisted conception are equally worrying. The first surviving IVF quadruplets were born in Australia in 1984 (Clay 1989) and the first IVF quintriplets in the UK in 1986 (Clay 1989).

Of the pregnancies achieved as a result of IVF in the UK in 1987, 77.6 per cent were singletons, 16 per cent were twins, 6.1 per cent triplets and 0.23 per cent quadruplets. The more embryos that are transferred the greater are the chances of a pregnancy (Table 15.1). Not surprisingly, the risk of a multiple pregnancy also increases with more embryos. There have even been reports of two consecutive triplet pregnancies (Kingsland *et al.* 1989). Broadly similar figures, which are still probably underestimates, are emerging amongst GIFT treatment pregnancies. In 1987 72 out of 141 triplet pregnancies in the UK arose from either IVF or GIFT treatments. An unknown but substantial proportion occurred as a result of ovulation-stimulating drugs alone. Thus, well over half of the triplets now born in the UK each year occur as a result of medical intervention. Collins and Bleyl (1990) found that 94 per cent of 71 quadruplet pregnancies in California resulted from assisted conception.

Table 15.1   Pregnancy and multiple pregnancy rates per pre-embryo or gamete transfer

No. pre-embryos or eggs transferred	IVF		GIFT	
	Pregnancy rate (%)	Multiple pregnancy rate (%)	Pregnancy rate (%)	Multiple pregnancy rate (%)
One	6.5	1.7	1.7	
Two	11.8	10.5	10.4	11.8
Three	21.0	22.4	18.6	18.7
Four	21.9	30.5	18.9	23.9
Five +	3.9	55.6	37.2	28.3

Source: From Interim Licensing Authority (1990) with permission.

In 1989 there were 52 units in the UK who performed either IVF or GIFT, or both. Eighteen more were hoping to start soon. There is every indication that these numbers will continue to climb.

The Interim Licensing Authority (ILA—formerly the Voluntary Licensing Authority) was set up to regulate the activities of clinics practising techniques of IVF and other related procedures. The ILA has issued guidelines that recommend that a maximum of three embryos should be transferred in IVF, and only exceptionally four. Otherwise there would be a disproportionately greater increase in multiple pregnancies relative to the increased success in achieving a pregnancy at all. In 1989 the guidelines were extended to include GIFT (Interim Licensing Authority 1990).

These are only voluntary guidelines, but they must be followed by any clinic that wishes to continue to be licensed by the ILA. However, many people feel that the licensing authority should have legal backing, and a Human Fertilization and Embryology Bill, with provisions to set up a statutory Human Fertilization and Embryology Authority, is going through the UK Parliament (Human Fertilization and Embryology Bill 1989). Unfortunately GIFT is not, so far, scheduled to be included in the Act. This is particularly worrying because GIFT is likely to become a more widely used procedure, often in units that lack the expertise and technical backup essential to the running of an IVF unit.

The ethics of new reproductive techniques

New treatments for infertility have meant that many previously childless couples have the joy of a baby. However, as has been discussed, to achieve these pregnancies we have had to accept a large and still increasing number of higher order pregnancies. There is therefore a high price to be paid by their families, by society and often by the children themselves (Bryan *et al.* 1991; Levene 1991).

A triplet pregnancy is hazardous to the mother and to the infants. Midtrimester abortions are not uncommon and are extremely distressing to the couple (yet they do not appear in the perinatal mortality figures). Because of the high incidence of prematurity, triplets are at high risk of neonatal complications and death.

Despite the fact that a large proportion of higher order birth infants are conceived as a result of treatment in the private sector, it is the National Health Service that has to carry the high cost of their neonatal care. Higher order babies often block the intensive care cots of a tertiary unit for many months, so that admission to many single babies has to be refused (Levene 1986). Furthermore, the financial and practical stresses of caring for three or more babies at the same time are such that most families need help from the Social Services Department (see p. 201). For those with a disabled child there will be a considerable long-term cost (see p. 206).

Triplets, therefore, bring a combination of financial, practical and emotional stress to many families. Inevitably many of the children will suffer from lack of individual attention. A recent study of IVF children in Israel found significantly lower developmental quotients amongst multiple birth children than singletons (Gershoni–Baruch *et al.* 1991). Care must be taken when making comparisons between children of infertility couples and spontaneously conceived children—the National Triplet Study has shown that there are many compounding factors (Macfarlane *et al.* 1990b). For example, infertile couples were of higher socio-economic status, less likely to be unemployed and, not surprisingly, had fewer children.

Selective reduction of pregnancy

A selective reduction of a higher order multiple pregnancy has been advocated as a way of allowing a woman to have the normal, near term, delivery of a singleton or twins instead of three or even more babies (Berkowitz *et al.* 1988). This procedure is now widely practised (Kanhai *et al.* 1986; Keown 1987; Berkowitz *et al.* 1988; Evans *et al.* 1988; Golbus *et al.* 1988; Itskovitz *et al.* 1989; Wapner *et al.* 1990) and has been used to reduce pregnancies from as large as octuplets (Evans *et al.* 1988).

The timing of the reduction procedure is controversial (Alvarez and Berkowitz 1990). It can be done as early as 7–8 weeks but this allows less time to detect an abnormal fetus and less time for spontaneous losses to occur (Goldman *et al.* 1989). However, as these losses are relatively uncommon after 11–12 weeks, there is no point in postponing the procedure further. The techniques most commonly used are transcervical aspiration of one or more sac or transabdominal intrathoracic injection of potassium chloride.

The decision as to which fetus should be terminated is usually made on the grounds of technical access with a preference for leaving the fetus nearest to the cervix untouched to avoid rupture of the presenting membranes. At this stage prenatal diagnosis is not reliable and selection because of sex or genetic abnormality is not yet possible.

Despite the general agreement that adverse perinatal outcome is directly related to the number of fetuses, there is much debate about both the number of fetuses needed to justify reduction and the appropriate number of fetuses to leave. Berkowitz and colleagues (1988) have suggested that women with four or more fetuses are suitable candidates for reduction, whereas in France some units routinely recommend reduction of triplet pregnancies.

Although singletons are recognized to have a better prognosis than twins, most people prefer reducing to twins on the grounds that these are much wanted babies and the prognosis for twins is still relatively good.

Because of the uncertain legal situation in Britain (selective feticide is not included in its present Abortion Act) and the danger of litigation, many obstetricians in the UK are currently refusing to perform selective reductions of pregnancy (Bryan 1990). The perverse consequence is that some patients are having reluctantly to proceed to a termination of the entire pregnancy.

An obstetrician may sometimes be asked by parents to reduce a twin pregnancy when he considers there are no medical grounds for it. He may refuse to do it but the couple may then insist that the only other option acceptable to them is the termination of the whole pregnancy. The obstetrician may then feel that he is left with no choice but to comply with their wishes so that he can avoid a second unnecessary death (Wapner *et al.* 1990).

The balance of risk and advantage will be different for each couple but for all there will be a sense of responsibility and much anxiety. Not surprisingly, partners sometimes disagree about what to do. There can be no simple 'right' solution, whatever final decision is arrived at there will be elements of compromise either between the partners or between rival desiderata in each of them.

The main concern of most people will be for the healthy survival of the babies. Parents' concern about the physical, emotional and financial demands of so many children will vary greatly from couple to couple and will not necessarily correlate with their socio-economic situation (Contrepas 1989).

Many parents are understandably distressed by the idea of a seemingly arbitrary choice as to who should live and who should die. Careful counselling is essential and this should be from the very beginning, before treatment for infertility is ever started. Not only should the risk of multiple pregnancies be realistically discussed at that stage but also the possibility of selective reduction of a higher order pregnancy. Some couples have not even heard of the procedure until after triplets or quads have been diagnosed; some are horrified by the idea (Hallett 1991).

The known risks of the procedure include inducing an abortion, introducing infection and doing physical damage to the remaining fetuses. The long-term effect on parents in terms of bereavement and guilt are as yet unknown, as is the psychological effect on the surviving siblings. The recognized phenomenon of 'survivor guilt' following a mass disaster could well be echoed in such people.

One of the most basic and sensitive questions is how many embryos or gametes should be transferred? Many people, including the interim Licensing Authority, would now say a maximum of three. Some would say only two, at least for the first trial. Have we any right to risk imposing triplets or more on parents? Many couples desperate for children will feel that triplets would be better than nothing (Contrepas 1989). Indeed some may persuade their obstetrician to transfer more embryos than he would normally recommend (Kingsland *et al.* 1989). Few can realistically imagine what it means to have three babies at the same time (Hallett 1991). Moreover, would-be parents are often making these choices in periods of exceptional emotional stress.

We can only hope that further research will improve the chances of a single pregnancy without couples being exposed to all the problems attached to a higher order pregnancy.

16

Higher order births II: Pregnancy and delivery

Pregnancy

In the past information about higher order births was largely derived from studies involving only small numbers, individual case histories and personal impressions. The results of the first comprehensive national study were published in 1990 and much of the information presented here comes from it. The United Kingdom National Study of Triplet and Higher Order Briths (Botting *et al.* 1990) consisted of a series of linked surveys covering medical and social aspects from the time of conception. The project was undertaken by the Office of Population, Censuses and Surveys, the National Perinatal Epidemiology Unit and the Child Care and Development Group at Cambridge University. Information was collected relating to higher order births between 1979 and 1985 (with the exception of 1981 when there was a strike involving those collecting birth statistics), although the survey of parents included births up to the end of 1988.

The reaction of parents told that they are to have triplets or more is, not surprisingly, even more ambivalent than that of parents of twins. They tend to be excited by the novelty and prestige, even if they are apprehensive about the likely publicity. Most of them are worried by the practical and financial implications. Those that are not are either unrealistic or blessed with exceptional financial and practical support.

The chance of losing some, if not all, the babies is high and most parents realize this. Many of the couples will have had several years of infertility behind them and thus the prospect of a ready-made family is particularly attractive. On the other hand, their fear for the babies' safety is bound to be all the greater because of the difficulty they have had in conceiving at all.

A triplet pregnancy is physically uncomfortable at the very least. Complications are common and all those discussed in Chapter 3 are even more likely to occur in higher multiple pregnancies than in twin pregnancies. Most such mothers will need periods of bedrest, usually in hospital. All should be delivered in centres with facilities for intensive care of the infants.

Fetal hazards peculiar to multiple pregnancies, such as the fetofetal transfusion syndrome (Cortes 1964), monoamniotic placentation (Sinykin 1958; Wharton *et al.* 1968; Holcberg *et al.* 1982) and locking have all been reported amongst higher multiple births, as have the congenital malformations discussed below.

Diagnosis

It is clearly an advantage both to parents and to medical staff if a higher order pregnancy is diagnosed early. Since the advent of ultrasound scans many are now diagnosed in the first trimester and indeed, those resulting from assisted conception may be detected by 6 weeks—a very different situation to that of 20 years ago in the UK and to that still found in many less developed countries. In a study from South Africa and Namibia of 367 triplet pregnancies, three babies were expected in only 55 per cent of the cases (Deale and Cronje 1984). The correct number of fetuses, however, may not be detected on the first scan. In a quarter of the families in the UK Triplet Study the correct number was missed on the first scan and in a small number the correct number of fetuses was only found at delivery (Macfarlane *et al.* 1990b).

The news of triplets or more comes as a shock to the parents at whatever stage the diagnosis is made and should never be given lightly or frivolously. The first indication one mother had of quintuplets was the flippant question 'Are you good at knitting?' (Macfarlane *et al.* 1990a); she was not amused. It is vital that the news should be given sensitively and that information and support should be offered immediately (see p. 207).

Duration of pregnancy

Any factors that predispose to preterm delivery of twins have even greater effect in a higher multiple pregnancy. Despite the slower fetal growth during the third trimester, the uterine distension and the total fetal and placental weight in triplets or more will be considerably greater than in twins.

The average duration of pregnancy in triplets is between 33.5 and 35 weeks (Ron-el *et al.* 1981; Newman *et al.* 1989) and for quadruplets it is 31.4

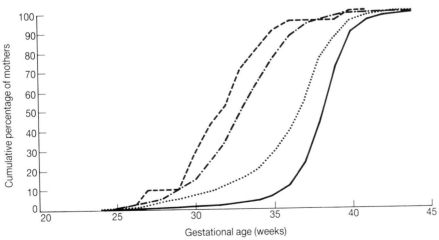

Fig. 16.1 Gestational age at delivery. From Macfarlane *et al.* (1990c) Reproduced with the permission of the controller of HMSO. — Singletons; ...... twins; ---- triplets; ————— quadruplets.

and 32 weeks (Collins and Bleyl 1990; Macfarlane *et al.* 1990c). About three-quarters of triplets are delivered prematurely (Itzkowic *et al.* 1979; Syrop and Varner 1985; Newman *et al.* 1989; Macfarlane *et al.* 1990c; Fig. 16.1).

In the UK Triplet Study almost half of the quadruplets were born before 32 weeks, compared with one-quarter of triplets, just under 10 per cent of twins and 1 per cent of singletons. Mothers who had had treatment for infertility tended to deliver earlier (Macfarlane *et al.* 1990c).

Delivery

In the UK Triplet Study about two-thirds of twins, triplets and quadruplets went into spontaneous labour. The others were induced for a number of reasons, including maternal complications, fetal growth retardation or because of relatively prolonged pregnancy. Some units have strict policies of not allowing multiple pregnancies to continue beyond a certain duration.

Caesarean sections for higher order deliveries have become much more common in recent years. In the UK between 1980 and 1986 65 per cent of triplets and 74 per cent of quadruplets were delivered by caesarean section, compared with 28 per cent of twins and 10 per cent of singletons. There is still strong debate, however, as to whether this should be routine practice. Some units perform caesarean sections in all except very premature deliveries (Michelwitz *et al.* 1981; Deale and Cronje 1984; Pons *et al.* 1988). Others would take a breech presentation of the first baby as an automatic indication for caesarean section. On the other hand Thiery *et al.* (1988) would advocate a vaginal delivery whenever possible. Pemkovsky and Vintzileos (1989) reviewed the literature and came to the conclusion that the lack of randomized trials and the very different results from both routes precluded any firm conclusion. The Dionne quintuplets were remarkable in all being delivered spontaneously at home, with no apparent complications (MacArthur 1938).

Women who have had infertility treatment are more likely to have caesarean sections (Derom *et al.* 1989; Macfarlane *et al.* 1990c). It has been suggested that these are less due to medical complications than to parental and medical anxiety about the safe delivery of such particularly precious babies.

The birth of triplets and quadruplets is not only a momentous event for the parents but also for the hospital staff and it is not uncommon for over 30 people to be in the delivery room. Many mothers are uncomfortable at being on such public view and it is important that the role of all personnel should be explained to her and her permission sought for the presence of any who are merely 'observers'. In many cases it seems that the father (or companion) is unnecessarily excluded (Macfarlane *et al.* 1990c). This is especially unfortunate, as the father's role will be crucial and the more fully he is involved from the start the better.

As birth asphyxia and prematurity are common in higher multiple births it is crucial that the resuscitation teams have been thoroughly briefed well before the babies are likely to arrive. Cooke (1991) describes the detailed preparations for the delivery of the Walton sextuplets. A list of all personnel was kept with their availability at any particular time in the preparatory weeks. At the time of the caesarean section six numbered resuscitation teams, each consisting of a paediatrician with full resuscitation equipment, a nurse and a runner, were present for the delivery. The runner collected the baby from the obstetrician and brought her to the allocated stand for resuscitation in an adjoining room. When the baby was in a stable condition she was transferred by her own team to the neonatal unit and was administered by them until her condition was stable enough to hand over to the resident neonatal staff.

Birth weight

McKeown and Record (1952) were the first to point out that the greater the number of babies, the lower their average individual birth weights. They found that the average birth weight for triplets was 1.8 kg and for quadruplets 1.4 kg. Others have reported similar results (Bulmer 1970; Holcberg *et al.* 1982; Newman *et al.* 1989; Macfarlane *et al.* 1990d; Fig. 16.2). Half the number of quadruplets born weigh less than 1500 g compared with a quarter of triplets, 9 per cent of twins and 1 per cent of singletons (Macfarlane *et al.* 1990d).

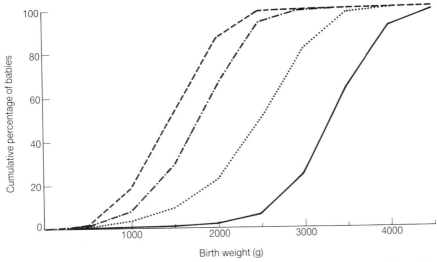

Fig. 16.2 Birthweight distributions of singleton and mutliple births. From Macfarlane *et al.* (1990d) Reproduced with the permission of the controller of HMSO. — Singletons; ...... twins; ---- triplets; ————quadruplets.

Whatever the number of fetuses it seems that all grow at a similar rate to singletons until the latter part of the second trimester. Only then does growth slow down in direct relation to the number of fetuses that the uteroplacental circulation must supply.

In contrast to twins (see p. 98), some studies have found that there is some correlation between birth order of higher order birth infants and weight, with the firstborn being the heaviest (Itzkowic 1979; Macfarlane *et al.* 1990d) and the thirdborn lightest. However, this was not supported by the work of Holcberg and colleagues (1982).

Congenital malformations

Many instances have been described in which one or more members of a higher multiple set is malformed (Little and Bryan 1988). Burnell (1974) reported two anencephalics in a set of otherwise normal septuplets and all three fetuses have been affected in MZ triplets (Scott and Paterson 1966). A conjoined pair may have a normal third partner (Tan *et al.* 1971a; Vestergaard 1972). An acardiac monster may be part of a monochorionic pair with a third dichorionic unaffected fetus (Benirschke and Kim 1973).

Placentation

Accurate descriptions of placentae in higher multiple births tend to be limited to case reports. There have been detailed descriptions of several types, including the placenta of septuplets (Cameron *et al.* 1969; Fig. 16.3). Little attention, however, has been given to the frequency of the various

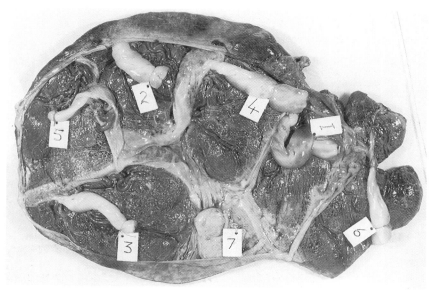

Fig. 16.3 Placenta from a septuplet pregnancy. None of the six liveborn infants were monozygotic and seven chorionic sacs were present. There were three females and four males, one of whom was a fetus papyraceus. From Cameron *et al.* (1969) by permission of the authors and the editors of *Journal of Obstetrics and Gynaecology of the British Commonwealth*.

chorion types as in most studies the numbers, even of triplets, are too small.

Following the pattern described for twins in Chapter 6 the placentae of all TZ triplets will be trichorionic and one-third of DZ triplets should also have three chorions, whereas two-thirds will be dichorionic. On the same grounds one-ninth of MZ triplets should be trichorionic, four-ninths dichorionic and four-ninths monochorionic.

The actual number of each chorion type will, of course, depend on the proportions of TZ triplets in the population (see Fig. 16.4). In a total of 23 sets of Caucasian triplets collected from the literature there were equal numbers (eight) of trichorionic and dichorionic placentae and three monochorionic (Nylander and Corney 1971). In Nigeria, as would be expected, the percentage of trichorionic placentae is much higher than in the UK. In 40 sets of triplets 29 were trichorionic, 10 were dichorionic and only one was monochorionic.

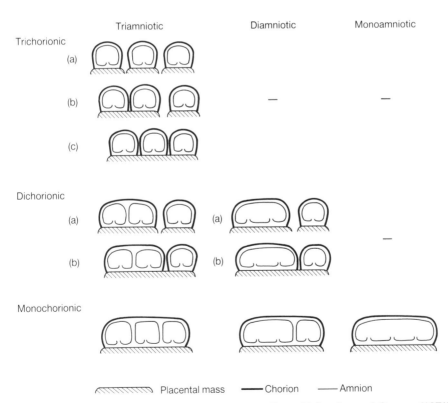

Fig. 16.4 The different types of triplet placentae. From Nylander and Corney (1971) by permission of the authors and the editors of *Annals of Human Genetics*.

Newborn 'Supertwins'

For all parents of 'supertwins' the first weeks are a strain. The mother is recovering from what is likely to have been a tiring pregnancy and a difficult delivery. She may well have medical complications (Macfarlane *et al.* 1990d). Furthermore, there is nearly always medical concern about at least one of the babies and sometimes about all of them.

The UK Triplet Study showed that only one-fifth of triplets and less than 5 per cent of quadruplets were able to stay with their mother on the general ward (Macfarlane *et al.* 1990d; Fig. 16.5). It is often some time before a mother can even see, let alone hold, her babies and photographs are an important means of bridging the gap.

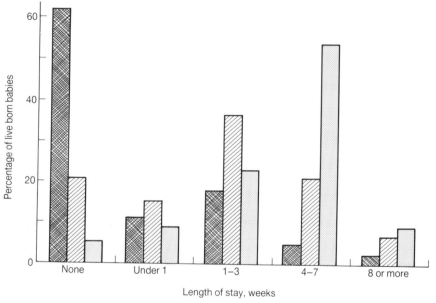

Fig. 16.5   Admission to special care and length of stay. From Macfarlane *et al.* (1990d) Reproduced with the permission of the controller of HMSO.   Twins; triplets; quadruplets.

The mother may well try, consciously or unconsciously, to prevent herself becoming attached to the babies to save herself from grief should they die. Many mothers have to lament the loss of one baby, either as a stillbirth or as a neonatal death, while remaining anxious for the life of the others. The uncertainty of the first days or weeks as one baby after another dies can be an intolerable strain. For those parents who are left with one or more survivors there is a complex process of celebrating the lives of some and grieving the death of others (see Chapter 14).

Perinatal mortality

The perinatal mortality rate amongst higher multiple births is, of course, very high (Fig. 16.6). So far there have probably been only seven sets of sextuplets to survive the neonatal period (see p. 183). Whole quintuplet sets are rare and sets of quadruplets are often incomplete. Perinatal mortality rates in these higher multiple births are bound to be inaccurate because of the small numbers involved, but there is no doubt that they are much higher than in twins and even triplets (Botting *et al.* 1987).

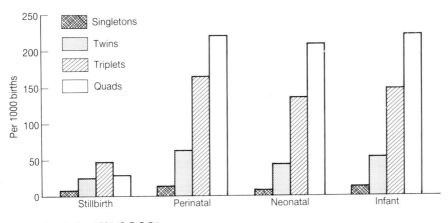

* excluding 1981 (O.P.C.S.)

Fig. 16.6 Mortality rates for singletons and multiple births in England and Wales 1975–1986 (excluding 1981). Source: Office of Population Censuses and Surveys.

The perinatal mortality of twins in England and Wales between 1975 and 1986 was 4.6 times that of singletons, the mortality of triplets was 12 times and the mortality of quadruplets 16 times that of singletons, with a higher rate amongst thirdborn than firstborn. However, the figures vary greatly between units and some have much better results than these (Kingsland *et al.* 1990). Zygosity is rarely recorded but the perinatal mortality is higher in like-sex than mixed sets—52 of 86 stillborn triplets were from like-sex sets (Botting *et al.* 1987).

As a number of higher order pregnancies are lost during the second trimester the true loss of children is higher than that reflected in perinatal mortality figures. Until 1991, in the UK, these figures did not include infants who were stillborn or miscarried before 28 weeks gestation (see p. 172).

The main complications described in Chapter 7, including the fetofetal transfusion syndrome, which may affect two or all three of the infants (Fisk *et al.* 1990; Pons *et al.* 1990), apply at least as often to higher multiple birth infants.

Most, if not all, parents will be aware of the high risk associated with a multiple pregnancy. For many this will be a constant if often unspoken anxiety throughout their pregnancy—a pregnancy that is already likely to be distressing due to complications or, at least, discomfort. Some have to face the loss of all their babies, a particularly cruel blow to those couples who have waited a long time for their pregnancy (Burnell 1974).

Cost

The rapidly increasing numbers of higher order births is putting an enormous financial and physical strain on many neonatal units (p. 105) (Levene 1986). Papiernik (1991) has calculated that the neonatal care of a quadruplet infant costs the National Health Service on average 42 times that of a single child, and therefore a set of quadruplets costs about 168 times that of a singleton. (There is also, of course, a higher cost for the pregnancy itself, as well as a continuing greater expenditure on the care of multiple births not least if one or more child is disabled, see p. 165). Furthermore, singleton babies may be displaced from intensive care units if cots become blocked by higher order infants (Bryan *et al.* 1991).

17

Higher order births III: The children and their families

The needs of triplets and their families are going to affect far more caring professionals than in the past. Not only is there a rapid increase in the number of triplet births but there is an even greater increase in the number of surviving triplet children. Many of these would never have survived before the recent improvements in neonatal care. These would, for example, include sets of triplets born at 26 weeks who in the past would have been classed as a miscarriage.

Management

Some mothers cope adequately, even well, with twins on their own. But with triplets help is essential during the first year at least. Even if a mother can manage the numerous practical needs of three babies, her inability to respond simultaneously to their demands makes the emotional burden impossible for her to carry alone. Two babies can be comforted at the same time; there is no arm left for a third.

The UK Triplet Study repeatedly found that help for families had been completely inadequate in amount and often slow to arrive. Too often the parents became ill and exhausted before help was provided. This then meant that even more help was required. A mother cannot and should not have to attempt to look after three babies at once. For many helpers, as well as parents, the practicalities of caring for so many babies is daunting. It is not just exhausting: there are not enough hours in the day. A study by the Australian Multiple Births Association showed that it took 197.5 hours per week just to care for baby triplets and do the necessary household tasks; unfortunately a week has only 168 hours (Australian Multiple Births Association 1984).

If the babies are poor sleepers, as many preterm babies seem to be, this can be the last straw (Berg *et al.* 1983). A night nurse for just one or two nights a week can save the mother from complete exhaustion but these are rarely provided. Thus, arrangements for regular help are a first priority with triplets.

Attempts to arrange this should be started early in the pregnancy because in many places help is difficult to find. Unlike some countries, such as Belgium, the UK provides no statutory rights to help for families with triplets and some Social Services Departments will need convincing of the need (Price 1990a). Many professionals assume that the extended family will help. Yet over 30 per cent of multiple birth parents had no family help on which they could rely and very few had sufficient.

Feeding

There is no way a mother can feed more than two babies at the same time (except by propping the bottles, a dangerous practice that should be strongly discouraged). Help with at least some feeds, is essential if the mother is not to spend most of her day on feeding rounds. Many mothers have partially breast-fed their triplets. Very occasionally they have been entirely breast-fed, as has one set of quadruplets (Noble 1990). Some mothers will breast-feed two of the babies at each feed whilst a helper gives a bottle to the third baby.

One mother of quadruplets chose to breast-feed one baby only at each feed. This meant that all four babies had their mother's undivided attention for at least half an hour each day. She felt that this was the only way she could develop a strong relationship with each baby. She was, of course, fortunate in having a willing team to feed the other three.

Transport

Transport of the babies is always a problem. Initially a large twin pram will suffice, with two babies at one end. Some mothers prefer to carry one of the babies in a sling at both the pram and early pushchair stage. Apart from the convenience, this allows the mother a little extra time for physical contact, which is always in short supply.

There are now a number of triple and quadruple pushchair/prams on the market and a triplet buggy can be formed by clipping a single onto a twin buggy.

It is difficult, indeed sometimes impossible, to keep an eye on three active babies. For this reason many mothers restrict triplets more than they would a single child. Goshen–Gottstein (1980) found that triplets were confined to playpens or even cots for long periods of the day. Many children therefore missed out on the early exploration that is an important part of any child's development (Fig. 17.1).

Cost

It is sometimes assumed that families with supertwins must become rich from commercial sponsorship. The UK Triplet Study completely disproved this idea. Although 75 per cent of families with triplets received national or local press coverage, few derived financial benefit from it.

For many parents the publicity can be very intrusive, particularly for those used to leading a quiet life and disliking the limelight. No couple asks for triplets yet many parents have been distressed by the thoughtless or intrusive comments by friends or strangers. Critical comments are more likely to be directed at those whose babies result from infertility treatment.

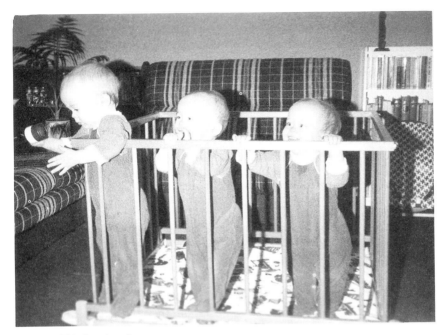

Fig. 17.1 Triplets in playpen.

The implication of such criticisms is that the parents have 'asked for it'—a particularly cruel accusation to a couple who may have been trying desperately for many years to have just one child.

Few people appreciate the enormously greater financial cost of triplets compared to three single children and for many parents this adds another major stress (Berg *et al.* 1983). One of the worst aspects is that clothes and equipment cannot be handed down. Three high chairs, three cots, three car seats and so on demand what for most families is a huge financial outlay and this is often on top of the cost of a larger home or car or both. With a family that is growing only gradually, there is less urgency: with triplets everything is needed at once.

Furthermore, a working mother is likely to take much longer to get back to work and the father may be torn between working extra hours and spending more time at home helping with the babies.

Mothers' attitudes

Even if their initial reaction to the idea of twins was negative most mothers happily accept their two babies by the time they are born—or at least soon afterwards. But Goshen–Gottstein (1980) found that this was not necessarily so with mothers of 'supertwins'. Seven out of ten Israeli mothers of triplets and quadruplets remained upset throughout the early months. However, several of these mothers already had large families when the 'supertwins' arrived. In the UK, where families tend to be smaller, more mothers have a positive approach. However, the greater the number of babies the harder it is for a mother to relate closely to each individually.

Many find this takes much longer than with singletons and they are inevitably hampered by the babies being handled by so many different carers. Many mothers, whilst appreciating the help, resent the positive responses given by their babies to other people and feel the more deprived in consequence.

Responding to the particular needs of each baby at the same time is an enormous strain. Many parents resort to treating them all alike with no regard for their different personalities. They tend to assume that their needs must be the same: that all should eat the same amount, that if one is tired then they all must be. Mothers may make little effort to distinguish the babies either by name or dress. To dress all babies differently demands imagination and energy.

There seem to be advantages in being the child who is 'odd-one-out' whether in sex or zygosity. This child has more chance of being treated as an individual. Many mothers treat like-sexed and in particular MZ children as a unit and refer to them as the 'twins', whereas the opposite-sexed child is named. Some mothers with like-sexed DZ triplets dress only the MZ pair alike, thereby actually accentuating the similarity (Goshen–Gottstein 1980).

When several children are competing for their mother's attention the loudest and most persistent tends to win. The noise, particularly during the second and third years, may be deafening. Many mothers find this in itself a great strain. The price of peace is often the loss of normal discipline and reasoning. Parents tend to swing from appeasement to reprimand without explanation.

Most parents admit to regimenting their children far more than they would a single child. Strict routines may be essential if the family is to function well or even adequately.

Many triplet children have little opportunity to mix with other children, or indeed to escape from each other. Biting, fighting and hair-pulling between 2- and 3-year-old triplets are common problems. Such children will benefit from early admission to nursery or playgroup, so that they have the chance to relate to other children and to dilute their own intense relationships.

Siblings

A little-recognized problem is the effect on other children in the family. Being the brother or sister of triplets is a most unenviable position. The triplets are not only very demanding, they get far more attention than their older siblings from relatives, friends and passers-by. Life is especially hard for the toddler who has been the centre of the family and is then displaced by an attention-attracting trio.

Illness

Even the most competent mother may find she reaches the end of her tether when one or more are ill. The extra demands of miserable children plus the knowledge that they need and deserve extra love and attention tries the most patient mother.

Although the incidence of illness is probably no higher amongst triplets than in any group of infants of similar gestation, the impact on the family is far worse. When three frail children are ill at the same time the worry for parents is enormous. It appears that some family doctors and health visitors are aware of this and give excellent support. Others are quite unrealistic in their expectations of parents sometimes, for instance, expecting the family to come to the surgery with several ill children (Price 1990b).

Even when all the children are well, visits to clinics are difficult and sometimes perilous and home visits for immunizations and weighing are greatly appreciated.

In the UK Triplet Study 21 per cent of children were admitted to hospital in the first 2 years, but amongst those under 1500 g the rate was 31 per cent. A surprising finding was that of a five-fold increase in pyloric stenosis (Macfarlane *et al.* 1990e).

Long-term development

There is no doubt that many members of triplet, quadruplet and even quintuplet sets become healthy adults of normal intelligence. However, there have been no large studies that compared overall development or incidence of disability in 'supertwins' with those of singletons. In such studies as have been made the numbers are inevitably small.

Miettinen and Gronroos (1965) studied the 225 members of 75 complete sets of triplets, many of whom had been born long before neonatal intensive care was available. Their ages ranged from 3 to 45 years. Nevertheless, they found that all but 4 per cent were of normal intelligence. Of these eight, five had a moderate degree of intellectual impairment and three were severely mentally retarded.

The growth of the group as a whole was similar to that of the singleton population. A further finding was that of a two-fold increase in left-handedness in triplets when compared with singletons.

The large Birmingham Study of children taking the eleven-plus examination in the 1950s included 33 triplets. The mean IQ of these children was 91.6, compared with 95.7 in twins and 100.1 in singletons.

As an increasingly large proportion of higher order birth children result from assisted conception it is clearly important to know whether their development differs from that of spontaneously conceived children. The first study of such children was carried out in Israel. It was found that there was no difference between the assisted conception group of multiple birth (twins and triplets) children compared with matched controls but that multiple birth children, both study and controls, had lower developmental quotients than single born children (Gershoni–Baruch *et al.* 1991).

No detailed study of language development in triplets has been reported. It would not be surprising if language delay in triplets was even greater than that found in twins. Not only do triplets communicate less with their mother but they are also deprived of the one-to-one relationship found in a pair of twins. It would be interesting to compare the progress of single surviving triplets, members of a pair of surviving triplets and members of a complete set. The continuing disadvantage of being brought up a twin is likely to be magnified for a triplet, who has two other companions competing for attention.

Disability

In the UK Triplet Study the incidence of cerebral palsy was 17.4 per 1000 compared with 2 per 1000 in the general population (Macfarlane *et al.* 1990e). In those with a birth weight of under 1500 g the incidence was 68 per 1000. However, the study did not include sets where less than three children had survived, so the incidence in the total population of triplet born children is probably higher. In the Australian Cerebral Palsy Register 1966–85 the prevalence of cerebral palsy was 31.6 among triplets (this included children from sets where some had died) compared with 6.3 amongst twins and 2.4 per 1000 live births amongst singletons. (Petterson *et al.* 1990).

Quadruplets and quintuplets

Although there is now more information on twins and triplets, there is very little documented information on quadruplets and quintuplets, except for individual case histories (Clay 1989). A recent follow-up study of 29 triplets, quadruplets and quintuplets found only one child with a major handicap (Gonen *et al.* 1990).

Inevitably small numbers mean that data takes time to gather but two useful studies from London and Munich are now available. In London five sets of quadruplets, one set of quintuplets and one set of sextuplets were followed (Stewart 1991). Fifty-three per cent of the children had no detectable impairment, 17 per cent had trivial problems, 20 per cent had minor impairments that did not cause disability and 10 per cent had major, disabling impairments. The proportion of minor and major impairments was similar to those found in singletons from the same unit of comparable gestation. The type of impairments were also similar, except in retinopathy of prematurity, which occurred in 13 per cent of the children.

In Munich, 11 sets of higher order births (three quintuplet and eight quadruplets) were followed (Rhein *et al.* 1991). Twelve per cent had major disability and 14 per cent had retinopathy of prematurity, which was about 20 times the incidence found amongst single babies of comparable gestation. This clearly needs further study. Attention in the Munich study was focussed on the lightest born twin, whose progress was compared to that of their larger siblings. None of the lightest suffered from a major disability and in general they did as well as the remainder of the set. This finding confirmed those of the London group that gestation, rather than birth weight, was the most important factor in the prognosis of these children.

One of the most worrying findings in the London group was that psychiatric referral was thought necessary in six out of seven families because of behavioural disturbances in 53 per cent of the children. All the elder siblings showed signs of behavioural disturbance within 2 years of the higher order births.

Support for parents

When a couple first hears they are expecting triplets, the chances of them knowing another family with triplets to whom they can turn for information and advice is remote; they feel very alone. The sooner they can be introduced to other families the better. In the UK the Supertwins Group, a section of TAMBA, has a country-wide network of families with triplets and produces a regular newsletter. There are a few similar organizations in other countries, notably Germany (see Appendix 2).

The Multiple Births Foundation runs a Supertwins Clinic (see Appendix 1) where families can have individual appointments with a paediatrician and then join in an informal lunch with twenty or more other families in a large hall. Expectant parents are welcomed at the clinic.

Appendix 1 The Multiple Births Foundation twins clinics

Twins clinics

The first Twins Clinic in Britain was established by the author in 1987 at Queen Charlotte's and Chelsea Hospital, London. Since then Twins Clinics have been started in three other centres in the UK (Birmingham, York and Middlesborough) as well as four Special Clinics in London (see below).

Referrals to a Twins Clinic may be made by the parents themselves (granted permission from their own doctor) or by any professional carer. The clinics are also used as a teaching forum for professionals.

The general twins clinics

These are run by two paediatricians, a nurse, a secretary/administrator and several volunteers. Families can bring their twins for a routine check or to discuss a particular worry.

A room is also provided where volunteers give practical help, support and information. The volunteers often look after the children to enable the parents to have an undisturbed talk with the paediatrician. They also look after the remaining twin and other siblings so that each twin in turn may be seen individually.

The volunteers are all parents of twins themselves and attend on a rota basis organized by the Volunteer Coordinator. Their work is supervised by a Volunteer Project Director who also provides training and study days.

Special clinics

Supertwins clinic

A 3-monthly Supertwins Clinic for triplets or more is run on the same lines as the Twins Clinic. In addition an informal lunch is provided for all the families in a large hall. Some of the families will come for the mutual support provided by the lunchtime meeting without requiring an appointment with the paediatrician. All the volunteers have triplets or quadruplets themselves. Couples expecting triplets are encouraged to come to the lunch.

Special needs clinic

A Special Needs Clinic for families who have one or more child with special needs is held 3-monthly. This is run on the same lines as the Supertwins Clinic. Families have an opportunity to discuss any concerns about either the disabled or the healthy twin.

Bereavement clinic

A Bereavement Clinic is held 3-monthly for parents who have lost one or both of their twins. Parents, together with surviving children, meet for an informal lunch and then divide into groups (whilst the children are entertained by a volunteer) according to their loss. This may be a single newborn death, the loss of all babies, a cot death or a later childhood death. Individual appointments with a paediatrician/counsellor are available on the same day or at other times by arrangement.

Education clinic

The Education Clinic is held 3-monthly for families who want to discuss the schooling of their children or problems that have already arisen. This is run jointly by a paediatrician and a teacher. A volunteer looks after the children.

Prenatal meetings

These are held in three centres with an illustrated talk by a paediatrician and discussion. They are primarily for parents (or grandparents) who are expecting twins or more but professionals are always welcome.

Appendix 2 Organizations concerned with multiple births

AUSTRALIA
Australian Multiple Birth Association Inc., P.O. Box 105, Coogee, NSW 2034, Australia.
Abbreviated title: AMBA   Contact: Joy Jacq   Telephone: 03-726-5579
AMBA was founded in 1974 and is a self-help voluntary organization, concerned with the well-being of multiple birth children and their families.

Australian NHMRC Twin Registry, The University of Melbourne, 151 Barry Street, Melbourne, VIC 3053, Australia.
Abbreviated title: ATR   Contact: Dr John Hopper   Telephone: 61-3-3472983   Fax: 61-3-344 7014
NHMRC (National Health & Medical Research Council) funded national registry of over 20 000 pairs of volunteer twins established in 1980. A resource for studies in medicine and science.

The La Trobe Twin Study, Department of Psychology, La Trobe University, Bundoora, Victoria, Australia.
Contact: Dr David Hay   Telephone: 03-479-2259   Fax: 03-478-0603

BELGIUM
Association Francophone d'Entraide Pour Naissances Multiples, Avenue Hulet 17, 1332, Genval, Belgium.
Abbreviated title: 'Naissances Multiples'   Contact: Madeleine Bouche
Telephone: 02.652.01.81
Support for families of multiple births through contact and exchanged experiences, list of discounts and free gifts.

CANADA
Parents of Multiple Births Association of Canada Inc. 4981 Hwy. East, Unit 12a, Suite 161, Markham, Ontario, L3R 1NI, Canada.
Abbreviated title: POMBA   Contact: Norinne Gratopp
Non-profit service organization for parents of twins, triplets and quadruplets. Provides information, liaison, publishing and research.

ETHIOPIA
Ethiopian Gemini Trust, PO Box 3547, Addis Ababa, Ethiopia.
Contact: Dr Carmela Abate   Telephone: 151947
An integrated urban development programme catering for needy families with twins. Integrated intervention offering primary health care, supplementary feeding, family support, job creation, day care and house upgrading.

FRANCE
Association Nationale d'Entr'aide des parents a naissances multiples, 8 place Alfred Sisley, 95430 Auvers sur Oise, France.

Abbreviated title: ANEPNM Contact: Mme C Lebatard Telephone: 16(1)30-36-19-67

Providing information on material help, on social services and psychological support to 3000 families organized in 22 subgroups.

GERMANY
ABC Club eV, Internationale Drillings und Mehrlingsinitiative, Strohweg 55, D-6100, Darmstadt, Germany.

Abbreviated title: ABC Club Contact: Helga Grutzner Telephone: 06151/55430

Gives counsel and benefit of experience to families with triplets and higher multiples, primarily in german speaking countries. Provides political representation and collects information for research.

INDONESIA
Nakula-Sadewa Indonesia Twins Foundation, Jl. Teuku Cik Ditiro No. 32 Jakarta 10310, Indonesia.

Abbreviated title: YNS Contact: Mr Seto Mulyadi Telephone: (021) 310 6177

A social foundation to help problems of multiple births and sharing of twins experience, also to aid in scholarship.

ITALY
Gemelli and Piu, Casella Postale 121, 95100 Catania, Via Marchesana 54, ACI S. Antonio, Italy.

Contact: Alfio Pizzone Telephone: 095/7921181

Magazine distributed amongst club members which number 600 throughout Italy.

International Society for Twin Studies, The Mendel Institute, Piazza Galeno 5, 00162 Rome, Italy.

Abbreviated title: ISTS Contact: Prof. Paulo Parisi Telephone: 864 658

An international, non-political, non-profit, multidisciplinary, scientific organization to further research and public education in all fields related to twins and twin studies, for the mutual benefit of the twins and their families and of scientific research in general.

JAPAN
The Japanese Association of Twins' Mothers, 5-5-20 Minami Aoyama, Minatoku, Tokyo, Japan 107.

Contact: Yukiko Amau Telephone: 03-400-0838

An association linking clubs and individual members throughout Japan. Newsletter and books published, local and national meetings held.

NETHERLANDS
Nederlands Tweelingen Register, Vrije Universiteit, de Boelelaan 1111, 1081 HV Amsterdam.

Contact: Mrs AJM Jonker Telephone: 020-5483863 Fax: 020-548 4443

Register of twins born since 1986 with information about behavioural and health characteristics, birth weight and smoking and drinking habits. Studies on health and behaviour development being carried out.

Nederlanse Vereniging Van/Tweeline, 2582 NV's Gravenhage, Johan V. Oldernbarneveltlaan 56.

NEW ZEALAND
New Zealand Multiple Birth Association, PO Box 1258, Wellington, NZ.
  Abbreviated title: NZMBA   Contact: Carla Wild   Telephone: WGTN (04) 769281
  National organization of multiple birth clubs of which there are approximately 45 throughout New Zealand. Lobby government, produce publications including a quarterly newsletter and have set up a National Multiple Birth Register.

NORWAY
Club for Families of Triplets and More, Bjaalandsgaten 1, N-4016 Stavanger, Norway.
  Abbreviated title: TRILOGI   Contact: Irene G. Svela   Telephone: 02-55 92 44
  Organization founded in 1989 to support families that are expecting or that already have higher multiples (triplets or more) in Norway. Members receive information about how to promote a healthy pregnancy and reduce risks and share feelings. Trilogi is also the name of the newsletter, produced three times a year.

Tvillingforeldreforeningen, Abinsgt. 7. 0253 Oslo 2, Norway.
  Abbreviated title: TFF   Contact: Ingun Ulven Lie   Telephone: 04582967
  TFF is a national organization with approx. 1000 members divided into about 60 local clubs. Support families of twins, triplets or more. Information to professionals and the public about the special needs of multiple birth families.

SOUTH AFRICA
South African Multiple Birth Association, PO Box 785070, Sandton 2146, South Africa.
  Abbreviated title: SAMBA   Contact: Jillian Bosman   Telephone: 27 11 789 4897
  SAMBA was established to serve the interests of multiples—twins and supertwins—and of their families. It is multiracial, bilingual, interdenominational, non-profitmaking and non-partisan.

SWEDEN
Svenska Tvillingklubben, Hermel insvagen 8, S-433 70 Partille, Sweden.
  Contact: L & A Ekelund   Telephone: 031 267083
  For twins of all ages, with activities, regular newsletter and local twin clubs.

Swedish Twin Registry, Department of Epidemiology, Inst. of Environmental Medicine, The Karolinska Institutet, Box 60208. S-10401, Stockholm.
  Contact: Dr Nancy Pedersen
  A collection of databases for the purpose of conducting epidemiological studies on morbidity and mortality.

UNITED KINGDOM
Maudsley Hospital Psychiatric Twin Register, Institute of Psychiatry (Genetics Section), De Crespigny Park, Denmark Hill, London SE5 8AF
  Contact: Alison Macdonald   Telephone: 071 703 5411 ex. 3416
  A register of all twins seen at the hospital since 1948 used for psychiatric genetic research and a volunteer twin register used for twin research on a wide range of illnesses, behaviours and psychological measures.

Multiple Births Foundation, Queen Charlotte's and Chelsea Hospital, Goldhawk Road, London, W6 0XG.
   Abbreviated title: MBF   Contact: Dr Elizabeth Bryan   Telephone: 081 748 4666 ext. 5201   Fax: 081 748 4666 ex. 5281
   Providing advice and professional support to families, information and advice to members of the caring professions, workshops, seminars, quarterly newsletter, resource centre for research workers and information service for the media.

The Twins Clinics, c/o MBF
   General Twins Clinics and four Special Clinics (Supertwins, Bereavement, Education, Special Needs) are held in three centres in the UK.

The Lone Twin Network, c/o MBF
   A register is kept to allow adult bereaved twins to be in contact with each other by telephone, letter and group meetings.

Twins and Multiple Births Association, PO Box 30, Little Sutton, L66 1TH
   Abbreviated title: TAMBA   Contact: Gina Siddons   Telephone: 051 3480020
   Supports families with twins, triplets and more, individually through local twins clubs and specialist support groups. Range of leaflets produced on many aspects; of the management of multiples, *Twins Triplets and More* magazine published three times a year. Annual conference and study days. Local twins clubs provide parent to parent support, clothes and equipment sales, day time and evening meetings.

Adopted Twins Register, c/o TAMBA
   For parents adopting twins or more, providing support and information around the time of adoption.

Bereavement Support Group, c/o TAMBA
   Provides support for parents bereaved of one or both twins, or one or more of a multiple set as a result of miscarriage, stillbirth, neonatal difficulties, cot death or other causes. Quarterly newsletter, support meetings, regional contact, Memorial service and Book of Remembrance.

Health and Education Group, c/o TAMBA
   Parents of multiples with a particular interest in research and specialist information on twins or more, many professionally qualified. Responsible for production of leaflets, study days, specialist support and advice to parents. Bulletin published twice yearly.

Single Parent Group, c/o TAMBA
   For those parents bringing up multiples alone, providing a support network.

Supertwins Group, c/o TAMBA
   For parents of triplets, quads, quins and sextuplets, providing support network, advice on breastfeeding and transport, practical help and study days. *Supernews* published three times during the year.

TAMBA Twinline, c/o TAMBA
   Telephone helpline for families with multiples to provide listening ear by trained volunteer parents of twins or more.

Twins with Special Needs, c/o TAMBA
   For parents of twins or more where one or both has special needs. Newsletter, contact with other parents.

UNITED STATES OF AMERICA

The Center for Study of Multiple Birth, 333 East Superior Street, Suite 464, Chicago, Illinois 60611.
Contact: Linda Neglia and Louis G. Keith, MD Telephone: (312) 266-9093
Dissemination of information regarding the medical risks of multiple birth, social costs and special problems encountered. Sponsors scientific conferences on care of multiple births, encourages funding for the support of medical and social research and operates the 'One Stop Twin Book Shop'.

Louisville Twin Study, Child Development Unit, Health Sciences Centre, University of Louisville, KY 40292.
Contact: Prof. Adam Matheny

Minnesota Center for Twin and Adoption Research, Department of Psychology, Elliott Hall, 75 East River Road, University of Minnesota, Minneapolis, MN 55455.
Contact: Prof. TJ Bouchard Telephone: (612) 625-4067 Fax: (612) 626-2079
Includes the Minnesota Study of Twins reared apart. Staff serve as resource for twins and adoptees who are in search of biological relatives. Source for information about twins and adoption.

Miss Helen Kirk, Supertwin Statistician, PO Box 254, Galveston, Texas 77553-0254.
Abbreviated title: Miss Helen Contact: Helen Kirk Telephone: 409 762-4792
Assistance is given to expectant parents, families with multiple births, news media, etc.

National Organisation of Mothers of Twins Clubs, Inc. PO Box #23188, Albuquerque, New Mexico 87192-1188.
Abbreviated title: NOMOTC Contact: Lois Gallmeyer Telephone: (505) 275-0955
13000 members in more than 380 clubs forming a non-profit organization founded in 1960 to cooperate with and participate in research projects. To educate parents, teachers and professionals involved in multiple birth. Publish quarterly newspaper and hold annual convention.

Our Newsletter: Support for Multiple Birth Loss, PO Box 1064, Palmer AK (Alaska) 99645.
Contact: Jean Kollantai Telephone: 907 745-2706

Triplet Connection, PO Box 99571, Stockton, CA 947709 USA.

The Twins Foundation, PO Box 6043, Providence, RI 02940-6043.
Contact: Anne R Gardner and Kay Cassill Telephone: (401) 274-TWIN
Non-profit membership organization founded in 1983. Maintains a National Twin Registry, publishes a quarterly newsletter, provides an informational clearing house on matters relating to multiples, facilitates research focusing on and using twins. Referral center for the National Research Council's Medical Follow up Agency.

Twin Services, PO Box 10066, Berkeley, CA 94709.
Contact: Patricia Malmstrom Telephone: (415) 524-0863
Non-profit health, education and social service agency providing publications and telephone advice, information and referral to parents and expectant parents of multiples throughout US. Research on twin care and development and resource for health and social workers.

World Multiple Organization, 1120 Linden Drive, Aurora, IL 60506.

USSR

Twins Club 'I/am/You', Harchenko Str. d.3 Kw.3, Leningrad 194100.
Abbreviated title: I am You Contact: Dr TB Morozova

Club meets every 4th Sunday in the month. The Founders, Dr TB Morozova an her sister, run children's section of the club and do scientific research into th development and social upbringing of twins.

ZIMBABWE
Zimbabwe Multiple Births Association, Charleigh, 3 Hillmorton Road, Meyrick Parl Harare, Zimbabwe.
Abbreviated title: ZIMBA   Contact: Mrs C Goddard

References

Aberg A, Mitelman F & Cantz M. (1978) Cardiac puncture of fetus with Hurler's disease avoiding abortion of unaffected co-twin. *Lancet*; *ii*: 990–1.

Abraham JM. (1967) Intrauterine feto-fetal transfusion syndrome. *Clin Pediatr*; **6**: 405–10.

Abraham JM. (1969) Character of placentation in twins, as related to haemoglobin levels. *Clin Pediatr*; **8**: 526–30.

Abrams RH. (1957) Double pregnancy. Report of a case with 35 days between deliveries. *Obstet Gynecol*; **9**: 435–8.

Adams DL & Fetterhoff CK. (1971) Locked twins. A case report. *Obstet Gynecol*; **33**: 53–60.

Addy HL. (1975) The breast-feeding of twins. *J Trop Pediatr Env Ch Health*; **21**: 231–9.

Adeleye JA. (1972) Retained second twin in Ibadan: its fate and management. *Am J Obstet Gynecol*; **114**: 204–7.

Aherne W & Dunnill MS. (1966) Quantitative aspects of placental structure. *J Path Bact*; **91**: 123–39.

Aherne W, Strong SJ & Corney G. (1968) The structure of the placenta in the twin transfusion syndrome. *Biol Neonat*; **12**: 121–35.

Aiken RA. (1969) An account of the Birmingham 'sextuplets'. *J Obstet Gynaecol Brit Cwlth*; **76**: 684–91.

Alberman ED. (1964) Cerebral palsy in twins. *Guys Hospital Report*; **113**: 285–95.

Allen G. (1981) The twinning and fertility paradox. In *Twin research 3: Twin biology and multiple pregnancy*; ed. W. Nance, pp. 1–13. New York, Alan R Liss.

Allen G. (1988) Frequency of triplets and triplet zygosity types among US births. *Acta Genet Med Gemellol*; **37**: 299–306.

Allen G & Kallmann FJ. (1962) Etiology of mental subnormality in twins. In *Expanding goals of genetics in psychiatry*; ed FJ Kallmann, ch. 21. London, Grune and Stratton.

Allen G & Parisi P. (1990) Trends in monozygotic and dizygotic twinning rates by maternal age and parity—further analysis of Italian data, 1949–1985, and rediscussion of US data, 1964–1985. *Acta Genet Med Gemellol*; **39**: 317–28.

Allen G & Schachter J. (1970) Do conception delays explain some changes in twinning rates? *Acta Genet Med Gemellol*; **21**: 30–4.

Allen JP. (1972) Twin transfusion syndrome. *Northwest Med*; **71**:, 296–8.

Allen MG, Pollin W & Hoffer A. (1971) Parental birth and infancy factors in infant twin development. *Am J Psychiatry*; **127**: 1597–604.

Allen MG, Greenspan SI & Pollin W. (1976) The effect of parental perceptions on early development in twins. *Psychiatry* **39**: 65–71.

Alm I. (1953) The long term prognosis for prematurely born children. *Acta Paediatr*; **42**: Suppl. 94, 9–116.

Alvarez M & Berkowitz R. (1990) Multifetal gestation. *Clin Obstet Gynecol*; **33**: 1045–50.

Anderson RC. (1977) Congenital cardiac malformations in 109 sets of twins and triplets. *Am J Cardiol*; **39**: 1045–50.

Anderson WJR. (1956) Stillbirth and neonatal mortality in twin pregnancy. *J Obstet Gynaecol Br Emp*; **63**: 205–15.

Antsaklis A, Politis J, Karagiannopoulos C & Kaskarelis D. (1984) Selective survival of only the healthy fetus following prenatal diagnosis of thalassaemia major in binovular twin pregnancy. *Prenat Diagn*; **4**: 289–96.

Archer CR. (1973) Twins in Papua. *Nursing Mirror*; **137**: 34–8.

Archer J. (1810) Facts illustrating a disease peculiar to the female children of negro slaves; and observations showing that a white woman by intercourse with a white man and a negro may conceive twins, one of which shall be white and the other a mulatto: and that, vice versa, a black woman by intercourse with a negro and a white man may conceive twins, one of which shall be white and the other a mulatto. *Med Reposit NY*; **1**: 319–23.

Arey LB. (1923) The cause of tubal pregnancy and tubal twinning. *Am J Obstet Gynecol*; **5**: 163–7.

Asher P & Schonell FE. (1950) A survey of 400 cases of cerebral palsy in childhood. *Arch Dis Child*; **25**: 360–79.

Atlay RD & Pennington GW. (1971) The use of clomiphene citrate and pituitary gonadotrophin in successive pregnancies. The Sheffield Quadruplets. *Am J Obstet Gynecol*; **109**: 402–7.

Australian Multiple Births Association (1984) Proposal submitted to the federal government concering 'Act of Grace' payments for triplet and quadruplet families. Coogee, Australia, Australian Multiple Births Association.

Avery LJ. (1972) *The Lact aid supplementer*; Denver, Colorado.

Avni A. *et al.* (1983) Down's syndrome in twins of unlike sex. *J Med Genet*; **20**: 94–6.

Babson SG & Phillips DS. (1973) Growth and development of twins dissimilar in size at birth. *N Engl J Med*; **298**: 937–40.

Baker VV & Doering MC. (1982) Fetus papyraceous, an unreported congenital anomaly of the surviving infant. *Am J Obstet Gynecol*; **142**: 234.

Bakwin H. (1973) Reading disability in twins. *Devel Med Child Neurol*: **15**: 184–7.

Banchi MT. (1984) Triplet pregnancy with second trimester abortion and delivery of twins at 35 weeks gestation. *Obstet Gynecol*; **64**: 728–30.

Barnes SE, Bryan EM, Harris D & Baum JD. (1977) Oedema in the newborn. *Molecular Aspects of Medicine*; **1**: No. 1.

Barss VA, Benacerraf BR & Frigoletto FD. (1985) Ultrasonographic determination of chorion type in twin gestation. *Obstet Gynecol*; **66**: 779–83.

Bass M. (1989) The fallacy of the simultaneous sudden infant death syndrome in twins. *Am J Forensic Med Pathol*; **10**: 200–5.

Bayani-Sioson PS, Cruz IT & Sioson C. (1967) Twinning characteristics of the contemporary Filipino population. *Acta Medica Philippina*; **4**: 56–63.

Beal S. (1983) Some epidemiological factors about sudden infant death syndrome (sids) in South Australia. In *Sudden infant death syndrome*, eds Tildon JT, Roeder LM & Steinschneider A. pp. 15–28. New York, Academic Press.

Beck L. *et al.* (1981) Twin pregnancy abortion of one fetus with Down's Syndrome by sectio parva the other delivered mature and healthy. *Eur J Obstet Gynecol Reprod Biol*; **12**: 257–9.

Behrman SJ. (1965) Hazards of twin pregnancies. *Postgrad Med*; **38**: 72–7.

Beischer NA, Pepperell RJ & Barrie JU. (1969) Twin pregnancy and erythroblastosis. *Obstet Gynecol*; **34**: 22–9.

Benda CE. (1952) *Developmental disorders of mentation and cerebral palsies*. pp. 221–91. Grune and Sratton, New York.

Bender S. (1952) Twin pregnancy, a review of 472 cases. *J Obstet Gynaecol Br Emp*; **59**: 510–17.

Benirschke K. (1961) Accurate recording of twin placentation. A plea to the obstetrician. *Obstet Gynecol*; **18**: 334–7.

Benirschke K. (1972) Prenatal cardiovascular adaptation. In *Comparative pathophysiology of circulatory disturbance. 3. Advances in experimental medicine and biology 22*, ed. CM Bloor. New York, Plenum Press.

Benirschke K. (1981) Lessons from multiple pregnancies in mammals. *Prog Biol Clin Res*; **69A**: 135–9.

Benirschke K. (1990) The placenta in twin gestation. *Clin Obstet Gynecol*; **33**: 18–31.

Benirschke K & Driscoll SG. (1967) *The pathology of the human placenta*; New York, Springer–Verlag.

Benirschke K & Kim CK. (1973) Multiple pregnancy—part 2. *N Engl J Med*; **288**: 1329–36.

Beral V, Doyle P, Tan SL, Mason BA & Campbell S. (1990) Outcome of pregnancies resulting from assisted conception. *Br Med Bull*; **46**: 753–68.

Berg JM & Kirman BH. (1960) The mentally defective twin. *Br Med J*; **1**: 1911–7.

Berg G, Finnstrom O, Selbing A. (1983) Triplet pregnancy in Linkoping, Sweden 1973–1981. *Acta Genet Med Gemellol*; **32**: 251–6.

Bergsma D. (1967) Conjoined twins. *Birth Defects Original Article*, Series 3, No. 1. New York, The National Foundation.

Berkowitz RL, Lynch L, Chitkara U, Wilkins TA & Mehalek KE. (1988) Selective reduction of multifetal pregnancies in the first trimester. *N Engl J Med*; **318**: 1043–7.

Bernabei P & Levi G. (1976) Psychopathologic problems in twins during childhood. *Acta Gent Med Gemellol*; **25**: 381–3.

Bernstein BA. (1980) Siblings of twins. *Psychoanal Study Child*; **35**: 135–54.

Bessis R & Papiernik E. (1981) Echographic imagery of amniotic membranes in twin pregnancies. Twin Research 3. *Twin Birth and Multiple Pregnancy*, ed. W. Nance, pp. 183–7. New York, Alan R Liss.

Betton JP & Loester LS. (1983) The impact of twinship—observed and perceived differences in mothers and twins. *Child Study J*; **13**: 85–93.

Bhargava I. (1976) Blood vessels of the twin placenta in relation to zygosity. *Acta Genet Med Gemellol*; **25**: 121–4.

Bhettay G, Nelson, MM & Beighton P. (1975) Epidemic of conjoined twins in Southern Africa. *Lancet*; **ii**: 741–3.

Bieber FR, Nance WE, Morton CC, Brown JA, Redwine FO, Jordan RL & Mohanakumar T. (1981). Genetic studies of an acardiac monster, evidence of polar body twinning in man. *Science*; **214**: 775–7.

Bildhaiya GS. (1978) A study of twin births. *Indian Pediatrics*; **15**: 931–4.

Bishop N, King FJ, Ward P, Rennie JM & Dixon AK. (1990) Paradoxical bone mineralisation in the twin-twin transfusion syndrome. *Arch Dis Child*; **7**: 705–10.

Blake A, Stewart A & Turcan D. (1975) Parents of babies of very low birthweight, long term follow up. In *Parent–infant interaction*; pp. 271–81. Ciba Foundation Symposium 33. Amsterdam, Elsevier.

Bleisch VR. (1964) Diagnosis of monochorionic twin placentation. *Am J Clin Path*; **42**: 277–84.

Bleker OP, Kloosterman GJ, Huidekoper BL & Breur W. (1977) Intrauterine growth of twins as estimated from birthweight and the fetal biparietal diameter. *Eur J Obstet Gynecol Reprod Biol*; **7**: 85–90.

Bleker OP, Breur W & Huidekoper BL. (1979) A study of birthweight, placental weight and mortality of twins as compared to singletons. *Br J Obstet Gynaecol*; **86**: 111–8.

Blickstein I. *et al.* (1989) Ultrasonic prediction of growth discordancy by intertwin difference in abdominal circumference. *Int J Gynaecol Obstet*; **29**: 121–4.

Bluglass K. (1980) Psychiatric morbidity after cot death. *Practitioner*; **224**: 533–9.

Boklage CE. (1986) Twinning, nonrighthandedness and fusion malformations: evidence for heritable causal elements held in common. *Acta Genet Med Gemellol*; **35**: Abstra., 44.

Bonnelykke B. (1990) Social class and human twinning. *J Biosoc Sci*; **22**: 381–6.

Bosma JF. (1954) Autotransfusion between two twins. *Am J Dis Child*; **88**: 509.

Botting B, Macdonald-Davis I & Macfarlane A. (1987) Recent trends in the incidence of multiple births and their mortality. *Arch Dis Child*; **62**: 941–50.

Botting BJ, Macfarlane AJ & Price FV. (1990). *Three, four and more: a study of triplet and higher order births*. London, HMSO.

Bourne GH. (1962). *The human amnion and chorion*. London, Lloyd-Luke.

Bourne S. (1968) the psychological effects of stillbirths on women and their doctors. *J Roy Coll Gen Pract*; **16**: 103–12.

Bowlby J. (1980). *Attachment and Loss, III Loss sadness and depression*. London, Hogarth Press.

Bowman E, Doyle LW, Murton LJ, Roy RND & Kitchen W. (1988) Increased mortality of preterm infants transferred between tertiary perinatal centres. *Br Med J*; **297**: 1098–1100.

Boyd JD & Hamilton WJ. (1970) *The human placenta*. Cambridge, Heffers.

Bracken MB. (1979) Oral contraception and twinning: an epidemiologic study. *Am J Obstet Gynecol*; **133**: 432–4.

Brandes JM. *et al.* (1989) Reduction of the number of embryos in a multiple pregnancy: quintuplet to triplet. *Fertil Steril*; **48**: 326–7.

Breslau N & Prabucki K. (1987) Siblings of disabled children: effects of chronic stress in the family. *Arch Gen Psychiatry*; **44**: 1040–6.

Brewster DP. (1979) Nursing twins. In, *You can breastfeed your baby . . . even in special situations*, pp. 399–414. Emmaus, Pennsylvania, USA, Rodale Press.

Brion L, Alexanders, Clercy A, Avni EG, Kirkpatrick C, Vermeylen D, Determmerman D & Pardou A. (1986) Fatal urea plasma infection in second twin born 60 days after delivery of the first in a patient with recurrent spontaneous abortion—a case report. *J Perinat Med*; **14**: 201–4.

British Medical Journal (1976) Koluchova's twins (editorial). *Br Med J*; 897–8.

Broadbent, B. (1985) Twin trauma *Nursing Times*, 28–30.

Brock, DJH, Barron L, Watt, M. & Scrimgeour, JB, (1979) The relation between maternal plasma alphafetoprotein and birthweight in twin pregnancy. *Br. J. Obstet. Gynaecol.*, **86**, 710–12.

Brown, B. (1977) Placentation effects on birthweight IQ in MZ twins. Presented to the Society for Research in Child Development, New Orleans.

Bryan EM. (1976) *Serum immunoglobulins in twin pregnancy with particular reference to the fetofetal transfusion syndrome*. London, MD Thesis.

Bryan EM. (1977a) Twins are a handful. How can we help? *Mat Child Health*; 348–53.

Bryan EM. (1977b) IgG deficiency in association with placental oedema. *Early Hum Devel*; **1**: 133–43.

Bryan EM. (1986) Are They Identical? The importance of determining zygosity. *Mat Child Health*; **11**: 171–6.

Bryan EM. (1989) The response of mothers to selective feticide. *Ethic Probs. Reprod. Med.*, **1**, 28–30.

Bryan EM. (1990) I don't want so many babies. *Multiple Births Foundation Newsletter*; **7**: 3.

Bryan EM. (1992) *Twins, triplets and more*. Harmondsworth, Middlesex, Penguin.

Bryan EM & Kohler H. (1974) The missing umbilical artery prospective study based on a maternity unit. *Arch Dis Child*; **49**: 844–51.

Bryan E. & Slavin B. (1974) Serum IgG levels in feto-fetal transfusion syndrome. *Arch. Dis. Child.*, **49**, 908–10.

Bryan EM, Slavin B & Nicholson E. (1976) Serum immunoglobulins in multiple pregnancy. *Arch Dis Child*; **51**: 354–9.

Bryan EM, Little J & Burn J. (1987) Congenital anomalies in twins. *Bailliere's Clin Obstet Gynecol*; **1**: 697–721.

Bryan E, Higgins R & Harvey D. (1991) Ethical dilemmas. In, *The stress of multiple births*, eds. Harvey D & Bryan E. London, Multiple Births Foundation.

Buckler JMH & Buckler JB. (1987) Growth characteristics in twins and higher order births. *Acta Genet Med Gemellol*; **36**: 197–208.

Buckler JMH & Robinson A. (1974) Matched developmen of a pair of monozygotic twins of grossly different size at birth. *Arch Dis Child*; **49**: 472–6.

Bulmer MG. (1958) The repeat frequency of twinning. *Ann Hum Genet*; **23**: 31–5.

Bulmer MG. (1959a) The effect of parental age, parity and duration of marriage on the twinning rate. *Ann Hum Genet*; **23**: 454–8.

Bulmer MG. (1959b) Twinning rate in Europe during the war. *Br Med J*; 29–30.

Bulmer MG. (1960) The twinning rate in Europe and Africa. *Ann Hum Genet (Lond)*; **24**: 121–5.

Bulmer MG. (1970) *The biology of twinning in man*. Oxford, Clarendon Press.

Burke MS. (1990) Single fetal demise in twin gestation. *Clin Obstet Gynecol*; **33**: 69–78.

Burlingham D. (1952) *Twins: a study of three pairs of identical twins*. New York, International Press.

Burn J. (1988) Monozygotic twins. *Contemporary Obstetric and Gynaecology*, pp. 161–75. ed. G Chamberlain. London, Butterworths.

Burn J. (1991) Disturbance of morphological laterality in humans. In *Biological asymmetry and handedness*; pp. 282–99. Ciba Foundation Symposium. Chichester, John Wiley and Sons.

Burn J & Corney G. (1984) Congenital heart defects and twinning. *Acta Genet Med Gemellol*; **33**: 61–9.

Burn J & Corney G. (1988) Zygosity determination and the types of twinning. In, *Twinning and Twins*. pp 7–26 eds I MacGillivray, Campbell DM & Thompson B. Wiley, Chichester.

Burn J, Povey S, Boyd Y, Munro EA, West L, Harper K & Thomas D. (1986) Duchenne muscular dystrophy in one of monozygotic twin girls. *J Med Genet*; **23**: 494–500.

Burnell GM. (1974) Maternal reaction to the loss of multiple births. A case of septuplets. *Arch Gen Psychiatry*; **30**: 183–4.

Bustamante SA & Stumpff LC. (1978) Fetal hydantoin syndrome in triplets: a unique experiment of nature. *Am J Dis Child*; **132**: 978–9.

Butler NR & Alberman ED. (1969) Perinatal problems—the second report of the 1958 British Perinatal Mortality Survey; **7**: 122–47. Edinburgh, E and S Livingstone Ltd.

Cameron AH, Robson EB, Wade-Evans J & Wingham J. (1969) Septuplet conception: placental and zygosity studies. *J Obstet Gynaecol Br Cwlth*; **76**: 692–8.

Cameron AH, Edwards JH, Derom R, Thiery M & Boelaert. (1983) The value of twin surveys in the study of congenital malformations. *Europ J Obstet Gynecol Reprod Biol*; **14**: 347–56.

Campbell M. (1961) Twins and congenital heart disease. *Acta Genet Med Gemellol*; **10**: 443–55.

Campbell S & Dewhurst CJ. (1970) Quintuplet pregnancy diagnosed and assessed by ultrasonic compound scanning. *Lancet*; **i**: 101–3.

Campbell DM, Campbell AJ & MacGillivray I. (1974) Maternal characteristics of women having twin pregnancies. *J Biosoc Sci*; **6**: 463–70.

Campbell DM, MacGillivray I & Thompson B. (1977) Twin zygosity and pre-eclampsia. *Lancet*; **ii**: 97, letter.

Campbell DM & MacGillivray I. (1988) Management of labour and delivery. In *Twinning and twins*, pp. 143–60. eds I MacGillivray, DM Campbell & B Thompson. Chichester, John Wiley and Sons.

Carey HM. (1976) Induction of ovulation resulting in nonuplet pregnancy. *Australian & New Zealand J Obstet Gynaecol*; **16**: 200.

Carothers AD, Frackiewicz A, de Mey R, Collyer S, Polani PE, Ostovics M, Horvath

K, Papp Z, May HM & Ferguson-Smith MA. (1980) A collaborative study of the aetiology of Turner Syndrome. *Ann Hum Genet*; **43**: 355–68.

Carpenter RG. (1965) Sudden death in twins. *MOH Rep Pub Hlth Med Subjects*; **113**: 51–2.

Carpenter RG, Gardner A, Pursall E, McWeeny PM & Emery JL. (1979) Identification of some infants at immediate risk of dying unexpectedly and justifying intensive study. *Lancet*; **ii**: 343–46.

Carr SR, Aronson MP & Coustan DR. (1990) Survival rates of monoamniotic twins do not decrease after 30 weeks gestation. *Am J Obstet Gynecol*; **163**: 719–22.

Carter CO. (1965) The inheritance of common congenital malformations. In *Progress in medical genetics*; pp 59–84 eds AG Steinberg & AG Bearn, London, Heinemann.

Cederlof R, Friberg L, Johnson E & Kay K. (1961) Studies on similarity diagnosis in twins with the aid of mailed questionnaires. *Acta Genet*; **11**: 338–62.

Ceelie N. (1985) Eenelige tweelinger en congenitale afwijkingen. *Tijdschr Kindergeneeskd*; **53**: 142–5.

Cetrulo C. (1986) The controversy of mode of delivery in twins: the intrapartum management of twin gestation (part I). *Semin Perinatol*; **10**: 39–43.

Chamberlain RN & Simpson RN. (1977) Cross-sectional studies of physical growth in twins postmature and small-for-dated children. *Acta Paediatr Scand*; **66**: 457–63.

Chang C. (1990) Raising twin babies and problems in the family. *Acta Genet Med Gemellol*; **39**: 501–5.

Cheng YJ, Chen CJ & Chang C. (1986) Twinning rates in Taiwan. *Acta Genet Med Gemellol*; **35**: 52.

Chitkara U, Berkowitz GS, Levine R, Riden DJ, Fagerstron RM, Chervenak FA & Berkowitz RL. (1985) Twin pregnancy: routine use of ultrasound examination in the prenatal diagnosis of intrauterine growth retardation and discordant growth. *Am J Perinatol*; **2**: 49–54.

Christoffel KK & Salafsky I. (1975) Fetal alcohol syndrome in dizygotic twins. *J Pediatr*; **87**: 963–7.

Churchill JA & Henderson W. (1974) Perinatal factors affecting fetal development—twin pregnancy. In *Birth defects and fetal development*, ed KS Moghissi. Springfield, Illinois, Charles C Thomas.

Clark PM & Dickman Z. (1984) Features of interaction of infant twins. *Acta Genet Med Gemellol*; **33**: 165–171.

Clay MM. (1989) *Quadruplets and higher multiple births. Clinics in Developmental Medicine No. 107.* Oxford, MacKeith Press.

Clemetson CAB. (1956) The difference in birthweight in human twins. 2. Cord blood haemoglobin levels. *J Obstet Gynaecol Br Emp*; **63**: 9–14.

Cohen DJ, Dibble E, Grawe JM & Pollin W. (1975) Reliably separating identical from fraternal twins. *Arch Gen Psychiatry*; **32**: 1371–5.

Collier HL. (1972). *The psychology of twins.* Collier, Arizona.

Collins MS & Bleyl JA. (1990) Seventy-one quadruplet pregnancies: management & outcome. *Am J Obstet Gynecol*; **162**: 1384–91.

Conrad A & Weidinger. (1982) Successful prolongation of immature twin pregnancy by tocolysis and recerclage following unavoidable delivery of the first foetus after emergency cerclage. *Geburtshilfe Fraunleike*; **42**: 79–83.

Contrepas C. (1989) Information before pregnancy: the limits of enlightened consent. *Multiple Births Foundation Newsletter*; **5**: 2.

Conway D, Lytton H & Pysh F. (1980) Twin-singleton language differences. *Can J Behav Sci*; **12**: 264–72.

Cooke R. (1991) The newborn. In: *The stress of multiple births*, eds D Harvey & E. Bryan London, MBE.

Corballis MC & Morgan MJ. (1978) On the biological basis of human laterality.

Evidence of a maturational left to right gradient. *Behav and Brain Sci*; 2: 261–9.

Corey LA, Nance WE, Kang KW & Christian JC. (1979) Effects of type of placentation on birth weight and its variability in monozygotic and dizygotic twins. *Acta Genet Med Gemellol*; 28: 41–50.

Corney G. (1966) *The Twin Transfusion Syndrome*. University of Liverpool, MD Thesis.

Corney G. (1975a) Mythology and customs associated with twins. In *Human multiple reproduction*; pp 1–15 eds I MacGillivray, PPS Nylander & G Corney. London, WB Saunders.

Corney G. (1975b) Placentation. In *Human multiple reproduction*; pp 40–76 eds I MacGillivray, PPS Nylander & G Corney. London, WB Saunders.

Corney G & Robson EB. (1975) Types of twinning and determination of zygosity. In *Human multiple reproduction*; pp 16–39 eds I MacGillivray, PPS Nylander & G Corney. London, WB Saunders.

Corney G, Robson EB & Strong SJ. (1972) The effect of zygosity on the birth weight of twins. *Ann Hum Genet*; 36: 45–59.

Corney G, Seedburgh D, Thompson B, Campbell DM, MacGillivray I & Timlin D. (1979) Maternal height and twinning. *Ann Hum Genet*; 43: 55–9.

Corney G, MacGillivray I, Campbell DM, Thompson B & Little J. (1983) Congenital anomalies in twins in Aberdeen and North-East Scotland. *Acta Genet Med Gemellol*; 28: 31–35.

Corston J McD. (1957) Twin survival. A comparison of mortality rates of the first and second twin. *Obstet Gynecol*; 10: 181–3.

Cortes RL. (1964) Quadruples con transfusion de feto a feto un producto con anemia otro con policitemia. *Revista Medica de Costa Rica*; 21: 89–99.

Costello AJ. (1978) Deprivation and family structure with particular reference to twins. In *The Child in the family. Vulnerable Children*, eds EJ Anthony, C Koupernik and C Chiland vol. 4. Wiley, New York.

Cotton M, Cotton G & Goodall J. (1981) A brother dies at home. *Mat Child Health*; 6: 288–92.

Craft MJ, Lakin JA, Opplinger RA, Clancy GM & Vanderlinden DW. (1990) Siblings as change agents for promoting the functional status of children with cerebral palsy. *Devel Med Child Neurol*; 32: 1049–1057.

Crane JP, Tomich PG & Kopta M. (1980) Ultrasonic growth patterns and discordant twins. *Obstet Gynecol*; 55: 678–83.

Crawford JA. (1975) An appraisal of lumbar epidural blockade in labour in patients with multiple pregnancy. *Br J Obstet Gynaecol*; 82: 929–35.

Crawford JA. (1987) A prospective study of 200 consecutive twin deliveries. *Anaesthesia*; 42: 33–43.

Crowther CA, Neilson JP, Verkuyl DAA, Bannerman C & Ashurst HM. (1989) Preterm labour in twin pregnancies, can it be prevented by hospital admission? *Br J Obstet Gynaecol*; 96: 850–3.

Czeizel A & Acsadi G. (1971) Demographic characteristics of multiple births in Hungary. *Acta Genet Med Gemellol*; 20: 301–13.

D'Alton ME & Dudley DK. (1989) The ultrasonographic prediction of chorionicity in twin gestation. *Am J Obstet Gynecol*; 160: 557–61.

D'Alton ME & Mercer BM. (1990) Antepartum management of twin gestation, ultrasound. *Clin Obstet Gynecol*; 33: 42–51.

D'Alton ME, Newton ER & Cetrulo CL. (1984) Intrauterine fetal demise in multiple gestation. *Acta Genet Med Gemellol*; 33: 43–9.

Dahlberg G. (1926). *Twin births and twins from a hereditary point of view*. Stockholm, AB Tidens Tryckeri.

Dahniya MH, Shoukry IF. Balami WI Fatukasi JI (1990). Simultaneous advanced extrauterine and intrauterine pregnancy. *Int J Gynecol Obstet*; 31: 61–5.

Danielson C. (1960) Twin pregnancy and birth. *Acta Obstet Gynaecol Scand*; **39**: 63–87.

Davenport CB. (1927) Does the male have an influence in human twin production? *Zeitschrift fur induktive Abstammungs and Vererbungslehre*; **46**: 85–6.

Davis EA. (1937) Linguistic skill in twins, singletons and siblings and only children from age five to ten years. University Minnesota. *Instit Child Welfare, Monograph Series*; No. 14.

Dawood MY, Ratnam SS & Lim YC. (1975) Twin pregnancy in Singapore. *Aust N Z J Obstet Gynecol*; **15**: 93–8.

Day E. (1932) The development of language in twins I. A comparison of twins and single children. *Child Dev*; **3**: 179–99.

Deale CJC & Cronje HS. (1984) A review of 367 triplet pregnancies. *S African Med J*; **66**: 92–4.

Deem HE. (1931) Observations on the milk of New Zealand women. *Arch Dis Child*; **6**: 53–62.

De Lia, JE. (1991) Laser treatment of severe twin-twin transfusion syndrome. Presented at the seventh workshop on multiple pregnancy. Berlin.

De Lia, JE, & Cruikshank, DP. (1990) Fetoscopic neodymium: YAG laser occlusion of placental vessels in severe twin transfusion syndrome. *Obstet. Gynecol*; **75**, 1046–53.

De La Torre Verduzco R. *et al.* (1976) Hyaline membrane disease in twins. *Am J Obstet Gynecol*; **125**: 668–671.

Derom C, Bakker E, Vlietinck R, Derom R, Van den Berghe, Thiery M & Pearson P. (1985) Zygosity determination in newborn twins using DNA variants. *J Med Genet*; **22**: 279–82.

Derom C, Vlietinck R, Derom R, Van den Berghe H & Thiery M. (1987) Increased monozygotic twinning rate after ovulation induction. *Lancet*; **i**: 1236–8.

Derom R, Vlietinck R, Derom C & Thiery M. (1989) Comparative study of outcome and zygosity in spontaneous and induced multiple pregnancies. Presented at the Sixth International Congress of Twin Studies. Rome.

Derom C, Derom R, Vlietinck R & Van den Berghe H. (1991) *Zygosity in a population-based registry of triplets*. Presented at the seventh workshop on multiple pregnancy. Berlin.

Donnenfeld AE, Glazerman LR, Cutillo DM, Librizzi RJ & Weiner S. (1989) Fetal exsanguination following intrauterine angiographic assessment and selective termination of a hydrocephalic, monozygotic co-twin. *Prenat Diagn*; **9**: 301–8.

Dorgan LT & Clarke PE. (1956) Uterus didelphys with double pregnancy. *Am J Obstet Gynecol*; **72**: 663–6.

Douglas B. (1958) The role of environmental factors in the etiology of 'so-called' congenital malformations I and II. *Plast Reconstr Surg*; **22**: 94–108, 214–29.

Douglas JE & Sutton A. (1978) The development of speech and mental processes in a pair of twins: A case study. *J Child Psychol Psychiatry*; **19**: 49–56.

Doyle PE, Beral V, Botting B & Wake CJ. (1991) Congenital malformations in twins in England and Wales. *J Epidemiol Health*; **45**: 43–48.

Drillien CM. (1964) *The growth and development of the prematurely born infant*. Edinburgh, E and S Livingstone Ltd.

Drucker P, Finkel J & Savel LE. (1960) Sixty-five day interval between the births of twins. A case report. *Am J Obstet Gynecol*; **80**: 761–3.

Dubowitz LMS, Dubbowitz V & Goldberg C. (1970) Clinical assessment of gestational age in the newborn infant. *J Pediatr*; **77**: 1–10.

Dudley DKL & D'Alton ME. (1966) Single fetal death in twin gestation. *Sem Perinatol*; **10**: 65–72.

Durkin MV, Kaveggia EG, Pendleton E, Neuhauser G & Opitz JM. (1976) Analysis of etiologic factors in cerebral palsy with severe mental retardation. Analysis of gestational parturitional and neonatal date. *Eur J Pediatr*; **123**: 67–81.

Eastman NJ. (1961) Editorial comments on uterine overdistension. *Obstet Gynecol Survey*; **16**: 185.

Eastman NJ, Kohl SG, Maisel JE & Kavaler F. (1962) The obstetrical background of 753 cases of cerebral palsy. *Obstet Gynecol Survey*; **17**: 459–97.

Edmond A, Golding J & Peckham C. (1989) Cerebral palsy in two national cohort studies. *Arch Dis Child*; **64**: 848–52.

Edmonds HW. (1954) The spiral of the normal umbilical cord in twins and in singletons. *Am J Obstet Gynecol*; **67**: 102–20.

Edmonds LD & Layde PM. (1982) Conjoined twins in the United States 1970–1977. *Teratology*; **25**: 301–8.

Edwards J. (1938) Season and rate of conception. *Nature (Lond.)*; vol. 1 142.

Edwards JH, Dent T & Kahn J. (1986) Monozygotic twins of different sex. *J Med Genet*; **3**: 117–23.

Edwards RG, Mettler L & Walters DE. (1986) Identical twins and in vitro fertilization. *J in Vitro Fertilization and Embryo Transfer*; **3**: 114–17.

Eisen S, Neunam R, Goldberg J, Rice J & True W. (1989) Determining zygosity in the Vietnam Era Twin Registry, an approach using questionnaires. *Clin Genet*; **35**: 423–32.

Elejalde BR & Elejalde MM. (1984) Further comments on amniocentesis in twin gestations. *Am J Med Genet*; **17**: 699–701.

Elias S, Gerbie AB, Simpson JL, Nadler HL, Sabbagha RE & Shkolnik A. (1980) Genetic amniocentesis in twin gestations. *Am J Obstet Gynecol*; **138**: 169–74.

Elliman A, Bryan E, Elliman AD & Starte D. (1986) Low birthweight babies at 3 years of age. *Child Care, Health and Development*; **12**: 287–311.

Ellis RG, Berger GS, Keith L & Depp R. (1979) The Northwestern University Multihospital Twin Study. II Mortality of first versus second twins. *Acta Genet Med Gemellol*; **28**: 347–52.

Elwood JM. (1973) Changes in the twinning rate in Canada 1926–1970. *Br J Prev Soc Med*; **27**: 236–41.

Elwood JM. (1978) Maternal and environmental factors affecting twin births in Canadian cities. *Br J Obstet Gynaecol*; **85**: 351–8.

Elwood JM & Elwood JH. (1980) *Epidemiology of anencephalus and spina bifida*. Oxford, Oxford University Press.

Emanuel I, Huang SW, Gutman LT, Yu FC & Linn CC. (1972) The incidence of congenital malformation in a Chinese population: the Taipei collaborative study. *Teratology*; **5**: 159–69.

Emery AEH. (1986) Identical twinning and oral contraception. *Journal of Eugenics Society*; **3**: 23–7.

Emery JL. (1979) Cot death. *Maternal and Child Health*; **4**: 374–8.

Eng HL. *et al.* (1989) Fetus in fetu, a case report and review of the literature. *J Pediatr Surg*; **24**: 296–9.

Eriksson AW & Fellman J. (1967) Twinning in relation to the marital status of the mother. *Acta Genet (Basel)*; **17**: 385–98.

Eriksson AW & Fellman JO. (1973) Differences in the twinning trends between Finns and Swedes. *Am J Hum Genet*; **25**: 141–5.

Eriksson AW, Eskola MR & Fellman JO. (1976) Retrospective studies on the twinning rate of Scandinavia. *Acta Genet Med Gemellol*; **25**, 29–35.

Evans MI, Fletcher JC, Zador IE, Newton BW Quigg, MH & Struyk CD. (1988) Selective first-trimester termination in octuplet and quadruplet pregnancies, clinical and ethical issues. *Obstet Gynecol*; **71**: 289–300.

Falkner F. (1978) Implications for growth in human twins. In *Human growth. I principles and prenatal growth*; eds F Falkner and JM Tanner, pp. 397–413. London, Bailliere Tindall.

226   *References*

Farge P, Dallaire L, Potier M & Melancon SB. (1985) Prenatal diagnosis of trisomy IO P in a twin pregnancy. *Prenat Diagn*; **5**: 199–203.
Farooqui MO, Grossman JH & Shannon RA. (1973) A review of twin pregnancy and perinatal mortality. *Obstet Gynecol Survey*; **28**: 144–53.
Farr V. (1975) Prognosis for the babies, early and late. In *Human multiple reproduction*; eds I MacGillivray, PPS Nylander & G Corney, pp. 118–211, London, WB Saunders.
Farrell AGW. (1964) Twin pregnancy: a study of 1000 cases. *S Af J Obstet Gynaecol*; **2**: 35–41.
Feichtinger W, Breitenecker G & Frohlich H. (1989) Prolongation of pregnancy to survival of twin B after loss of twin A at 21 weeks gestation. *Am J Obstet Gynecol*; **161**: 891–3.
Fellman JO & Eriksson AW. (1990) Standardization of the twinning rate. *Hum Biol*; **62**: 803–16.
Felszer M. (1979) The incidence of twins in the Kingdom of Tonga and maternal and perinatal complication. *Fiji Medical Journal*; **7**: 156–62.
Fenner A, Malm T & Kusserow U. (1980) Intrauterine growth of twins. A retrospective analysis. *Eur J Pediatr*; **133**: 119–21.
Ferguson WF. (1964) Perinatal mortality in multiple gestations. A review of perinatal deaths from 1609 multiple gestations. *Obstet Gynecol*; **23**: 861–70.
Ferguson-Smith MA. (1966) Kleinfelter's syndrome and mental deficiency. In *Sex chromatin*, ed. Moore KL, pp. 277–315. Philadelphia, WB Saunders.
Field T & Widmayer S. (1980) Early development of term and preterm twins. University of Miami Medical School. Paper presented at New Haven (unpublished).
Filkins K, Russo J, Brown T, Schmerler S & Searle B. (1984) Genetic amniocenteses in multiple gestations. *Prenat Diagn*; **4**: 223–6.
Finberg HJ & Birnholz JC. (1979) Ultrasound observations in multiple gestation with first trimester bleeding, the blighted twin. *Radiology*; **132**: 137–42.
Fisk NM, Borrel A, Hubinot C, Tannirandorn Y, Nicolini U & Rodeck CH. (1990) Feto-fetal transfusion syndrome: do the neonatal criteria apply *in utero*? *Arch Dis Child*; **65**: 657–61.
Fliegner JR & Eggers TR. (1984) The relationship between gestational age and birthweight in twin pregnancy. *Aust NZ J Obstet Gynaecol*; **24**: 192–7.
Foglmann R. (1976) Monoamniotic twins. *Acta Genet Med Gemellol*; **26**: 62–5.
Foong JC. (1971) Further study of twinning in Singapore. *J Singapore Paediatr Soc*; **13**: 85–90.
Forrester RM, Lees VT & Watson GH. (1966) Rubella syndrome, escape of a twin. *Br Med J*; **1**: 1403.
Fox H. (1978) The placenta in multiple pregnancy. In *Pathology of the placenta*; pp. 73–94, London, WB Saunders.
Fraser FC & Nora JJ. (1975) *Genetics of man*, p. 177. Lea & Febiger, Philadelphia.
Friedman EA & Sachtleben MR. (1964) The effect of uterine distention on labor. 1. Multiple pregnancy. *Obstet Gynecol*; **23**: 164–72.
Froggatt P, Lynas MA & McKenzie G. (1971) Epidemiology of sudden unexpected death in infants 'cot death' in Northern Ireland. *Br J Prev Soc Med*; **25**: 119–134.
Frutiger P. (1969) Zum problem der akardie. *Acta Anat (Basel)*; **74**: 505–31.
Fujikura T & Froehlich LA. (1971) Twin placentation and zygosity. *Obstet Gynecol*; **37**: 34–43.
Fujikura T & Froehlich LA. (1974) Mental and motor development in monozygotic co-twins with dissimilar birthweights. *Pediatrics*; **53**: 884–9.
Fusi L & Gordon H. (1990) Twin pregnancy complicated by single intrauterine death. Problems and outcome with conservative management. *Br J Obstet Gynaecol*; **97**: 511–6.

Gabrielcyzk MR. (1987) Personal view. *Br Med J*; **295**: 209.

Gaehtgens G. (1936) Klinischer beitrag zur pathogenese des akuten hydramnions. *Monatsschrift fur Geburtschilfe und Gynakologie*; **103**: 40–48.

Garrett WJ. (1960) Uterine overdistension and the duration of labour. *Med J Aust*; **2**: 376–7.

Gedda L. (1961) *Twins in history and science*. Springfield, Illinois, Charles Thomas.

Geeves RC. (1928) an armorphous 'Siamese' twin and its separation from a normal foetus. *Med J Aust*; **i**: 617–8.

Gershoni-Baruch R, Schert A, Itskovitz J, Thaler I & Brandes JM. (1991) The physical and psychomotor development of children conceived by IVF and exposed to high-frequency vaginal ultrasonography (6.5 MHz) in the first trimester of pregnancy. *Ultrasound Obstet Gynecol*; **1**: 21–8.

Geyer E. (1940) Ein Zwllingsparchen mit zwei Vatern nachgewiesne Uberschwangerung beim Menschen—A pair of twins with 2 fathers. *Arch Rassenbiol*; **34**: 226–36.

Ghodsian M. (1989) Personal communication to Redshow R & Rutter M. Growing up as a twin: twin–singleton differences in psychological development. In *The stress of multiple births*, eds D Harvey & E Bryan, Multiple Births Foundation, London.

Ghosh S & Ramanujacharyulu TKTS. (1979) Study of twin births in an urban community of Delhi. *Indian J Med Res*; **701**: 70–7.

Gifford S, Murawski BJ, Brazelton TB & Young GC. (1966) Differences in individual development within a pair of identical twins. *Int J Psychoanalysis*; **47**: 261–8.

Gigon U, Moser H & Aufdermauer P. (1981) Zwillingsschwangershaft mit operativeer Entfernung eines feten mit mosaik 46XX45x0 und geburt eines kindes 46XY am geburtstermin. Twin pregnancy with operative removal of one fetus with chromosomal mosaicism 46XX45XO and term delivery of a healthy baby. *Z Geburtshilfe Perinatol*; **185**: 365–6.

Giles WB, Trudinger BJ, Cook CM & Connelly AJ. (1990) Doppler umbilical artery studies in the twin–twin transfusion syndrome. *Obstet Gynecol*; **76**: 1097–99.

Giovannucci-Uzielli ML, Vecchi C, Donzelli GP, Levi D'Ancona V & Lapi E. (1981) The history of the Florentine Sextuplets, Obstetric and genetic considerations. *Twin Res*; **3** Twin Biology & Multiple Pregnancy 217–20. New York, Alan R Liss.

Gleeson C, Hay DA, Johnston CJ & Theobald TM. (1990) 'Twins in school'. An Australian-wide program. *Acta Genet Med Gemellol*; **39**: 231–44.

Golbus MS, Cunningham N & Goldberg J. (1988) Selective termination of multiple gestation. *Am J Med Genet*; **31**: 339–48.

Goldgar DE & Kimberling WJ. (1981) Genetic expectations of polar body twinning. *Acta Genet Med Gemellol*; **30**: 257–66.

Golding J. (1986) Social class and twinning. *Acta Genet Med Gemellol*; **35**: 29.

Goldman GA, Dicker D, Feldberg D, Ashkenazi J, Yeshaya A & Goldmar JA. (1989) The vanishing foetus. A report of 17 cases of triplets & quadruplets. *J Perinat Med*; **17**: 157–62.

Gonen R, Heyman E, Asztalos EV, Ohlsson A, Pitson LC, Shennan AT & Milligan JE. (1990) The outcome of triplet, quadruplet and quintuplet pregnancies managed in a perinatal unit: obstetric, neonatal and follow-up data. *Am J Obstet Gynecol*; **162**: 454–9.

Goplerud EP. (1964) Monoamniotic twins with double survival. *Obstet Gynecol*; **23**: 289–90.

Goshen-Gottstein ER. (1980) The mothering of twins, triplets and quadruplets. *Psychiatry*: **43**: 189–204.

Goshen-Gottstein ER. (1981) Differential maternal socialization of opposite-sexed twins, triplets and quadruplets. *Child Dev*; **52**: 1255–64.

Goswami HK & Wagh KV. (1975) Twinning in India. *Acta Gen Med Gemellol*; **24**: 347–50.

228 *References*

Grant P & Pearn JH. (1969) Foetus-in-foetu. *Med J Aust*; **1**: 1016–19.

Green QL, Schanck GP & Smith JR. (1961) Normal, living twins in uterus didelphys with 38-day interval between deliveries. *Am J Obstet Gynecol*; **82**: 340–2.

Greenspan L & Deaver GG. (1953) Clinical approach to the etiology of cerebral palsy. *Arch Phys Med Rehab*; **34**: 478–85.

Grennert L, Persson PH, Gennser G, Kullander S & Thorelli J. (1976) Ultrasound and human-placental-lactogen screening for early detection of twin pregnancies. *Lancet*; **1**: 4–6.

Greulich WW. (1934) Heredity in human twinning. *Am J Phys Anthropol*; **19**: 391–431.

Griffiths M. (1967) Cerebral palsy in multiple pregnancy. *Dev Med Child Neurol*; **9**: 713–31.

Griffiths MI. (1981) The hospital treatment of twins in childhood. In *Twins Research (Birmingham 1968–72)*. *Vol. 2*, ed CJ Phillips. Centre for Child Study, University of Birmingham, Part IV, pp. 225–41.

Groenewegen KJ & Van de Kaa DJ. (1967) *Resultaten van het demografisch enderzoek westellijk Nieun-Guinea. Deel 6: de progenituur van Papoes viouwen.* The Hague, Government Printing and publishing office.

Groothuis JR, Altemeir WA, Robarge JP, O'Connor S, Sandler H, Vietze P & Lustig JV. (1982) Increased child abuse in families with twins. *Pediatrics*; **70**: 769–73.

Gross RE, Clatworthy HW & Meeker JA. (1951) Sacrococcygeal teratomas in infants and children. *Surg Gynecol*; **92**: 341–54.

Gruenwald P. (1970) Environmental influences on twins apparent at birth, a preliminary study. *Biol Neonat*; **15**: 79–93.

Grutzner-Konnecke H et al. (1990) Higher order multiple births, natural wonder or failure of therapy. *Acta Genet Med Gemellol*; **39**: 491–5.

Gunther M. (1973) Infant feeding. London, Penguin Books.

Gutowitz HE, Baillie P, Harrison V & Zief S. (1974) Sextuplet gestation, a case report. *S African Med J*; **48**: 1449–52.

Guttmacher AF. (1939) An analysis of 573 cases of twin pregnancy. *Am J Obstet Gynecol*; **38**: 277–88.

Guttmacher AF & Kohl SG. (1958) The fetus of multiple gestations. *Obstet Gynecol*; **12**: 528–41.

Guttmacher AF & Nichols BL. (1967) Teratology of conjoined twins. In *Conjoined twins. Birth defects*; Original Article Series 3, no. 1, pp. 3–9. ed D Bergsma. New York, The National Foundation.

Guyton AC. (1981) Pre-pregnancy reproductive function of the female and the female hormones. In *Textbook of medical physiology*, p. 1016. Philadelphia, WB Saunders.

Haigh J & Wilkinson L. (1989) Care and management of twins. *Health Visitor*; **62**: 43–45.

Hall JG, Reed SD, McGillivray BC, Herrman J, Partington MW, Schinzel A, Shapiro J & Weaver DD. (1983) Part II. Amyoplasia, twinning in amyoplasia—a specific type of arthrogryposis with an apparent excess of discordantly affected identical twins. *Am J Med Genet*; **15**: 591–9.

Hallett F. (1991) Counting the cost, when assisted conception results in triplets. *Multiple Births Foundation Newsletter*; **10**: 2.

Hamon A & Dinno N. (1978) Dicephalus dipus tribrachius conjoined twins in a female infant. *Birth Defects*; **14**: 213–8.

Hanson JW. (1975) Incidence of conjoined twinning. *Lancet*; **2**: 1957.

Harlap S, Shahar S & Baras M. (1985) Overripe ova and twinning. *Am J Hum Genet*; **37**: 1206–15.

Harrison KA & Rossiter CE. (1985) Child bearing health and social priorities. A survey of 22774 consecutive hospital births in Zaria, northern Nigeria. *Br J Obstet Gynaecol*; **92**: Suppl. 5(7), 49–60.

Harvey MAS, Huntley RMC & Smith DW. (1977) Familial monozygotic twinning. *J Pediatr*; **90**: 246–7.

Hay DA & O'Brien PJ. (1984) The role of parental attitudes in the development of temperament in twins at home, school and test situations. *Acta Genet Med Gemellol*; **33**: 191–204.

Hay DA & O'Brien PJ. (1987) Early influences on the school social adjustments of twins. *Acta Genet Med Gemellol*; **36**: 239–248.

Hay DA, Prior M, Collett S & Williams M. (1987) Speech and language development in preschool twins. *Acta Genet Med Gemellol*; **36**: 213–222.

Hay DA, McIndoe R, O'Brien PJ. (1988) The older sibling of twins. *Aus J Early Child*; **13**: 25–8.

Hay DA, Gleeson C, Davies C, Lorden B, Mitchell D & Paton L. (1990) What information should the multiple birth family receive before, during and after the birth? *Acta Genet Med Gemellol*; **39**: 259–69.

Hay S & Wehrung DA. (1970) Congenital malformations in twins. *Am J Hum Genet*; **22**: 662–78.

Heifetz SA. (1984) Single umbilical artery a statistical analysis of 237 autopsy cases and review of the literature. *Perspect Pediatr Pathol*; **8**: 345–78.

Hellin D. (1895) *Die Ursache det multiparitat der unipaaren tiere uberhaupt und der Zwillingsschwangerschaft beim menschen insbesondere*, Munchen, Seltz and Schamer.

Hemon D, Berger C & Lazar P. (1979) The etiology of human dizygotic twinning with special reference to spontaneous abortions. *Acta Genet Med Gemellol*; **28**: 253–8.

Hemon D, Berger C & Lazar P. (1982) Interaction between twinning and maternal factors associated with small for datedness. Presented at the International Workshop on Multiple Pregnancy, Paris.

Hendricks CH. (1966) Twinning in relation to birthweight mortality and congenital anomalies. *Obstet Gynecol*; **27**: 47–53.

Henrichsen L, Skinhoj K & Anderson GE. (1986) Delayed growth and reduced intelligence in 9–17 year old intrauterine growth retarded children compared with their monozygous co-twins. *Acta Paediatr Scand*; **75**: 31–5.

Henriksen JB, Flugsrud LB & Orstavik I. (1968) Cytomegali hos en nyfodt tvilling pavist ved isolation av cytomegalvirus. *Tidsskr Nor Laegeforen*; **88**: 81.

Herlitz G. (1941) Zur kenntnis der anamischen und polyzytamischen zustande bei neugenborenensowie des icterus gravis neonatorum. *Acta Paediat*; **29**: 211–53.

Hewitt D & Stewart A. (1970) Relevance of twin data to intrauterine selection. *Acta Genet Med Gemellol*; **19**: 83–6.

Hibbard BM. (1959) Hydrops foetalis in one of uniovular twins. *J Obstet Gynaecol Br Emp*; **66**: 649–53.

Hill, AVS & Jeffreys AJ. (1985) Use of minisatellite DNA probes for determination of twin zygosity at birth. *Lancet*; **2**: 1394–5.

Hodgkinson V. (1987) It should never have happened. *The Independent*, 23 August.

Hoefnagel D & Benirschke K. (1962) Twinning in Klinefelter's Syndrome. *Lancet*; **2**: 1282.

Hoffman EL & Forrest CB. (1990) Birth Weight less than 800 grams, changing outcomes and influences of gender and gestation number. *Pediatrics*; **86**: 27–33.

Holcberg G, Biale Y, Leweinthal H & Insler V. (1982) Outcome of pregnancy in 31 triplet gestations. *Obstet Gynecol*; **59**: 427–7.

Hollenbach KA & Hickok DE. (1990) Epidemiology and diagnosis of twin gestation. *Clin Obstet Gynecol*; **33**: 3–9.

Hollingworth MJ & Duncan C. (1966) The birthweight and survival of Ghanaian twins. *Ann Hum Genet*; **30**: 13–24.

Holmes GE, Miller HC, Hassanein K, Lansky SB & Goggin JE. (1977) Post natal somatic growth in infants with a typical fetal growth pattern. *Am J Dis Child*; **131**: 1078–83.

Holt SB. (1968) *The genetics of dermal ridges*. Springfield, Illinois, Charles C Thomas.
Howie P, Forsyth JS, Ogston SA, Clark A & du V Florey C. (1990) Protective effect of breast feeding against infection. *Br. Med. J.* **300**, 11–16.
Howie PW, Forsyth JS, Ogston SA, Clark A & du V Florey C. (1990) Protective effect of breast feeding against infection. *Br. Med. J.*, **300**, 11–16.
Human Fertilisation and Embryology Bill (1989) London, HMSO.
Hunter AG, & Cox DM, (1979) Counselling problems when twins are discovered at genetic amniocentesis. *Clin. Genet.*, **16**, 34–42.
Husen T. (1959) *Psychological twin research*. Stockholm, Almquist and Wiksell.
Husen T. (1961) Abilities of twins. *Acta. Psychol.*, **19**, 736–8.
Husen T. (1963) Intra-pair similarities in the school achievements of twins. *Scand. J. Psychol.*, **4**, 108–14.
Hyrtl J. (1870) *Die Blutgefasse der Menschlichen Nachgeburt*. The blood vessels of the human placenta. W. Braumuller, Vienna.
Idelberger K. (1929) Die zwillings pathologie des angeborenen klumpfuss. *Beilagehft zur Zeitschrift fur Ornithologie and praktische Geflugelzucht*, **69**.
Idelberger K. (1951) *Der erb pathologie der segamaunter angeborenen heift vervenkung*. Munchen, Berlin, Urban and Schwarzenberg.
ILA Report. (1990) *The fifth report of the voluntary licensing authority for human in vitro fertilisation and embryology*. London, Interim Licensing Authority.
Illingworth RS & Woods GE. (1960) The incidence of twins in cerebral palsy and mental retardation. *Arch Dis Child*; **35**: 333–4.
Imaizumi Y. (1978) Concordance and discordance of anencephaly in 109 twin pairs in Japan. *Jap J Human Genet*; **23**: 389–93.
Imaizumi Y. (1990) Triplets and higher order multiple births in Japan. *Acta Genet Med Gemellol*; **39**: 295–306.
Imaizumi Y & Inouye E. (1984) Multiple birth rates in Japan. Further analysis. *Acta Genet Med Gemellol*; **33**: 107–14.
Imaizumi Y, Asaka A & Inouye E. (1980) Analysis of multiple birth rates in Japan. V Seasonal and social class variations in twin births. *Jap J Hum Genet*; **25**: 299–307.
Imaizumi Y, Inouye E & Asaka A. (1981) Mortality rate of Japanese twins: Infant deaths of twins after birth to one year of age. *Soc Biol*; **28**: 228–38.
Imperato PJ. (1971) Twins among the Bambara and Malinke of Mali. *J Trop Med Hygiene*; **74**: 154–9.
Inouye E & Imaizumi Y. (1981) Analysis of twinning rates in Japan. In *Twin Research 3: Twin biology and multiple pregnancy*, ed W Nance, pp. 21–33. New York, Alan R Liss.
Itskovitz J, Boldes R, Thaler I, Bronstein M, Erlik Y & Brandes JM. (1989) Transvaginal ultrasonography-guided aspiration of gestational sacs for selective abortion in multiple pregnancy. *Am J Obstet Gynecol*; **160**: 215–7.
Itzkowic D. (1979) A survey of 59 triplet pregnancies. *Br J Obstet Gynaecol*; **86**: 23–8.
Jackson EW, Norris FD & Klauber MR. (1969) Childhood leukaemia in California-born twins. *Cancer*; **23**: 913–19.
James WH. (1972) Secular changes in dizygotic twinning rates. *J Biosoc Sci*; **4**: 427–34.
James WH. (1975) The secular decline in dizygotic twinning rates in Italy. *Acta Genet Med Gemellol*; **24**: 9–14.
James WH. (1977) The sex ratio of monoamniotic twin pairs. *Ann Hum Biol*; **4**: 143–53.
James WH. (1978a) A hypothesis on the declining dizygotic twinning rates in developed countries. *Prog Clinic Biol Res*; **24**: 81–8.
James WH. (1978b) A note on the epidemiology of acardiac monsters. *Teratology*; **16**: 211–6.
James WH. (1980a) Sex ratio and placentation in twins. *Ann Hum Biol*; **7**: 273–76.
James WH. (1980b) Seasonality in twin and triplet birth. *Ann Hum Biol*; **7**: 163–75.

James WH. (1986a) Dizygotic twinning, cycle day of insemination, and erotic potential of Orthodox Jews. *Am J Hum Genet*; **39**: 542–4.

James WH. (1986b) Recent secular trends in dizygotic twinning. *J Biosoc Sci*; **18**: 497–504.

James WH. (1987) The human sex ratio. Part 2: a hypothesis and a program of research. *Hum Biol*; **59**: 873–900.

James WH. (1988) Anomalous X chromosome inactivation: the link between female zygotes, monozygotic twinning and neural tube defects? *J Med Genet*; **25**: 213–14.

Jandial V. *et al.* (1979) The value of measurement of pregnancy-specific proteins in twin pregnancies. *Acta Genet Med Gemellol*; **28**: 319–25.

Janovski NA. (1962) Fetus in fetu. *J Pediatr*; **61**: 100–4.

Jarvis GJ. (1979) Diagnosis of multiple pregnancy. *Br Med J*; **2**: 593–4.

Jaschevatzky OE, Shalit A, Levy Y & Grunstein S. (1977) Epidural analgesia during labour in twin pregnancy. *Br J Obstet Gynecol*; **84**: 327–31.

Jaschevatsky OE, Goldman B, Kampf D, Wexler H & Grunstein S. (1980) Etiological aspects of double monsters. *Eur J Obst Gynaecol Reprod Biol*; **10**: 343–49.

Javert CT. (1957) *Spontaneous and habitual abortion* New York, Blakiston.

Jeanneret O & MacMahon B. (1962) Secular changes in rates of multiple births in the United States. *Am J Hum Genet*; **14**: 410–25.

Jelliffe DB & Jelliffe EFP. (1975) Human milk, nutrition and the world resource crisis. *Science (NY)*; **188**: 557–61.

Jelliffe DB & Jelliffe EFP. (1978) *Human milk in the modern world (psychosocial, nutritional, and economic significance)*. Oxford, Oxford University Press.

Johnston C, Prior M & Hay D. (1984) Prediction of reading disability in twin boys. *Dev Med Child Neurol*; **26**: 588–95.

Jones KL & Benirschke K. (1983) The developmental pathogenesis of structural defects: the contribution of monozygotic twins. *Seminars in Perinatology*; **7**: 239–43.

Jorgensen G, Bettren AJ & Stoermer J. (1971) Genetische untersuchungen bei verschiedenen typen angeborener herzfehler. *Mschr Kinderhelk*; **119**: 417–21.

Junnarkar AR & Nadkarni MG. (1979) Incidence of multiple births in an Indian rural community. *J Epidemiol Comm Hlth*; **33**: 305–6.

Junqueira LCU de C Pinto, VA. (1951) 'Foetus in foetu' a cardico. Consideracoes em torno de um caso. Acardiac Foetus in foetu. *Rev Paul Med*; **38**: 118–22.

Kaelber CT & Pugh TF. (1969) Influence of intrauterine relations on the intelligence of twins. *N Engl J Med*; **280**: 1080–4.

Kamimura K. (1976) Epidemiology of twin births from a climatic point of view. *Br J Prev Soc Med*; **30**: 175–9.

Kang YS & Cho WK. (1962) The sec ratio at birth and other attributes of the newborn from maternity hospitals in Korea. *Human Biology*; **34**: 38–48.

Kanhai HHH, Van Rijssel EJC, Meerman RJ & Bennebroek-Gravenhorst J. (1986) Selective termination in quintuplet pregnancy during first trimester. *Lancet*; **i**: 1447.

Kaplan M & Eidelman AI. (1983) Clustering of conjoined twins in Jerusalem Israel: an epidemiologic survey. *Am J Obstet Gynecol*; **145**: 636–7.

Karn, MN & Penrose LS. (1952) Birth weight and length of gestation of twins together with maternal age, parity, and survival rate. *Ann Eugen*; **16**: 365–77.

Karp L, Bryant JI, Tagatz G, Giblett E & Fialkow PJ. (1975) The occurrence of gonadal dysgenesis in association with monozygotic twinning. *J Med Genet*; **12**: 70–8.

Kasriel J & Eaves L. (1976) The zygosity of twins, further evidence of the agreement between diagnosis by blood groups and written questionnaires. *J Biosoc Sci*; **8**: 263–6.

Kaufman MH. (1985) *Experimental aspects of monozygotic twinning. Implantation of the human embryo*. London, Academic Press.

Kaufman MH & O'Shea KS. (1978) Induction of monozygotic twinning in the mouse. *Nature (Lond)*; **276**: 707–8.

Kauppila A, Jouppila P, Koivisto M, Moilanen I & Ylikorkala O. (1975) Twin Pregnancy. A clinical study of 335 cases. *Acta Obstet Gynecol Scand*; Suppl. **44**: 5–12.

Keay AJ. (1958) The significance of twins in mongolism in the light of new evidence. *J Ment Defic Res*; **2**: 1–7.

Keet MP, Jaroszewicz AM, Lombard CJ. (1986) Follow-up study of physical growth of monozygous twins with discordant within-pair birth weights. *Pediatrics*; **77**: 336–43.

Keet MP, Jaroszewicz AM, & Liebenberg A Le R. (1974) Assessment of gestational age in twins. *Arch Dis Child*; **49**: 741–2.

Kenna AP, Smithells RW & Fielding DW. (1975) Congenital heart disease in Liverpool: 1960–69. *Q J Med*; **154**: 17–44.

Kennell JH, Klaus MH, Sosa R & Urrutia J. (1976) Early neonatal contact: effect on growth breastfeeding and infection in the first year of life. *Pediatr Res*; **10**: 426.

Keown J. (1987) Selective reduction of multiple pregnancy. *New Law Journal*; **137**: 1165–6.

Kerenyi TD & Chitkara U. (1981) Selective birth in twin pregnancy with discordancy for Down's Syndrome. *N Engl J Med*; **304**: 1525–27.

Kerr MG & Rashad MN. (1966) Autosomal trisomy in a discordant monozygotic twin. *Nature*; **212**: 726–7.

Khanna KK, Roy PB & Bhat VP. (1969) Female pseudohermaphroditism in conjoined twins. *Indian J Med Sci*; **23**: 201–5.

Khoo SK & Green K. (1975) Twin pregnancies, influence of antenatal complications, hospital bed rest, and misdiagnosis on prematurity and perinatal mortality. *Aust N Z J Obstet Gynecol*; **15**: 84–92.

Khoury MJ & Erikson TD. (1983) Maternal factors in dizygotic twinning: evidence from inter-racial classes. *Ann Hum Biol*; **10**: 409–15.

Khunda S. (1972) Locked twins. *Obstet Gynecol*; **39**: 453–9.

Kim CC, Dales RJ, Connor R, Walter J & Witherspoon R. (1969) Social interaction of like-sex twins and singletons in relation to intelligence, language and physical development. *J Genet Psychol*; **114**: 203–14.

Kimmel DL, Moyer EK, Peale AR, Winborne LW & Gotwals JE. (1950) Cerebral tumour containing five human foetuses: a case of fetus in fetu. *Anatomical Record*; **106**: 141–65.

Kindred JE. (1944) Twin pregnancies with one twin blighted. *Am J Obstet Gynecol*; **48**: 642–82.

King MC, Friedman GD, Lattanzio D, Rogers G, Lewis AM, Dupuy ME & Williams H. (1980) Diagnosis of twin zygosity by self-assessment and by genetic analysis. *Acta Genet Med Gemellol*; **29**: 121–6.

Kingsland CR, Smith SJ & Mason BA. (1989) Consecutive triplet pregnancies following in-vitro fertilization and embryo transfer. Two case reports. *Hum Reprod*; **4**: 473–4.

Kingsland CR, Steer CV, Pampiglione JS, Mason BA, Edwards RG & Campbell S. (1990) Outcome of triplet pregnancies resulting from IVF at Bourn Hallam 1984–1987. *Eur J Obstet Gynecol*; **34**: 197–203.

Kinsey VE. (1956) Retrolental fibroplasia: Cooperative study of retrolental fibroplasia and the use of oxygen. *Arch Ophthalmol*; **56**: 481–543.

Klaus MH & Kennell JH. (1970) Mothers separated from their newborn infants. *Pediatr Clin North Am*; **17**: 1015–37.

Klebe JG & Ingomar CJ. (1972) The fetoplacental circulation during parturition illustrated by the interfetal transfusion syndrome. *Pediatrics*; **49**: 112–6.

Klingberg WG, Jones B, Allen WM & Dempsey E. (1955) Placental parabiotic circulation of single ovum human twins. *Am J Dis Child*; **90**: 519–20.

Kloosterman GJ. (1963) The 'third circultion' in identical twins. *Ned Tijdschr Verloskd Gynaecol*; **63**: 395–412.

Knight GJ, Kloza EM, Smith DE & Haddow JE. (1981) Efficiency of human placental lactogen and alpha-fetoprotein measurement in twin pregnancy detection. *Am J Obstet Gynecol*; **141**: 585–6.

Knox EG. (1970) Fetus-fetus interaction—a model aetiology for anencephaly. *Develop Med Child Neurol*; **12**: 167–77.

Knox EG. (1974) Twins and neural tube defects. *Br J Prev Soc Med*; **28**: 73–80.

Knox G & Morley D. (1960) Twinning in Yoruba women. *J Obstet Gynaecol Br Cwlth*; **67**: 981–4.

Koch HL. (1966) *Twins and twin relations*. Chicago, University of Chicago Press.

Koivisto M, Jouppila P, Kauppila A, Moilanen I & Ylikorkala O. (1975) Twin pregnancy. Neonatal morbidity and mortality. *Acta Obstet Gynaecol Scand*; **44**: 21–9.

Koluchova J. (1972) Severe deprivation of twins: a case study. *J. Child. Psychol. Psychiat.*, 13, 107–14.

Koluchova J. (1976) The further development of twins after severe and prolonged deprivation: a second report. *J Child Psychol Psychiatr*; **17**: 181–8.

Koranyi G & Kovacs J. (1975) Uber das Zwillingstransfusion syndrom. *Acta Paed Acad Sci Hung*; **16**: 119–25.

Kranitz MA & Welcher DW. (1971) Behavioural characteristics of twins. *J Hopkins Med J*; **129**: 1–5.

Kraus JF & Borhani NO. (1972) Post-neonatal sudden unexplained death in California: a cohort study. *Am J Epid*; **95**: 497–510.

Kyu H, Thu A & Cook PJL. (1981) Human genetics in Burma. *Human Heredity*; **31**: 291–5.

Lachelin GCL, Brant HA, Swyer GIM, Little V & Reynolds EOR. (1972) Sextuplet pregnancy. *Br Med J*; **1**: 787–90.

Landy HJ, Keith L & Keith D. (1982) The vanishing twin. *Acta Genet Med Gemellol*; **31**: 179–94.

Landy HJ, Weiner S, Corson SL, Batzer FR & Bolognese RJ. (1986) The 'vanishing twin': ultrasonographic assessment of fetal disappearance in the first trimester. *Am J Obstet Gynecol*; **155**: 14–19.

Law RG. (1967) *Standards of obstetric care: the report of the West Metropolitan Regional Obstetric Survey 1962–64. Part II*, pp. 92–204. Edinburgh, E & S Livingstone.

Layde PM, Erickson JD, Falek A & McCarthy BJ. (1980) Congenital malformations in twins. *Am J Hum Genet*; **32**: 69–78.

Lazar P, Berger C & Hemon D. (1981) Preconceptional prediction of twin pregnancies. In *Twin research 3. Twin biology and multiple pregnancy*, ed. W Nance, pp. 175–81. New York, Alan R Liss.

Le Marec B, Roussey M, Oger J & Senecal J. (1978) Excess twinning in the parents of spina bifida. *Prog Clin Biol Res*; **24b**: 121–3.

Lee DA. (1979) Munchausen syndrome by proxy in twins. *Arch Dis Child*; **54**: 646–7.

Lee EYC. (1965) Foetus in foetu. *Arch Dis Child*; **40**: 689–93.

Lemli L & Smith DW. (1963) The XO syndrome: a study of differential phenotype in 25 patients. *J Pediatr*; **63**: 597–601.

Lenz W. (1966) Malformations caused by drugs in pregnancy. *Am J Dis Child*; **112**: 99–106.

Leonard LG. (1982) Breastfeeding twins: maternal–infant nutrition. II JOGN. *Nurs*; **11**: 148–53.

Leonard MR. (1959) Problems in identification and ego development in twins. Presented to the American Psychoanalytic Association, Philadelphia.

Leroy B, Lefort F & Jeny R. (1982) Uterine height and umbilical perimeter curves in twin pregnancies. *Acta Genet Med Gemellol*; **31**: 195–8.

Leroy F. (1985) Early embryology and placentation of human twins. In *Implantation of the human embryo*, pp. 393–409. eds RG Edwards, JM Purdy, PC Steptoe. London: Academic Press.

Levene MI. (1986) Grand multiple pregnancies and demand for neonatal intensive care. *Lancet*; **ii**: 347–8.

Levene M. (1991) Assisted reproduction and its implications for paediatrics. *Arch Dis Child*; **66**: 1–3.

Leveno KJ, Santos-Ramos R, Duenhoelter JH, Reisch JS & Whalley PJ. (1979) Sonar cephalometry in twins: a table of biparietal diameters for normal twin fetuses and a comparison with singletons. *Am J Obstet Gynecol*; **135**: 727–30.

Levi S. (1976) Ultrasonic assessment of the high rate of human multiple pregnancy in the first trimester. *J Clin Ultrasound*; **4**: 3–5.

Lewis E. (1979) Mourning by the family after a stillbirth or neonatal death. *Arch Dis Child*; **54**: 303–5.

Lewis E. (1983) Stillbirth: Psychological consequences and strategies of management. In *Advances in perinatal medicine 3*, ed, A Mulinsky, EA Friedman & I Gluck. New York, Plenum.

Lewis E & Bryan EM. (1988) Management of perinatal loss of a twin. *Br Med J*; **297**: 1321–3.

Lewis E & Page A. (1978) Failure to mourn a still birth: an overlooked catastrophe. *Br J Med Psychol*; **51**: 237–41.

Lin RS & Chen KP. (1968) A preliminary study in Taiwan. I. epidemiological aspects. *Journal of the Formosan Medical Association*; **67**: 329–42.

Lindsten J. (1963) *The nature and origin of X-chromosome aberrations in Turner's syndrome.* Stockholm, Amquist and Wiksell.

Linney J. (1980) The emotional and social aspects of having twins. *Nursing Times*; **76**: 276–79.

Linney J. (1983) The *management of multiple births*. Chichester, John Wiley.

Lipovestskaya NG & Yampol'skaya YA. (1975) Decrease in the birth rate of twins and multiple-pregnancy factors. *Genetika*; **11**: 150–7.

Little J & Bryan EM. (1988) Congenital anomalies in twins. In *Twinning and twins*. eds I MacGillivray, DM Campbell & B Thompson. pp. 207–40. Chichester, John Wiley.

Little J & Nevin NC. (1989) Congenital anomalies in twins in Northern Ireland. III: anomalies of the cardiovascular system 1974–79. *Acta Genet Med Gemellol*; **38**: 27–35.

Little J & Thompson B. (1988) Descriptive epidemiology. In *Twinning and twins*, pp. 207–40. eds I MacGillivray, DM Campbell, B Thompson, Chichester, John Wiley and Sons.

Livingstone JE & Poland BJ. (1980) A study of spontaneously aborted twins. *Teratology*; **21**: 139–48.

Ljung BO, Fischbein S & Lindgren G. (1977) Comparison of growth in twins and singleton controls of matched age longitudinally from 10–18 years. *Ann Hum Biol*; **4**: 405–15.

Loehlin JC & Nichols RC. (1976) *Heredity, environment and personality: a study of 850 sets of twins.* Austin, University of Texas Press.

Loughnan PM, Gold H & Vance JC. (1973) Phenytoin teratogenicity in man. *Lancet*; **i**: 70–2.

Lykken DT. (1978) The diagnosis of zygosity in twins. *Behaviour Genetics*; **8**: 437–73.

Lytton H. (1980) *Parent–child interaction. The socialization process observed in twin and singleton families.* New York, Plenum Press.

Lytton H, Conway D & Suave R. (1977) The impact of twinship on parent–child interaction. *J Personality and Social Psychology*; **35**: 97–107.

Macafee CAJ, Fortune DW & Beischer NA. (1970) Non immunological hydrops fetalis. *J Obstet Gynaecol Br Cmwlth*; **77**: 226–37.

MacDonald AD. (1964) Mongolism in twins. *J Med Genet*; **1**: 39–41.

Macfarlane AJ, Price FV & Daw EG. (1990a) Infertility drugs and procedures. In *Three, four and more*, pp. 46–58. eds BJ Botting, AJ Macfarlane & FV Price, London, HMSO.

Macfarlane AJ, Price FV & Daw EG. (1990b) Antenatal care. In *Three, four and more*, pp. 60–62. eds BJ Botting, Macfarlane AJ & EV Price. London, HMSO.

Macfarlane AJ, Price FV & Daw EG. (1990c) The delivery. In *Three, four and more*, pp. 80–97. eds BJ Botting, AJ Macfarlane & FV Price. London, HMSO.

Macfarlane AJ, Price FV & Daw EG. (1990d) Early days. In *Three, four and more*, pp. 99–128. eds BJ Botting, AJ Macfarlane & FV Price, London, HMSO.

Macfarlane AJ, Johnson A & Bower P. (1990e) Disabilities and health problems in childhood. In *Three, four and more*, pp. 153–60. eds BJ Botting, AJ Macfarlane & FV Price. London HMSO.

MacGillivray I. (1958) Some observations on the incidence of pre-eclampsia. *J Obstet Gynaecol Br Emp*; **65**: 536–9.

MacGillivray I. (1975a) Diagnosis of twin pregnancy. *In Human Multiple Reproduction*; pp 116–23. London: WB Saunders.

MacGillivray I. (1975b) Labour in multiple pregnancies. In *Human Multiple Reproduction*. pp. 147–64. eds I MacGillivray, PPS Nylander, G Corney. London: WB Saunders.

MacGillivray I. (1975c) Management of multiple pregnancies. In *Human multiple reproduction*, pp. 124–36. Eds I MacGillivray, PPS Nylander & G Corney. London: WB Saunders.

MacGillivray I. (1982) Preterm labour in twin pregnancies. Presented at the International Workshop on Multiple Pregnancy, Paris.

MacGillivray I. (1984) The Aberdeen contribution to twins. *Acta Genet Med Gemellol*; **33**: 5–11.

MacGillivray I. (1986) Epidemiology of twin pregnancy. *Semin Perinatol*; **10**: 4–8.

MacGillivray I. (1990) Disability in twins. *Multiple Births Foundation Newsletter*; **9**: 1.

MacGillivray I & Campbell DM. (1981) The outcome of twin pregnancies in Aberdeen. In *Twin Research 3. Twin biology and multiple pregnancy*, pp. 203–6. eds L Gedda, P Parisi & WE Nance. New York: Alan R Liss.

MacGillivray I & Campbell DM. (1988) Management of twin pregnancies. In *Twinning and twins*, 111–42 eds I MacGillivray, DM Campbell & B Thompson. Chichester, John Wiley.

MacGillivray I, Campbell DM & Thompson B. (1988a) *Twinning and twins*. Chichester, John Wiley.

MacGillivray I, Samphier M & Little J. (1988b) Factors affecting twinning. In *Twinning and twins*. 67–98 eds I MacGillivray, DM Campbell & B Thompson. Chichester, John Wiley.

Macourt DC, Stewart P & Zaki M. (1982) Multiple pregnancy and fetal abnormalities in association with oral contraceptive usage. *Aust NZ J Obstet Gynaecol*; **22**: 25–8.

Mahony BS, Filly RA & Callen PW. (1985) Amnionicity and chorionicity in twin pregnancies: prediction using ulstrasound. *Radiology*; **155**: 205–9.

Mahony BS, Petty CN, Nyberg DA, Luthy DA, Hickok DE & Hirsch JH. (1990) The 'stuck twin' phenomenon: ultrasonographic findings, pregnancy outcome, and management with serial amniocenteses. *Am J Obstet Gynecol*; **163**: 1513–22.

Majsky A & Kohl M. (1982) Another case of occurrence of two different fathers of twins by HLA typing. *Tissue Antigens*; **20**: 305.

Malmstrom PEM, Faherty T & Wagner P. (1988) Essential non-medical perinatal services for multiple birth families. *Acta Genet Med Gemellol*; **37**: 193–198.

Mannino FL, Jones KL & Benirschke K. (1977) Congenital skin defects and fetus papyraceus. *J Pediatr*; **91**: 559–64.

Marinho AO, Ilesanmi AO, Lodele OA, Asuni OH, Omigbodun A & Oyejide CO. (1966) A fall in the rate of multiple births in Ibadan and Igbo Ora Nigeria. *Acta Genet Med Gemellol*; **35**: 201–4.

Marlow N, Ellis AM, Roberts BL & Cooke RWI. (1990) Five year outcome of preterm sextuplets related to size at birth. *Arch Dis Child*; **65**: 451–2.

Mashiach S, Ben-Rafael Z, Dor J & Serr DM. (1981) Triplet pregnancy in uterus didelphys with delivery interval of 72 days. *Obstet Gynecol*; **58**: 519–22.

Matheny AP Jr & Brown AM. (1971) The behaviour of twins: effects of birth weight and birth sequence. *Child Dev*; **42**: 251–7.

Matheny AP, Brown AM & Wilson RS. (1971) Behavioural antecedents of accidental injuries in early childhood: a study of twins. *J Pediatr*; **79**: 122–4.

Matheny AP, Wilson RS & Dolan AB. (1976) Relations between twins' similarity of appearance and behavioural similarity: testing an assumption. *Behav Genet*; **6**: 343–51.

Mauriceau F. (1721) *Traite des maladies des femmes grosses*. Paris.

Mayer CF. (1952a) Sextuplets and higher multiparous births. Part 2, Sextuplets and higher births. *Acta Genet Med Gemellol*; **1**: 242–75.

Mayer CF. (1952b) Sextuplets and higher multiparous births. Part 1, Multiparity and sextuplets. *Acta Genet Med Gemellol*; **1**: 118–35.

McArthur JW. (1938) Genetics of quintuplets 1. Diagnosis of the Dionne quintuplets as a monozygotic set. *J Hered*; **29**: 323–9.

McCarthy BJ, Sachs BP, Layde PM, Burton A, Terry J & Rochat R. (1981) The epidemiology of neonatal deaths in twins. *Am J Obstet Gynecol*; **141**: 252–6.

McKeown T & Record RG. (1952) Observations on foetal growth in multiple pregnancy in man. *J Endocrinol*; **8**: 386–401.

McKeown T & Record RG. (1953) The influence of placental size on foetal growth in man with special reference to multiple pregnancy. *J Endocrinol*; **9**: 418–26.

McKeown T & Record RG. (1960) *Malformations in a population observed for five years*. CIBA Foundation Symposium on Congenital Malformations, pp. 2–21. London, Churchill, Livingstone.

McManus IC. (1980) Handedness in twins. A critical review. *Neuropsychologia*; **18**: 347–55.

McMullen P. (1986) Northern Ireland twin study (1983). *The Ulster Medical Journal*; **44**: 131–5.

Mead M. (1957) Changing patterns of parent–child relations in an urban culture. *Int J Psychoanal*; **38**: 369–78.

Meadow R. (1977) Munchausen syndrome by proxy—the hinterland of child abuse. *Lancet*; **ii**: 343–5.

Mehrotra SN & Maxwell J. (1949) The intelligence of twins: a comparative study of eleven-year-old twins. *Pop Stud*; **3**: 295–302.

Mellin GN & Katzenstein M. (1962) The saga of thalidomide. *N Engl J Med*; **267**: 1184–93, 1238–44.

Melnick M. (1977) Brain damage in survivor after death of monozygotic co-twin. *Lancet*; **ii**: 1287.

Melnick M & Myrianthopoulos NC. (1979) The effects of chorion type on normal and abnormal developmental variation in monozygous twins. *Am J Med Genet*; **4**: 147–56.

Menez-Bautista R, Fikrig SM, Pahwa S, Sarangadharan MG & Stoneburner RL. (1986) Monozygotic twins discordant for the acquired deficiency syndrome. *Am J Dis Child*; **140**: 678–9.

Merrell, Pharmaceuticals Ltd. (1981) Clomid. In *Data-sheet compendium*, pp. 770. London, Datapharm Publications.

Metrakos JD, Metrakos K & Baxter H. (1958) Clefts of the lip and palate in twins including a discordant pair whose monozygosity was confirmed by skin transplants. *Plast Reconstr Surg*; **22**: 109–22.

Meyer WC, Keith L & Webster A. (1970) Monoamniotic twin pregnancy with the transfusion syndrome. *Chicago Med Sch Quarterly*; **29**: 42–51.

Michaels L. (1967) Unilateral ischaemia of the fused twin placenta: a manifestation of the twin transfusion syndrome. *Can Med Assoc J*; **96**: 402–5.

Michelwitz H, Kennedy J, Kawada C & Kennison R. (1981) Triplet pregnancies. *J Reprod Med*; **26**: 243–6.

Miettinen M. (1954) On triplet and quadruplets in Finland. *Acta Paediatr*; **43**: Suppl. 99, 9–103.

Miettinen M & Gronroos JA. (1965) A follow-up study of Finnish triplets. *Ann Paediatr Fenniae (Helsinki)*; **11**: 71–83.

Mijsberg WA. (1957) Genetic-statistical data on the presence of secondary oocytary twins among non-identical twins. *Acta Genet*; **7**: 39–42.

Milham S. (1966) Symmetrical conjoined twins: an analysis of the birth records of 22 sets. *J Pediatr*; **69**: 643–7.

Millis J. (1959) The frequency of twinning in poor Chinese in the maternity hospital Singapore. *Ann Hum Genet*; **23**: 171–4.

Minde KK, Perrotta M & Corter C. (1982) The effect of neonatal complications in same-sexed premature twins on their mother's performance. *J Am Acad Child Psychiatry*; **21**: 446–52.

Minde K, Corter C, Goldberg S & Jeffers D. (1990) Maternal preference between premature twins up to age four. *J Am Acad Child & Adolesc Pyschiatry*; **29**: 367–74.

Minde K, Corter C & Goldberg S. (1984) The contribution of twinship and early biological impediment to early interaction and attachment between premature infants and their mother. *Frontiers of infant psychiatry*, pp. 160–76. eds JD Call, E Galenson, RL Tyson. New York: Basic Books.

Mitchell SC, Sellmann AH, Westphal MC & Park J. (1971) Etiologic correlates in a study of congenital heart disease in 56,109 births. *Am J Cardiol*; **28**: 653–7.

Mittler P. (1970) Biological and social aspects of language development in twins. *Dev Med Child Neurol*; **12**: 741–57.

Mittler P. (1971) *The study of twins*. London, Penguin Books.

Mittler P. (1976) Language development in young twins: biological genetic and social aspects. *Acta Genet Med Gemellol*; **25**: 359–65.

Modan B, Kallner H, Modan M & Nemser L. (1968) Differential twinning in Israeli major ethnic groups. *Am J Epidemiol*; **88**: 189–94.

Mogford K. (1988) Language development in twins. In *Language development in exceptional circumstances*, pp. 80–96 eds D Bishop & K Mogford. Edinburgh, Churchill Livingstone.

Molloy D et al. (1990) Multiple-sited (heterotopic) pregnancy after in vitro fertilization and gamete intrafallopian transfer. *Fertility & Sterility*; **53**: 1068–71.

Monni G, Rosatelli C, Falchi AM, Scalas MT, Addis M, Maccioni L, Di Tucci A & Tuvieri T. (1986) First trimester diagnosis of B thalassaemia in a twin pregnancy. *Prenatal Diagnosis*; **6**: 63–8.

Montgomery RC & Stockdell K. (1970) Congenital rubella in twins. *J Pediatr*; **7**: 772–3.

Moore CM, McAdams AJ & Sutherland J. (1969) Intrauterine disseminated intravascular coagulation: a syndrome of multiple pregnancy with a dead twin fetus. *J Pediatr*; **74**: 523–8.

Moore TR, Gale S & Benirschke K. (1990) Perinatal outcome of forty-nine pregnancies complicated by acardiac twinning. *Am J Obstet Gynecol*; **163**: 907–12.

Morales WJ, O'Brien WF, Knuppel RA, Gaylord S & Hayes P. (1989) The effect of mode of delivery on the risk of intraventricular hemorhage in nondiscordant twin gestations under 1500 g. *Obstet Gynaecol*; **73**: 107–10.

Morris N, Osborn SB & Wight HP. (1955) Effective circulation of the uterine wall in late pregnancy measured by ^{24}NaCl. *Lancet*; **i**: 323–4.

Morton NE. (1962) Genetics of interracial crosses in Hawaii. *Eugenics Quart*; **9**: 23–4.

Mucklow ES. (1990) Locked twins with survival of both. *J Obstet Gynecol*; **10**: 532–3.

Muller M. (1976) *The baby killer. A War on Want investigation into the promotion and sale of powdered baby milks in the Third World*, 3rd ed. London, War on Want.

Muller-Holve W, Saling E & Schwarz M. (1976) The significance of the time interval in twin delivery. *Perinat Med*; **4**: 100–5.

Munsinger H. (1977) The identical-twin transfusion syndrome: a source of error in estimating IQ resemblance and heritability. *Ann Hum Genet*; **40**: 307–21.

Myrianthopoulos NC. (1970) An epidemiologic survey of twins in a large prospectively studied population. *Am J Hum Genet*; **22**: 611–29.

Myrianthopoulos NC. (1975) Congenital malformations in twins: Epidemiologic survey. *Birth. Def Orig Art Ser XI*; No. 8, pp. 1–29. New York, Nat. Found. March. of Dimes.

Myrianthopoulos NC. (1978) Congenital malformations: the contribution of twin studies. *Birth Defects*; **14**: 151–65.

Myrianthopoulos NC & Melnick M. (1977) Malformations in monozygotic twins: a possible example of environmental influences on the developmental genetic clock. In *Gene–environmental interaction in common diseases*, pp. 206–20. Tokyo, University of Tokyo Press.

Myrianthopoulos NC, Churchill JA & Baszynski. (1971) Respiratory distress syndrome in twins. *Acta Genet Med Gemellol*; **20**: 199–204.

Myrianthopoulos NC, Nichols PL & Broman SH. (1976) Intellectual development of twins—comparison with singletons. *Acta Genet Med Gemellol*; **25**: 376–80.

Naeye RL. (1963) Human intrauterine parabiotic syndrome and its complications. *N Engl J Med*; **268**: 804–9.

Naeye RL. (1964a) Organ composition in newborn parabiotic twins with speculation regarding neonatal hypoglycaemia. *Pediatrics*; **34**: 415–8.

Naeye RL. (1964b) The fetal and neonatal development of twins. *Pediatrics*; **33**: 546–53.

Naeye RL. (1965) Organ abnormalities in a human parabiotic syndrome. *Am J Pathol*; **46**: 829–41.

Naeye RL & Letts HW. (1964) Body measurements of fetal and neonatal twins. *Arch Pathol*; **77**: 393–6.

Naeye RL, Benirschke K, Hagstrom JWC & Marcus CC. (1966) Intrauterine growth of twins as estimated from liveborn birthweight data. *Pediatrics*; **37**: 409–16.

Nageotte MP, Hurwitz SR, Kaupke CJ, Vaziri ND & Pandian MR. (1989) Atriopeptin in the twin transfusion syndrome. *Obstet Gynecol*; **73**: 867–70.

Nakamura I & Miura T. (1987) Seasonality of birth in mother of like-sexed and unlike-sexed twins. *Progress in Biometerology*; **5**: 51–60.

Nance WE. (1981) Malformations unique to the twinning process. In *Twin research 3: Twin biology and multiple pregnancy*; pp. 123–33. ed. W Nance, New York, Alan R Liss.

Nance WE & Uchida I. (1964) Turner's syndrome twinning and an unusual variant of glucose-6-phosphate dehydrogenase. *Am J Hum Genet*; **16**: 380–92.

Nance WE, Winter PM & Segreti WO. (1978) A search for evidence of hereditary superfetation in man. In *Twin research: biology and epidemiology*, pp. 65–70. eds WE Nance, G Allen & P Parisi. New York, Alan R Liss.

National Academy of Sciences. (1974) *Recommended dietary allowance*, 8th ed. Washington DC, National Academy of Sciences.

Neilson JP. (1981) *Detection of the small-for-dates twin fetus by ultrasound. Br J Obstet Gynaecol*; **88**: 27–32.

Nelson CMK & Bunge RG. (1974) Semen analysis: evidence for changing parameters of male fertility potential. *Fertil Steril*; **25**: 503–7.

New Zealand Yearbook (1982) Wellington, Department of Statistics.

Newman HH. (1928) Asymmetry reversal or mirror imaging in identical twins. *Biol Bull*; **5**: 298–315.

Newman RB, Hamer C & Miller CM. (1989) Outpatient triplet management: a contemporary review. *Am J Obstet Gynecol*; **161**: 547–3.

Nichols BL, Blattner RJ & Rudolph AJ. (1967) General clinical management of thoracopagus twins. *Birth Defects: Original Article Series*; **iii**: 38–51.

Nichols JB. (1954) Quintuplet and sextuplet births in the US. *Acta Genet Med Gemellol*; **3**: 143–52.

Nielsen J. (1970) Twins in sibships with Klinefelter's syndrome and the XYY syndrome. *Acta Genet Med Gemmellol*; **19**: 399–404.

Nielsen J & Dahl G. (1976) Twins in the sibships and parental sibships of women with Turner's syndrome. *Clin Genet*; **10**: 93–6.

Nissen ED. (1958) Twins: collision impaction, compaction and interlocking. *Obstet Gynecol*; **11**: 514–25.

Noble E. (1990) *Having Twins: A parent's guide to pregnancy, birth and early childhood.* Boston, Haughton Mifflin.

Noonan JA. (1978) Twins conjoined twins and cardiac defects. *Am J Dis Child*; **132**: 17–18.

Nora JJ, Gilliland JC, Sommerville RJ & McNamara DG. (1967) Congenital heart disease in twins. *N Engl J Med*; **227**: 568–71.

Norman RJ & Joubert SM. (1982) *Amniotic fluid phospholipids in twin pregnancies.* Presented at the International Workshop on Twin Pregnancies. Paris.

Nylander PPS. (1967) Twinning in West Africa. *World Med J*; **14**: 178–80.

Nylander PPS. (1969) The frequency of twinning in a rural community in Western Nigeria. *Ann Hum Genet*; **33**: 41–4.

Nylander PPS. (1970a) Twinning in Nigeria. *Acta Genet Med Gemellol*; **19**: 457–64.

Nylander PPS. (1970b) Placental forms and zygosity determination of twins in Ibadan Western Nigeria. *Acta Genet Med Gemellol*; **19**: 49–54.

Nylander PPS. (1970c) A simple method for determining monochorionic and dichorionic placentation in twins. *Niger J Sci*; **4**: 239–44.

Nylander PPS. (1971a) The incidence of triplets and higher multiple births in some rural and urban populations in Western Nigeria. *Ann Hum Genet*; **34**: 409–15.

Nylander PPS. (1971b) Biosocial aspects of multiple births. *J Biosoc Sci*; Suppl. 3, 29–38.

Nylander PPS. (1973) Serum levels of gonadotrophins in relation to multiple pregnancy in Nigeria. *J Obstet Gynaecol Brit Cwlth*; **80**: 651–3.

Nylander PPS. (1975a) The causation of twinning. In *Human multiple reproduction*, pp. 77–86. eds I MacGillivray, PPS Nylander & G Corney. London, WB Saunders.

Nylander PPS. (1975b) Factors which influence twinning rates. In *Human multiple reproduction*. pp. 98–106. eds I MacGillivray, PPS Nylander & G Corney. London, WB Saunders.

Nylander PPS. (1975c) Factors which influence twinning rates. In *Human multiple reproduction*, pp. 98–106. eds I MacGillivray, PPS Nylander & G Corney. London: WB Saunders.

Nylander PPS. (1978) Causes of high twinning frequencies in Nigeria. In *Twin research: biology and epidemiology*, pp. 35–43. eds WE Nance, G Allen & P Parisi. New York: Alan R Liss.

Nylander PPS. (1979) The twinning incidence in Nigeria. *Acta Genet Med Gemellol*; **28**: 261–3.

Nylander PPS. (1981) The factors that influence twinning rates. *Acta Genet Med Gemellol*; **30**: 189–202.

Nylander PPS & Corney G. (1971) Placentation and zygosity of triplets and higher multiple births in Ibadan, Nigeria. *Ann Hum Genet*; **34**: 417–26.

Nylander PPS & Corney G. (1977) Placentation and zygosity of twins in Northern Nigeria. *Ann Hum Genet*; **40**: 323–9.

Nylander PPS & MacGillivray I. (1975) Complications of twin pregnancy. In *Human multiple reproduction*, eds I MacGillivray, PPS Nylander & G Corney. pp. 137–46. London: WB Saunders.

Nylander PPS & Osunkoya BB. (1970) Unusual monochorionic placentation with heterosexual twins. *Obstet Gynecol*; **36**: 621–5.

Obladen M & Gluck L. (1977) RDS and tracheal phospholipid composition in twins: independent of gestational age. *J Pediatrics*; **90**: 799–802.

O'Connor MC, Murphy H, Dalrymple IJ. (1979) Double blind trial of Ritodrine and placebo in twin pregnancy. *Br J Obstet Gynaecol*; **86**: 706–9.

Olofsson P & Rhydstrom H. (1985) Twin delivery: how should the second twin be delivered? *Am J Obstet Gynecol*; **153**: 479–81.

Onyskowova Z, Dolezal A & Jedlicka V. (1971) The frequency and the character of malformations in multiple births: a preliminary report. *Teratology*; **4**: 496–7.

Orlebeke JF, Eriksson AW & Vlietinck R. (1989) Weinberg's rule reconsidered. *Acta Genet Med Gemellol*; **38**: 237–8.

Ornoy A, Navot D, Menashi M, Laufer N, Chemke J. (1980) Asymmetry and discordance for congenital anomalies in conjoined twins: A report of six cases. *Teratology*; **22**: 145–54.

Ozil JP. (1983) Production of identical twins by bisection of blastocysts in the cow. *J Reprod Fertil*: **69**: 463–8.

Palmer EA, Flynn JT, Hardy RJ. *et al.* (1991) Incidence and early course of retinopathy of prematurity. *Opthalmology*; **98**: 1628–40.

Papiernik E. (1991) Cost of multiple pregnancies. In *The stress of multiple births*, pp. 22–34. eds D Harvey & E Bryan. London: Multiple Births Foundation.

Papiernik E, Mussy MA, Vial M & Richard A. (1985) A low rate of perinatal deaths for twin births. *Acta Genet Med Gemellol*; **34**: 201–6.

Parisi P, Gatti M, Prinzi G & Caperna G. (1983) Familial incidence of twinning. *Nature*; **304** 626–8.

Parmar VT & Mulgund SV. (1968) Interlocking of twin pregnancy in uterus circuatus subseptus. *J Postgraduate Medicine*; **14**: 139–41.

Parsons PA. (1965) Birth weights and survival of unlike sexed twins. *Ann Hum Genet*; **28**: 1–10.

Partridge J. (1987) Telling parents about their twins' zygosity, presented to the British Paediatric Association, York (unpublished).

Patel N, Bowie W, Campbell DM, Howat R, Melrose E, Redford D, MacIlivaine G & Smalls M. (1984) *Scottish twin study 1983 report*. Social Paediatric and Obstetric Research Unit, University of Glasgow and Greater Glasgow Health Board.

Pedersen IK, Philip J, Seue V & Starup J. (1980) Monozygotic twins with dissimilar phenotypes and chromosome complements. *Acta Obstet Gynecol Scand*; **59**: 459–62.

Peller S. (1946) A new rule for predicting the occurrence of multiple births. *Am J Physical Anthropology*; **4**: 99–105.

Pemkovsky BM & Vintzileos AM. (1989) Management and outcome of multiple pregnancy of high fetal order: literature review. *Obstet and Gynecol Survey*; **44**: 578–84.

Penrose LS. (1937) Congenital syphilis in monovular twin. *Lancet*; **i**: 322.

Pepper CK. (1967) Ethical and moral considerations in the separation of conjoined twins. In *Conjoined twins*, Ed. D Bergsman. Birth Defects. Original Article Series: 1. New York, The National Foundation.

Perez LV & Gallo AD. (1965) Transfusion fetofetal. *Rev Chile Pediat*; **36**: 497–500.

Perlman EJ, Stetton G, Tuckmuller CM, Fauber RA & Blallenon, KJ (1990). Sexual discordance in monozygotic twins. *Am J Med Genet*; **3**: 551–7.

Pescia G, Ferrier PE, Wyss-Hutin D & Klein D. (1975) 45X Turner's syndrome in monozygotic twin sisters. *J Med Genet*; **12**: 390–6.

Petres RE & Redwine FO. (1981) Selective birth in twin pregnancy. *N Engl J Med*; **305**: 1218–9 (letter).

Petterson B, Stanley F & Henderson D. (1990) Cerebral palsy in multiple births in Western Australia. *Am J Med Genet*; **37**: 346–51.

Phillips CJ. (1981) Some observation of handedness in twin children. In *Twins research (Birmingham 1968–72)* vol 2, Part V, ed. CJ Phillips, pp. 243–72. Centre for Child Study, University of Birmingham.

Phillips CJ & Watkinson M. (1981) Characteristics of the families and similarity of environment within twin pairs. In *Twin research (Birmingham 1968–72)*; vol 2, Part 1, ed. CJ Phillips, pp. 2–57. Centre for Child Study University of Birmingham.

Ping YW & Chin CL. (1967) Incidence of twin births among the Chinese in Taiwan. *Am J Obstet Gynecol*; **98**: 881–4.

Piontelli A. (1989) A study on twins before and after birth. *Int Rev Psychol-Anal*; **16**: 413–26.

Plomin R, Willerman L & Loehlin JC. (1976) Resemblances in appearance and the equal environments assumption in twin studies of personality traits. *Behav Genet*; **6**: 43–52.

Pochedly C & Musiker S. (1970) Twin-to-Twin transfusion syndrome. *Postgrad Med*; **47**: 172–6.

Pollard GN. (1969) Multiple births in Australia 1944–63. *J Biosoc Sci*; **1**: 389–404.

Pons JC, Mayenga JM, PluG, Forman RG & Papiernik E. (1988) Management of triplet pregnancy. *Acta Genet Med Gemellol*; **37**: 99–103.

Pons JC *et al.* (1990) *Quadruplet pregnancy in France.* Presented at the 12th Congress of Perinatal Medicine, Lyons, 1990.

Porter R, Smith B, Ahiya K, Tucker M & Craft I. (1986) Combined twin ectopic pregnancy and intrauterine gestation following in vitro fertilization and embryo transfer. *Journal of In Vitro Fertilization and Embryo Transfer*, **3**: 330–2.

Portes L & Granjon A. (1946) Les presentations au cours des accouchments gemellaires. *Gynecologie et Obstetrique*; **87**: 566–77.

Potter AM & Taitz LS. (1972) Turner's syndrome in one of monozygotic twins with mosaicism. *Acta Paediatr Scand*; **61**: 473–6.

Potter EL. (1963) Twin zygosity and placental form in relation to the outcome of pregnancy. *Am J Obstet Gynecol*; **87**: 566–77.

Potter EL & Craig JM. (1976) *Pathology of the fetus and the infant*, 3rd edn. Chicago, Yearbook Medical Publishers, pp. 220–1.

Potter EL & Fuller H. (1949) Multiple pregnancies at the Chicago lying-in hospital, 1941–7. *Am J Obstet Gynecol*; **58**: 139–46.

Powell TJ. (1981) *Symptoms of postnatal (atypical) depression in mothers of twins.* MSc thesis University of Surrey.

Powers WF & Miller TC. (1979) Bed rest in twin pregnancy; identification of a critical period and its cost implications. *Am J Obstet Gynecol*; **134**: 23–30.

Price FV. (1990a) Who helps? In *Three, four and more. A study of triplet and higher order births*, pp. 131–150. Eds BJ Botting, AJ MacFarlane & FV Price. London: HMSO.

Price FV. (1990b) Consequences. In *Three, four and more. A study of higher order births*, pp. 161–76. Eds BJ Botting, AJ MacFarlane & FV Price. London: HMSO.

Prokop VO & Herrmann U. (1973) Blutgruppenbefunde bei Achtlingen. *Zentralblatt fur Gynakologi*; **95**: 1497.

Quigley JK. (1935) Monoamniotic twin pregnancy. *Am J Obstet Gynecol*; **29**: 354–62.

Race RR & Sanger R. (1975) Blood groups in twins and chimeras. In *Blood groups in man*, 6th edn, pp. 511–46. Oxford, Blackwell Scientific.

Radestad A & Thomassen PA. (1990) Acute polyhydramnios in twin pregnancy—a retrospective study with special reference to therapeutic amniocentesis. *Acta Obstet Gynecol Scand*; **69**: 297–300.

Rajegowda BK, Freedman MD, Falciglia H, Exconde M & Sukumaran T. (1975) Absence of respiratory distress syndrome following premature rupture of membranes in one sib of a set of twins in two cases. *Clin Res*; **23**: 600A.

Ramzin MS, Stucki D, Napflin S, Allemann F & Gamper S. (1982) *Early prenatal loss in twin pregnancies*. Presented at the International workshop on Multiple Pregnancy, Paris.

Rao PSS, Inbaraj SG & Muthurathnam S. (1983) Twinning rates in Tamilnadu. *J Epidemiol Comm Hlth*; **37**: 117–20.

Rausen AR, Seki M & Strauss L. (1965) Twin transfusion syndrome. Review of 19 cases studied at one institution. *J Pediatr*; **66**: 613–28.

Record RG, McKeown T & Edwards JH. (1970) An investigation of the difference in measured intelligence between twins and single births. *Ann Hum Genet*; **34**: 11–20.

Redford DHA. (1982) Ultrasound assessment of uterine growth in twin pregnancy. Presented at the Multiple Pregnancy Workshop. Paris.

Redshaw J & Rutter M. (1991) Growing up as a twin: twin-singleton differences in psychological development. In *The Stress of multiple births*, pp. 77–87. eds D Harvey & E Bryan. London: Multiple Births Foundation.

Reece EA, Petrie RH, Sirmans MF. *et al.* (1983) Combined intrauterine and extra-uterine gestations: A review. *Am J Obstet Gynecol*; **146**: 323.

Registrar General. (1989) *Birth statistics*, Series FMI No. 6. London, Offices of Population Census and Surveys, HMSO.

Registrar General for Scotland. (1983) *Annual Report*, no. 129, Edinburgh, HMSO.

Rehan NE, Sobrero AJ & Fertig JW. (1975) The semen of fertile men. Statistical analysis of 1300 men. *Fertil Steril*; **26**: 492–502.

Rein MS, Barbieri RL & Greene MF. (1990) The causes of high-order multiple gestation. *Int J Fertil*; **35**: 154–6.

Reisman LE & Pathak A. (1966) Bilateral renal cortical necrosis in the newborn. *Am J Dis Child*; **111**: 541–3.

Reisner SH, Forbes AE & Cornblath M. (1965) The smaller of twins and hypo-glycaemia. *Lancet*; 524–6.

Rempen A. (1988) Vaginal sonography in ectopic pregnancy: a prospective evaluation. *J Ultrasound Med*; **7**: 381–7.

Reveley AM, Gurling HMD & Murray RM. (1981) Mortality and psychosis in twins. In *Twin Research 3. Part B. Intelligence, personality and development*, pp. 175–8. eds L Gedda, P Parisi & WE Nance. New York, Alan R Liss.

Rhein R, Knitza R, Fendel T, Dworschak L, Hepp H & Versmold H. (1991) Outcome of 47 quadruplets and quintuplets. In *Obstetrics and neonatology up-to-date. The very low birthweight infant*. ed G Duc. Zurich (in press).

Rhine SA & Nance WE. (1976) Familial twinning: A case of superfetion in man. *Acta Genet Med Gemellol*; **25**: 66–9.

Riekhof PL, Horton WA, Harris DJ & Schimke RN. (1972) Monozygotic twins with the Turner Syndrome. *Am J Obstet Gynecol*; **112**: 59–61.

Rife DC. (1940) Handedness with special reference to twins. *Genetics*; **25**: 178–86.

Robertson EG & Neer KJ. (1983) Placental injection studies in twin gestation. *Am J Obstet Gynecol*; **147**: 170–4.

Robin M, Josse D & Tourette C. (1988) Mother-twin interaction during early childhood. *Acta Genet Med Gemellol*; **37**: 151–9.

Robinson HP & Caines JS. (1977) Sonar evidence of early pregnancy failure in patients with twin conceptions. *Br J Obstet Gynecol*; **84**: 22–5.

Robson KS & Moss HA. (1970) Patterns and determinants of maternal attachment. *J Pediatr*; **77**: 976–85.

Rodeck CH. (1984) Fetoscopy in the management of twin pregnancies discordant for a severe abnormality. *Acta Genet Med Gemellol*; **33**: 57–60.

Rodeck CH & Wass D. (1981) Sampling pure fetal blood in twin pregnancies by fetoscopy using a single uterine puncture. *Pren Diag*; **1**: 43–9.

Rodis JF, Egan JFX, Craffey A, Ciarleglio L, Greenstein RM & Scorza WE. (1990) Calculated risk of chromosomal abnormalities in twin gestations. *Obstet Gynecol*; **76**: 1037–41.

Rogers JG, Voullaire L & Gold H. (1982) Monozygotic twins discordant for Trisomy 21. *Am J Med Genet*; **11**: 143–6.

Rola-Janicki A. (1974) Multiple births in Poland 1949–71. In *Multiple births and twin care*, ed. P Parisi. *Acta Genet Med Gemellol*, Suppl 22.

Ron-el, R, Caspi E, Schreyer P, Weinraub Z, Arieli S & Golberg M. (1981) Triplet and quadruplet pregnancies and management. *Obstet Gynecol*; **57**: 458–63.

Rothman KJ. (1977) Fetal loss twinning and birth weight after oral contraceptive use. *N Engl J Med*; **297**: 468–71.

Rowe J, Clyman R, Green C, Mikkelsen C, Haight J & Ataide L. (1978) Follow up of families who experience a perinatal death. *Pediatrics*; **62**: 166–70.

Rudolph AJ, Michaels JP & Nichols BL. (1967) Obstetric management of conjoined twins. In: *Conjoined twins*. ed: D Bergsma. Birth Defects Original Articles Series 3 28–57.

Russell EM. (1961) Cerebral palsied twins. *Arch Dis Child*; **36**: 328–36.

Rutter M, Bolton P, Harrington R, Lecouteur A, Macdonald A & Simonoff E. (1990) Genetic factors in child pyschiatric disorders review and research strategies. *J Child Psychology and Psychiatry*; **31**: 3–37.

Rydhstrom H. (1990a) The effects of maternal age, parity and sex of the twins on twin perinatal mortality: A population based study. *Acta Genet Med Gemellol*; **39**: 401–8.

Rydhstrom H. (1990b) Prognosis for twins with birth weight <1500 g: the impact of cesarean section in relation to fetal position. *Am J Obstet Gynecol*; **163**: 528–33.

Rydhstrom H. (1991) Prognosis for a twin after antenatal death of its co-twin with long term follow-up. Presented at the seventh workshop on multiple pregnancy. Berlin.

Rydhstrom H & Ohrlander S. (1985) Twin deliveries in Sweden 1973–81. The value of an increasing caesarian section rate. *Arch Gynecol*; **237**: 168.

Sacks MO. (1959) Occurrence of anaemia and polycythemia in phenotypically dissimilar single ovum twins. *Pediatrics*; **24**: 604–8.

Saier F, Burden L & Cavanagh D. (1975) Fetus papyraceus; an unusual case with congenital anomaly of the surviving fetus. *Obstet Gynecol (New York)*; **45**: 217–20.

Saint L, Maggiore P & Hartmann PE. (1986) Yield and nutrient content of milk in eight women breast-feeding twins and one woman breast-feeding triplets. *Br J Nutr*; **56**: 49–58.

Salariya EM, Easton PM & Cater JI. (1978) Duration of breast-feeding after early initiation and frequent feeding. *Lancet*; **ii**: 1141–3.

Samm M, Curtis-Cohen M & Keller M. (1986) Necrotizing enterocolitis in infants of multiple gestation. *Am J Dis Child*; **140**: 937–9.

Savic S. (1980) How twins learn to talk. London: Academic Press.

Say B, Gungor E & Durmus Z. (1967) Twin births in Turkey (letter). *Lancet*; **i**: 52.

Scarr S. (1969) Effects of birth weight on later intelligence. *Soc Biol*; **16**: 249–56.

Schatz F. (1900) *Klinische beitrage zur physiologie des fotus.* (Clinical observations on the physiology of the foetus.) Berlin: A. Hirschwald.

Scheinfeld A. (1973) *Twins and supertwins*. Harmondsworth, Middlesex, Penguin Books.

Schinzel AAGL, Smith DW & Miller JR. (1979) Monozygotic twinning and structural defects. *J Pediatr*; **95**: 921–30.

Schmidt M & Salzano FM. (1980) Dissimilar effects of thalidomide in dizygotic twins. *Acta Genet Med Gemellol*; **29**: 295–7.

Schneider L. (1978) Echographic study of twin fetal growth: a plea for specific charts for twins. *Prog Clin Biol Res*; **24C**: 137–41.

Schneider L, Bessis R & Simmonet T. (1979) The frequency of ovular resorption during first trimester of twin pregnancy. *Acta Genet Med Gemellol*; **28**: 271–2.

Schwartz JL, Maniscalo WM, Lane AT & Currao WJ. (1984) Twin transfusion syndrome causing cutaneous erythropoiesis. *Pediatrics*; **74**: 527–9.

Scialli AR. (1986) The reproductive toxicity of ovulation induction. *Fertility and Sterility*; **45**: 315–23.

Scobie W. (1979) A language just for two. *Observer Magazine* **May 20th**: 67–8.

Scott JM & Ferguson-Smith MA. (1973) Heterokaryotypic monozygotic twins and the acardiac monster. *J Obstet Gynaecol Br Cwlth*; **80**: 52–59.

Scott JM & Paterson L. (1966) Monozygous anencephalic triplets—a case report. *J Obstet Gynaecol Br Cwlth*; **73**: 147–51.

Scottish Council for Research in Education. (1953) *Social implications of the 1947 Scottish mental survey*. London, University of London Press.

Scragg RFR & Walsh RJ (1970) A high incidence of multiple births in one area of New Britain. *Human Biology*; **42**: 442–9.

Segal NL. (1984) Cooperation competition and altruism within twin sets: a reappraisal. *Ethology and Sociobiology*; **5**: 163–77.

Segreti WO, Winter PM & Nance WE. (1978) Familial studies of monozygotic twinning. *Prog Clin Biol Res*; **24b**: 55–60.

Seller MJ. (1990) Conjoined twins discordant for cleft lip & palate. *Am J Med Genet*; **37**: 530–1.

Shah SB & Patel DN. (1984) Twinning and structural defects. *Indian Pediatrics*; **21**: 475–8.

Shapiro LR, Zemek L & Shulman MJ. (1978) Familial monozygotic twinning: an autosomal dominant form of monozygotic twinning with variable penetrance. *Prog Clin Biol Res*; **24**: 57–62.

Shorland J. (1971) Management of the twin transfusion syndrome. *Clin Pediatr*; **10**: 160–3.

Simpson CW, Olatunbosun OA & Baldwin VJ. (1984) Delayed interval delivery in triplet pregnancy: report of a single case and review of the literature. *Obstet Gynecol*; **64**: 85–115.

Sims CD, Cowan DB & Parkinson CE. (1976) The lecithin/sphingomyelin ratio in twin pregnancies. *Br J Obstet Gynaecol*; **83**: 447–51.

Sinha DP, Nandakumar VC, Brough AK & Beebeejaum MS. (1979) Relative cervical incompetence in twin pregnancy. *Acta Genet Med Gemellol*; **28**: 327–31.

Sinykin MB. (1958) Monoamniotic triplet pregnancy with triple survival. *Obstet Gynecol*; **12**: 78–82.

Skelly H, Marivate M, Norman R, Kenoyer G & Martin R. (1982) Consumptive coagulopathy following fetal death in a triplet pregnancy. *Am J Obstet Gynecol*; **142**: 595–6.

Skerlj B. (1939) Menarche une Umvelt. *Z Menschl Vererb-Konstit Lehre*; **23**: 299–359.

Smellie WA. (1752) *A treatise on the theory and practice of midwifery*; 2nd edn. pp. 100–1. London: Wilson & Durham.

Smith, SM & Penrose LS. (1955) Monozygotic and dizygotic twin diagnosis. *Am J Hum Genet*; **19**: 273–89.

Snyder T, DelCostillo J, Graff J, Hoxsey R & Hefti M. (1988) Heterotopic pregnancy after IVF and ovulatory drugs. *Ann Emergy Med*; **17**: 846–9.

Soltan HC. (1968) Genetic characteristics of families of XO and XXY patients including evidence of source of X chromosomes in 7 aneuploid patients. *J Med Genet*; **5**: 173–80.

Soma H, Takayama M, Kiyokawa I, Akaeda T & Tokoro K. (1975) Serum gonadotropin levels in Japanese women. *Obstet Gynecol*; **46**: 311–2.

Sorgo G. (1973) Das problem der supefoecundatio in vater schafsgutachten. *Beitr Gerichtl Med*; **30**: 415–21.

Spellacy WN, Cruz AC, Buhi WC & Birk SA. (1977) Amniotic fluid L/S ratio in twin gestation. *Obstet Gynecol*; **50**: 68.

Spiers PS. (1974) Estimated rates of concordancy for the sudden infant death syndrome in twins. *Am J Epidemiol*; **100**: 1–7.

Spillman JR. (1984) *The role of birthweight in maternal-twin relationships*. MSc Thesis, Cranfield Institute of Technology.

Spillman JR. (1985) 'You have a little bonus my dear' The effect on mothers of the diagnosis of mutliple pregnancy. *Br Med Ultrasound Soc Bull*; **39**: 6–9.

Spurway JH. (1962) The fate and management of the second twin. *Am J Obstet Gynecol*; **83**: 1377–88.

Stables J. (1980) Breastfeeding twins. *Nursing Times*; 1493–4.

Stanley FJ. (1979) An epidemiological study of cerebral palsy in Western Australia 1956–75. I. Changes in total incidence of cerebral palsy and associated factors. *Dev Med Child Neurol*; **21**: 701–13.

Stanley F. (1989) Cerebral palsy in multiple births. *Irish Medical Journal*; **82**: 97.

Stevenson AC, Johnston HA, Stewart MIP & Golding DR. (1966) Congenital malformations. A report of a study of a series of consecutive births in 24 centres. *Bull Wld Hlth Org*; **34**, Suppl 1–127.

Stewart A. (1991) The long term outcome. In *The stress of multiple births*, pp. 127–34. eds D Harvey & EM Bryan. London: Multiple Births Foundation.

Stockard CR. (1921) Developmental rate and structural expression: an experimental study of twins 'double monsters' and single deformities and the interaction among embryonic organs during their origin and development. *Am J Anat*; **28**: 115–277.

Storlazzi E, Vintzileos AM, Campbell WA, Nochimson BJ & Weinbaum PJ. (1987) Ultrasonic diagnosis of discordant fetal growth in twin gestations. *Obstet Gynecol*; **69**: 363–7.

Strong SJ & Corney G. (1967) *The placenta in twin pregnancy*. Oxford, Pergamon Press.

Strong TH Jr & Brar HS. (1989) Placenta praevia in twin gestation. *J Reprod Med*; **34**: 415–16.

Stucki D, Ramzin MS & Zehnder A. (1982) *Management of twin pregnancies*. Presented at the International Workshop on Multiple Pregnancy. Paris.

Sunday Times (1989) 25th June. A new life for Masha and Dasha.

Syrop CH & Varner MW. (1985) Triplet gestation: maternal and neonatal implications. *Acta Genet Med Gemellol*; **34**: 81–8.

Szendi B. (1939) Double monsters in light of recent biological experiments and investigations regarding hereditary contributions of sex. *J Obstet Gynaecol Brit Emp*; **46**: 836–47.

Szymonowicz W, Preston H & Yu VYH. (1986) The surviving monozygotic twin. *Arch Dis Child*; **61**: 454–8.

Tabsch K, Crandall B, Lebherz T & Howard J. (1985) Genetic amniocentesis in twin pregnancy. *Obstet Gynecol*; **65**: 843–5.

Tagawa T. (1974) Monoamniotic twins with a double survival. Report of a case with a peculiar cord complication. *Wis Med J*; **73**: 131–2.

Tan KL, Tock EPC, Dawood MY & Ratnam S. (1971a) Conjoined twins in a triplet pregnancy. *Am J Dis Child*; **122**: 455–8.

Tan KL, Goon SM, Salmon Y & Wee JH. (1971b) Conjoined twins. *Acta Obstet Gynaecol Scand*; **50**: 373–80.

Tan KL, Tan R, Tan SH & Tan AM. (1979) The twin transfusion syndrome. *Clin Pediat*; **18**: 111–14.

Tanimura M *et al.* (1990) Child abuse of one of a pair of twins in Japan. *Lancet*; **336**: 1298–9.

Tanner JM, Healy MJR, Lockhart RD, Mackenzie JD & Whitehouse RH. (1956) The prediction of adult body measurements taken each year from birth to 5 years. *Arch Dis Child*; **31**: 372–81.

Taylor EM & Emery JL. (1988) Maternal stress, family and health care of twins. *Children & Society*; **4**: 351–66.

Terasaki PI, Gjertson D, Bernoco D, Perdue S, Mickey MR & Bond J. (1978) Twins with two different fathers identified by HLA. *N Engl J Med*; **299**: 590–2.

Theron JP. (1969) A case of locked twins in a double uterus. *J Obstet Gynaecol Br Cwlth*; **76**: 750–1.

Thiery M, Kermans G & Derom R. (1988) Triplet and higher order births. What is the optimal delivery route? *Acta Genet Med Gemellol*; **37**: 89–98.

Thom H, Buckland CM, Campbell AGM, Thompson B & Farr Y. (1984) Maternal serum alpha fetoprotein in monozygotic and dizygotic twin pregnancies. *Prenatal Diagnosis*; **4**: 341–6.

Thomas PA *et al.* (1990) Paediatric acquired immuno deficiency syndrome: an unusually high incidence of twinning. *Pediatrics*; **66**: 774–7.

Thompson B, Pritchard C & Corney G. (1983) *Perinatal mortality in twins by zygosity and placentation.* Paper presented at 4th Congress of International Society for Twin Studies, London.

Thomsen RJ. (1978) Delayed interval delivery of a twin pregnancy. *Obstet Gynecol*; **52**: 357–405.

Thorpe K, Golding J, MacGillivray I & Greenwood R. (1991) Comparison of prevalence of depression in mothers of twins and mothers of singletons. *Brit Med J*; **302**: 875–8.

Timonen S & Carpen E. (1968) Multiple pregnancies and photoperiodicity. *Ann Chir Gynaec Fenn*; **57**: 135–8.

Tomasello M, Mannle S & Kruger AC. (1986) Linguistic environment of 1–2 year old twins. *Developmental Psychology*; **22**: 169–76.

Torgersen J. (1950) Situs inversus asymmetry and twinning. *Am J Hum Genet*; **2**: 361–70.

Tow SH. (1959) Fetal wastage in twin pregnancy. *J Obstet Gynaecol Br Emp*; **66**: 444–51.

Tresmontant R & Papiernik E. (1983) Economic anlaysis of the prevention of preterm births in twin pregnancies. *Eur J Obstet Gynecol Reprod Biol*; **15**: 277–9.

Turksoy RN, Toy BL, Rogers J & Papageorge W. (1967) Birth of septuplets following gonadotrophin administration in Chiari-Frommel syndrome. *Obstet Gynecol*; **30**: 692–8.

Tyson JE. (1976) In *Breastfeeding and the mother.* Ciba Foundation Symposium 45 (new series). p. 65. London, Elsevier.

Uchida IA, De Sa DJ & Whelan DT *et al.* (1983) 45x/46xx mosaicism in discordant monozygotic twins. *Pediatrics*; **71**: 413–7.

United Nations Department of Economic and Social Affairs. (1981) *Demographic yearbook.* New York, United Nations.

Urig MA, Clewell WH & Elliott JP. (1990) Twin-twin transfusion syndrome. *Am J Obstet Gynecol*; **163**: 1522–6.

Valaes T & Doxiadis SA. (1960) Intrauterine blood transfer between uniovular twins. *Arch Dis Child*; **35**: 503–5.

Van Allen MI, Smith DW & Shepard TH. (1983) Twin reversed arterial perfusion TRAP sequence: a study of 14 twin pregnancies with acardius. *Semin Perinatol*; **7**: 285–93.

Vandell DL, Owen MT, Wilson KS & Henderson VK. (1988) Social development in infant twins: peer & mother child relationships. *Child Devel*; **59**: 168–77.

Van Staey M, DeBie S, Matton MT & De Roose J. (1984) Familial congenital esophageal atresia. Personal case report and review of the literature. *Hum Genet*; **66**: 260–6.

Vandenberg SG & Falkner F. (1966) Hereditary factors in human growth. *Hum Biol*; **37**: 357–65.

Very PS & Van Hine NP. (1969) Effects of birth order upon personality development of twins. *J Genet Psychol*; **114**: 93–5.

Vestergaard P. (1972) Triplets pregnancy with a normal foetus and a dicephalus dibrachius sirenomelus. *Acta Obstet Gynaecol Scand*; **51**: 93–4.

Viljoen DL, Nelson MM & Beighton P. (1983) The epidemiology of conjoined twinning in Southern Africa. *Clin Genet*; **24**: 15–21.

Villena C, Gnir J, Ertan K, Boos R & Schmidt W. (1991) Prenatal diagnosis and monitoring of pregnancies with twin-twin transfusion syndrome. Presented at the seventh workshop on multiple pregnancy. Berlin.

Vlietinck R, Papiernik E, Derom C, Grandjean H, Thiery M & Derom R. (1988) The European Multiple Birth Study (EMBS). *Acta Genet Gemellol*; **37**: 27–30.

Wald NG, Cuckle H, Stirrat GM, Bennett MJ & Turnbull AC. (1977) Maternal serum alphafetoprotein and low birthweight. *Lancet*; **ii**: 268–70.

Wald NJ, Cuckle H, Stirrat GM & Turnbull AC. (1978) Maternal serum alphafetoprotein and birthweight in twin pregnancies. *Br J Obstet Gynaecol*; **85**: 582–4.

Wald NJ, Cuckle HS, Peck S, Stirrat GM & Turnbull AC. (1979) Maternal serum alphafetoprotein in relation to zygosity. *Br Med J*: **1**: 455.

Walker J & Turnbull EPN. (1955) The environment of the foetus in human multiple pregnancy. *Etudes Neonatales*; **4**: 123–36.

Walthers FJ & Ramaekers LHJ. (1982) Growth in early childhood of newborns affected by disproportionate intrauterine retardation. *Acta Paed Scand*; **71**: 651–6.

Wang LN, Wang YF, Hornec C & Shiao LC. (1990) Congenital rubella infection: escape of one monozygotic twin with two amnions, one chorion, and single placenta. *Taiwan-I-Hsueh-Hui-Tsa-Chih*; **89**: 30–3.

Wapner RJ, Davis GH, Johnson A, Weinblatt VJ, Fischer RL, Jackson LG, Chervenak FA & McCullough LB. (1990) Selective reduction of multifetal pregnancies. *Lancet*; **335**: 90–3.

Watts DA & Lytton H. (1980) *Twinship as handicap: fact or fiction? A longitudinal study.* Calgary, The University of Calgary.

Weekes ARL, Menzies DN & West CR. (1977a) Spontaneous premature birth in twin pregnancy. *Br Med J*; **2**: 14–17.

Weekes ARL, Menzies EN & de Boer CH. (1977b) The relative efficacy of bed rest, cervical suture and no treatment in the management of twin pregnancy. *Br J Obstet Gynaecol*; **84**: 161–4.

Weekes ARL, Cheridjian VE & Mwanje DK. (1977c) Lumbar epidural analgesia in labour in twin pregnancy. *Br Med J*; **2**: 730–2.

Weinberg W. (1902) Beitrage zur physiologie and pathologie der mehrlingsgeburten beim menschen. *Pflugers Archiv fur die gesamte physiologie de Menschen un de Tiers*; **88**: 346–430.

Weir PE, Ratten GJ & Beischer NA. (1979) Acute polyhydramnios a complication of monzygous twin pregnancy. *Br J Obstet Gynaecol*; **86**: 849–53.

Welch P, Black KN & Christian JC. (1978) Placental type and Bayley Mental Development scores in 18-month-old twins. *Prog Clin Biol Res*; **24**: 145–9.

Weller PH, Jenkins PA, Gupta J & Baum JD. (1976) Pharyngeal lecithin/sphingomylin ratios in newborn infants. *Lancet*; **i**: 12–15.

Wharton B, Edwards JH & Cameron AH. (1968) Monoamniotic twins. *J Obstet Gynaecol*; **75**: 158–63.

White C & Wyshak G. (1964) Inheritance of human dizygotic twinning. *N Engl J Med*; **271**: 1003–5.

Whitehouse DBB & Kohler HG. (1960) Vasa praevia in twin pregnancy: report of two cases. *J Obstet Gynaecol Br Emp*; **67**: 281–3.

Willerman L & Churchill JA. (1967) Intelligence and birth weight in identical twins. *Child Devel*; **38**: 623–9.

Williams B & Cummings G. (1953) Unusual case of twins: case report. *J Obstet Gynaecol Br Emp*; **60**: 319–21.

Wilson RS. (1974a) Growth standards for twins from birth to four years. *Ann Hum Biol*; **1**: 175–88.

Wilson RS. (1974b) Twins: mental development in the pre-school years. *Devel Psychol*; **10**: 580–8.

Wilson RS. (1978) Synchronies in mental development. An epigenetic perspective. *Science*; **202**: 939–47.

Wilson RS. (1979) Twin growth: initial deficit recovery and trends in concordance from birth to nine years. *Ann Hum Biol*; **6**: 205–20.

Wilson RS. (1981) Synchronized developmental pathways for infant twins. In *Twin research 3: Intelligence, personality and development*, pp. 199–209. ed. W Nance, New York, Alan R Liss.

Wilson R. (1983) The Louisville Twin Study. *Child Devel*; **54**: 298–316.

Wilson RS, Brown AM & Matheny AP. (1971) Emergence and persistence of behavioural differences in twins. *J Child Devel*; **42**: 1381–98.

Windham GC & Bierkedal T. (1984) Malformations in twins and their siblings. *Acta Genet Gemellol*; **38**: 87–95.

Winn HN, Gabrielli S, Reece EA, Roberts JA, Salafia C & Hobbins JC. (1989) Ultrasonographic criteria for the prenatal diagnosis of placental chorionicity in twin gestations. *Am J Obstet Gynecol*; **161**: 1540–2.

Winnicott DW. (1958) The capacity to be alone. In *The Maturational processes & facilitating environment*. London, Hogarth Press.

Wittmann BK, Farquaharson DF, Thomas WDS, Baldwin VJ & Wadsworth LD. (1986) The role of feticide in the management of severe twin transfusion syndrome. *Am J Obstet Gynecol*; **155**: 1023–6.

Wolkind S. (1981) Depression in mothers of young children. *Arch Dis Child*; **52**: 735–7.

Woods DL & Malan AF. (1977) Assessment of gestational age in twins. *Arch Dis Child*; **52**: 735–7.

Woodward J. (1988) The bereaved twin. *Acta Genet Med Gemellol*; **37**: 173–80.

Wyshak G. (1978) Menopause in mothers of multiple births and mothers of singletons only. *Soc Biol*; **25**: 52–61.

Wyshak G. (1981) Reproductive and menstrual characteristics of mothers of multiple births and mothers of singletons only: a discriminant analysis. In *Twin Research 3: Twin Biology and Multiple Pregnancy*, pp. 95–105. ed. W Nance, New York, Alan R Liss.

Wyshak G & White C. (1963) Birth hazard of the second twin. *J Am Med Ass*; **186**: 869–70.

Wyshak G & White C. (1965) Genealogical study of human twinning. *Am J Public Health*; **55**: 1586–93.

Ylitalo V, Kero P & Erkkola R. (1988) Neurological outcome of twins dissimilar in size at birth. *Early Hum Dev*; **17**: 245–55.

Yoshida K & Matoyoshi K. (1990) A study on prognosis of surviving co-twin. *Acta Genet Med Gemellol*; **39**: 383–7.

Yoshioka H, Kadomoto Y, Mino M, Morikawau Y, Kasubuchi Y & Kusunoki T. (1979) Multicystic encephalomalacia in liveborn twin with a stillborn macerated co-twin. *J Pediatr*; **95**: 798–800.

Yu VYH, Loke HL, Bajuk B. *et al*. (1986) Prognosis for infants born at 23–28 weeks' gestation. *Br Med J*; **293**: 1200–3.

Yue SJ. (1955) Multiple births in cerebral palsy. *Am J Phys Med*; **34**: 335–41.

Zake EZN. (1984) Case reports of 16 sets of conjoined twins from a Uganda Hospital. *Acta Genet Med Gemellol*; **33**: 75–80.

Zazzo R. (1960) *Les jumeaux: Le couple et la personne*. Paris, Presse Universitaire de France.

Zazzo R. (1979) The twin condition and the couple effects on personality development. *Acta Genet Med Gemellol*; **25**: 343–52.

Zimmerman AA. (1967) Embryologic and anatomic considerations of conjoined twins. *Birth Defects: Original Articles* Series 3: 1, 18–27.

Zuckerman H & Brzezinski A. (1961) Multiple pregnancies. *Israel Med J*; **20**: 251–8.

Index

morphological studies of 94
separate 73, 74
types of 82
ultrasonic scanning 95
Placentation 85
development and 162
in higher order births 196
onset of labour and 74
zygosity and 27
Plautus (250–184BC) 3
Pollution 25
Polyhydramnios
causes 54
in conjoined twins 61
in fetofetal transfusion syndrome 39, 101
incidence of 39
in multiple pregnancy 39
onset of labour and 74
Polymorphisms
zygosity and 27
Porencephaly 71
Positional defects 65
Prader–Willi syndrome 58
Prams 125, 202
Pre-eclampsia 38
Pregnancy
heterotopic 37
intrauterine and extrauterine 37
in higher order births 193
multiple *See Multiple pregnancy*
selective reduction of 189
Prematurity
breast-feeding and 113
effect on mother 108
effects of 74
physical growth and 153
retinopathy of 104
Prenatal meetings 242
Preparation for twins 43
Pre-school twin 133–45
behaviour 134
discipline 137
intrapair relationships 132
Presentation at delivery 75
Pre-term labour 74
Prevalence of twinning 9
among differing ethnic groups 20
contraceptive pill affecting 16, 23, 25
environmental factors 20
infertility treatment and 16, 24
international variation in 10, 11, 12, 13, 25
maternal age, parity and 20, 21
maternal height and weight and 22
in negroid races 20
nutrition and 22
seasonal variation 23
secular trends 25
social class and 23

in United Kingdom 14
Push chairs 125, 202

Quadriplegia 166
Quadruplets
birthweight 195
delivery 194
development 206
gestational age at birth 194
newborn 198
Quintuplets 183
development 206

Radiography 34
Reading 162
Relationships
intrapair 128, 133
mother–baby *See Mother–twin relationship*
siblings 130
Religious beliefs about twins 4
Respiratory distress syndrome 103
Retinopathy of prematurity 104
Retrolental fibroplasia 104
Rhesus isoimmunization 68
Romulus and Remus 2
Rubella virus infection 67
Rubinstein–Taybi syndrome 58

School 146–52
choice of 149
differing abilities at 147
pre- *See Preschool twin*
preparation for 150
separation at 147, 149, 151
sex differences in development 148
starting 151
together or apart? 146
Secret language 142
Separation at school 147, 149, 151
Septuplets 183
placentation in 196
survival 199
Sex
zygosity and 26
Sex ratio of twins 14
Sextuplets 183
Shakespeare, William (1564–1615) 3
Shopping 125
Siamese twins 61
See also Conjoined twins
Siblings
effect of triplets on 204
of disabled children 168, 169
reaction to death 178
relationship with twins 130
resent among 130
Sirenomelia 64
Situs inversus 139
Skin
erythroopoiesis 101

genetic markers 28
of higher order births 185
growth and development and
    157
laboratory investigation of 27

mental development 162, 163
in onset of labour 74
placentation and 27
polymorphisms and 27
skin grafts and 30